Physical Therapy of the Cervical and Thoracic Spine

Second Edition

Edited by

Ruth Grant, B.P.T., M.App.Sc., Grad.Dip.Adv.Man.Ther.

Professor of Physiotherapy
Dean, Faculty of Health and Biomedical Sciences
University of South Australia
Adelaide, South Australia
Australia

CHURCHILL LIVINGSTONE

New York, Edinburgh, London, Madrid, Melbourne, Milan, Tokyo

Library of Congress Cataloging-in-Publication Data

Physical therapy of the cervical and thoracic spine / edited by Ruth
Grant. — 2nd ed.
  p. cm. — (Clinics in physical therapy)
  Includes bibliographical references and index.
  ISBN 0-443-08918-3
  1. Neck pain—Physical therapy. 2. Backache—Physical therapy.
3. Cervical vertebrae—Diseases—Physical therapy. 4. Thoracic
vertebrae—Diseases—Physical therapy.   I. Grant, Ruth, M. App. Sc.
II. Series.
  [DNLM: 1. Cervical Vertebrae. 2. Thoracic Vertebrae. 3. Physical
Therapy. 4. Spinal Diseases—rehabilitation.   WE 725 P5775 1994]
RD768.P48 1994
617'.375062—dc20
DNLM/DLC
for Library of Congress   94-12194
                                                              CIP

Distributed in the United Kingdom by Churchill Livingstone, Robert Stevenson House, 1–3
Baxter's Place, Leith Walk, Edinburgh EH1 3AF, and by associated companies, branches, and
representatives throughout the world.

The Publishers have made every effort to trace the copyright holders for borrowed material. If
they have inadvertently overlooked any, they will be pleased to make the necessary
arrangements at the first opportunity.

Acquisitions Editor: *Carol Bader*
Copy Editor: *Elizabeth Bowman-Schulman*
Production Supervisor: *Patricia McFadden*

Printed in the United States of America

First published in 1994   7 6 5 4 3 2 1

Physical Therapy of the Cervical and Thoracic Spine
Second Edition

CLINICS IN PHYSICAL THERAPY

EDITORIAL BOARD

Otto D. Payton, Ph.D., **Chairman**
Louis R. Amundsen, Ph.D.
Suzann K. Campbell, Ph.D.
John L. Echternach, Ed.D.

Physical Therapy for the Cancer Patient
Charles L. McGarvey III, M.S., P.T., guest editor

Gait in Rehabilitation
Gary L. Smidt, Ph.D., guest editor

Physical Therapy of the Hip
John L. Echternach, Ed.D., guest editor

Physical Therapy of the Shoulder, 2nd Ed.
Robert Donatelli, M.A., P.T., guest editor

Pediatric Neurologic Physical Therapy, 2nd Ed.
Suzann K. Campbell, Ph.D., P.T., F.A.P.T.A., guest editor

Physical Therapy Management of Parkinson's Disease
George I. Turnbull, M.A., P.T., guest editor

Pulmonary Management in Physical Therapy
Cynthia Coffin Zadai, M.S., P.T., guest editor

Physical Therapy Assessment in Early Infancy
Irma J. Wilhelm, M.S., P.T., guest editor

Physical Therapy of the Low Back, 2nd Ed.
Lance T. Twomey, Ph.D., and James R. Taylor, M.D.,
Ph.D., guest editors

Temporomandibular Disorders, 2nd Ed.
Steven L. Kraus, P.T., guest editor

Forthcoming Volumes in the Series

Physical Therapy for Traumatic Brain Injury
Jacqueline Montgomery, P.T., guest editor

Physical Therapy of the Knee, 2nd Ed.
Robert E. Mangine, M.Ed., P.T., A.T.C., guest editor

Physical Therapy of the Foot and Ankle, 2nd Ed.
Gary C. Hunt, M.A., P.T., O.C.S., and
Thomas G. McPoil, Ph.D., P.T., A.T.C., guest editors

Contributors

David S. Butler, B. Phty., Grad.Dip.Adv.Man.Ther., M.M.P.A.A.
Adjunct Lecturer, School of Physiotherapy, Faculty of Health and Biomedical Sciences, University of South Australia; Private Practitioner, Slater, Butler and Shacklock Pty. Ltd., Manipulative Physiotherapists, Adelaide, South Australia, Australia

Nikolai Bogduk, M.D., Ph.D., B.Sc.(Med.), F.A.C.R.M.(Hon.)
Professor, Department of Anatomy, The University of Newcastle Faculty of Medicine; Director, Cervical Spine Research Unit, Mater Misericordiae Hospital, Newcastle, New South Wales, Australia

Judi Carr, A.U.A., Grad.Dip.F.E.
Senior Lecturer, School of Physiotherapy, Faculty of Health and Biomedical Sciences, University of South Australia, Adelaide, South Australia, Australia

Nicole Christensen, P.T., M.App.Sc.
Lecturer, Physical Therapy Department, Mount St. Mary's College, Los Angeles, California; Staff Physical Therapist, Camarillo Orthopaedic and Sports Therapy, Camarillo, California

Brian C. Edwards, B.Sc., B.App.Sc., Grad.Dip.Man.Ther.
Specialist Manipulative Physiotherapist and Honorary Fellow, Curtin University of Technology; Principal, Brian C. Edwards and Associates, Perth, Western Australia, Australia

Rodney N. Grant, Dip.P.T., A.D.P.(M.T.), Dip. M.T.
Research Physiotherapist, The McKenzie Institute International, Waikanae, New Zealand

Ruth Grant, B.P.T., M.App.Sc., Grad.Dip.Adv.Man.Ther.
Professor of Physiotherapy, and Dean, Faculty of Health and Biomedical Sciences, University of South Australia, Adelaide, South Australia, Australia

Vladimir Janda, M.D., D.Sc.
Professor and Director, Department of Rehabilitation Medicine, and School of Physiotherapy, Third Faculty of Medicine, Charles University; Professor and Director, Department of Rehabilitation Medicine, Postgraduate Medical Institute, Prague, Czech Republic

Helen Jones, B.App.Sc., Grad.Dip.Adv.Man.Ther., M.App.Sc.
Private Practitioner, Bayside Manipulative Physiotherapy, Glenelg, South Australia, Australia

Mark Jones, R.P.T., Grad.Dip.Adv.Man.Ther., M.App.Sc.
Senior Lecturer, School of Physiotherapy, Faculty of Health and Biomedical Sciences, University of South Australia, Adelaide, South Australia, Australia

Gwendolen A. Jull, M.Phty., Grad.Dip.Adv.Man.Ther., F.A.C.P.
Senior Lecturer, Department of Physiotherapy, The University of Queensland; Specialist Manipulative Physiotherapist, Chapel Hill Physiotherapy Clinic, Brisbane, Queensland, Australia

Diane Lee, B.S.R., M.C.P.A., C.O.M.P.
Instructor/Examiner, Orthopaedic Division, Canadian Physiotherapy Association, Toronto, Ontario, Canada; Instructor/Examiner, North American Institute of Orthopaedic Manipulative Therapy, United States; Private Practitioner, Delta Orthopaedic Physiotherapy Clinic, Delta, British Columbia, Canada

Geoffrey D. Maitland, M.B.E., A.U.A., F.C.S.P., F.A.C.P.(Monog.), F.A.C.P., M.APP.Sc. (Hon.)
Visiting Specialist Lecturer, School of Physiotherapy, Faculty of Health and Biomedical Sciences, University of South Australia; Specialist Manipulative Physiotherapist, Adelaide, South Australia, Australia

Mary E. Magarey, Dip.Tech. (Physio.), Grad.Dip.Adv.Man.Ther.
Lecturer, School of Physiotherapy, Faculty of Health and Biomedical Sciences, University of South Australia, Adelaide, South Australia, Australia

Robin A. McKenzie, O.B.E., F.C.S.P., F.N.Z.S.P.(Hon.), Dip. M.T.
International Director, The McKenzie Institute International, Waikanae, New Zealand

Barbara McPhee, Dip. Phty., M.P.H.
Senior Research Scientist, Ergonomics Unit, National Institute of Occupational Health and Safety; Senior Lecturer, Department of Occupational Health, The University of Sydney, Sydney, New South Wales, Australia

Shirley A. Sahrmann, Ph.D., F.A.P.T.A.
Associate Professor, Program in Physical Therapy and Department of Neurology, and Director, Program in Movement Science, Washington University School of Medicine, St. Louis, Missouri

Helen Slater, M.App.Sc., M.M.P.A.A.
Adjunct Lecturer, School of Physiotherapy, Faculty of Health and Biomedical Sciences, University of South Australia; Private Practitioner, Slater, Butler and Shacklock Pty. Ltd., Manipulative Physiotherapists, Adelaide, South Australia, Australia

James R. Taylor, M.D., Ph.D.
Associate Professor, Department of Anatomy and Human Biology, University of Western Australia Medical Faculty, Nedlands, Western Australia; Research Fellow, Department of Neuropathology, and Clinical Assistant, Sir George Bedbrook Spinal Unit, Royal Perth Hospital, Perth, Western Australia; Spinal Physician, Perth Pain Management Centre, Applecross, Western Australia, Australia

Patricia H. Trott, M.Sc., Grad.Dip.Adv.Man.Ther., F.A.C.P.
Associate Professor and Head, School of Physiotherapy, Faculty of Health and Biomedical Sciences, University of South Australia; Specialist Manipulative Physiotherapist, Adelaide, South Australia, Australia

Lance T. Twomey, Ph.D.
Deputy Vice-Chancellor and Professor of Physiotherapy and Clinical Anatomy, Curtin University of Technology, Perth, Western Australia, Australia

Fernando Valencia, B.Sc., M.Sc., M.Com., PostGrad.Dip.Physio.
Private Practioner, Randwick Physiotherapy Centre, Randwick, New South Wales, Australia

Steven G. White, Dip. Phyty., Dip.M.T.
Lecturer, New Zealand Manipulative Therapists Diploma of Manipulative Therapy; Private Practitioner, Auckland, New Zealand

David R. Worth, Ph.D., M.App.Sc.
Research Physiotherapist, Department of Radiology, Flinders Medical Centre, Bedford Park, South Australia; Senior Consultant, Rankin Occupational Safety and Health, North Adelaide, South Australia, Australia

Preface

Physical therapists involved in the management of patients with symptoms arising from the cervical and thoracic spine face no less of a challenge than they did six years ago when the first edition of *Physical Therapy of the Cervical and Thoracic Spine* was published. Indeed, headache and neck pain remain as ubiquitous today as they did then, still affecting two-thirds of the population, while the incidence of neck and upper extremity pain in the workplace shows little reduction (Ch. 18).

This second edition has expanded the volume from 15 to 19 chapters of which eight are new chapters or chapters containing entirely new material. All other chapters in the book show progression and change from the first edition, and many include significant new material.

The book is presented in three interrelated sections as before. The first part has been enhanced by chapters on the anatomy of the cervical spine and clinical biomechanics of the thorax.

The second part on examination and assessment builds upon the first edition with a chapter on examination and treatment by passive movement, and encourages the physical therapist to consider the patient's symptoms from a mechanism of symptoms approach (Chs. 6, 11, and 15). Physical therapists are now harnessing new knowledge from the pain sciences in their clinical reasoning, examination, and treatment of patients. The reader is introduced to four mechanisms of neurogenic pain: peripherally evoked, centrally evoked, autonomic involvement, and affective mechanisms, and to how these might be recognized.

Chapters in the third part on clinical management have been written to assist the practicing clinician in the assessment and management of patients with upper quarter dysfunction. This section includes two new chapters, one on a movement system balance approach to the management of musculoskeletal pain (Ch. 16) and one on a conceptual basis for the management of neural injury in the thoracic spine by manual therapy (Ch. 15).

The final chapter reminds us that science, art, and placebo are all integral parts of manual therapy and emphasizes that if the scientific basis of manual therapy is to continue to grow, it is likely that an upsetting of established beliefs will be part of the critical analysis that must continue to take place.

Ruth Grant, B.P.T., M.App.Sc., Grad.Dip.Adv.Man.Ther

Contents

I. Anatomy, Biomechanics, and Innervation

1. **Functional and Applied Anatomy of the Cervical Spine**   1
   James R. Taylor and Lance T. Twomey

2. **Biomechanics of the Cervical Spine**   27
   Nikolai Bogduk

3. **Biomechanics of the Thorax**   47
   Diane Lee

4. **Innervation and Pain Patterns of the Cervical Spine**   65
   Nikolai Bogduk

5. **Innervation and Pain Patterns of the Thoracic Spine**   77
   Nikolai Bogduk and Fernando Valencia

II. Examination and Assessment

6. **Clinical Reasoning in Orthopedic Manual Therapy**   89
   Mark Jones, Nicole Christensen, and Judi Carr

7. **Examination of the Cervical and Thoracic Spine**   109
   Mary E. Magarey

8. **Vertebral Artery Concerns: Premanipulative Testing of the Cervical Spine**   145
   Ruth Grant

9. **Combined Movements of the Cervical Spine in Examination and Treatment**   167
   Brian C. Edwards

10. **Muscles and Motor Control in Cervicogenic Disorders: Assessment and Management**   195
    Vladimir Janda

11. **The Upper Limb Tension Test Revisited**   217
    David S. Butler

12. Evaluation and Treatment by Passive Movement   245
Helen Jones, Mark Jones, and Geoffrey D. Maitland

III. Clinical Management

13. Headaches of Cervical Origin   261
Gwendolen A. Jull

14. Management of Selected Cervical Syndromes   287
Patricia H. Trott

**15. Neural Injury in the Thoracic Spine: A Conceptual
Basis for Manual Therapy**   313
David S. Butler and Helen Slater

**16. A Movement System Balance Approach to
Management of Musculoskeletal Pain**   339
Steven G. White and Shirley A. Sahrmann

**17. Mechanical Diagnosis and Therapy for the Cervical
and Thoracic Spine**   359
Rodney N. Grant and Robin A. McKenzie

18. Neck and Upper Extremity Pain in the Workplace   379
Barbara McPhee and David R. Worth

19. Manual Therapy: Science, Art, and Placebo   409
Ruth Grant

Index   421

1 | Functional and Applied Anatomy of the Cervical Spine

James R. Taylor
Lance T. Twomey

The human spine, as a whole, combines three important functions:

1. It forms a stable osteo-ligamentous axis for the neck and torso and for the support of the head and limbs.
2. It provides a wide variety and range of movements that are essential for human tasks related to positioning of the upper limbs and hands, varying the direction of vision, and contributing to locomotion.
3. It forms a protective conduit for the spinal cord and its nerves, conducting them as closely as possible to the points of distribution of the spinal nerves to the parts they innervate.

The cervical and thoracolumbar regions of the spine differ in the balance between the first two of these two functions: in the thoracolumbar spine stability is the primary requirement, while the cervical spine is specialized for mobility. It not only holds the head up but directs the gaze through a range of almost 180° in the horizontal plane and a range of about 120° in the vertical plane.[1] The severe handicap posed by neck stiffness in a car driver with ankylosing spondylitis illustrates the importance of rapid, wide-range mobility in the neck.

This functional contrast between the cervical spine and the rest of the spine is reflected by many differences in the shape, size, and structure of its vertebrae and its intervertebral joints. The first two cervical vertebrae are unique, and their synovial joints contribute about a third of the flexion–extension and over half of the axial rotation of the cervical spine. The remainder of the cervical spine, with its six motion segments (C2-3 to C7-T1), is also much more slender and more mobile than the six motion segments of the lumbar spine.[2] These cervical joints collectively provide a sagittal range of up to 90°, compared to 60° in the lumbar spine. The lower cervical joints allow a wide range of axial rotation, a movement that is very restricted in the lumbar spine.[3,4]

The structural features that contribute most to the contrasting functions of the two regions are the greater slenderness of the cervical spine and the marked difference in facet shape and orientation between the two regions. Another important contrast is the presence of prominent uncinate processes projecting up from the lateral margin of each cervical vertebral body and their complete absence from lumbar vertebrae.[5–7] The slender cervical spine carries the thickest part of the spinal cord in a wide spinal canal, and supports the head, which weighs about 3 kg.[8] The support of a heavy head on a slender, highly mobile stalk makes the neck vulnerable to injury. In our postmortem study of spinal injuries in 385 victims of road trauma, half of all the spinal injuries were to the cervical spine.[9] Control of the motor and sensory functions of the whole torso and all four limbs is transmitted through the cervical spinal cord. The blood vessels supplying the brain stem, cerebellum, and occipital lobes of the cerebrum also pass up through the cervical transverse processes. Therefore, the consequences of cervical injury are potentially more serious than those of injury in lower regions.

These general considerations make it abundantly clear that a sound and practical knowledge of the functional and applied anatomy of the cervical spine is essential for any health professional who would examine it and understand or treat cervical pain or dysfunction. This account begins by reviewing spinal development and growth, then describes adult anatomy and movements, common features of aging in the cervical spine, and the anatomy of injuries and of pain of cervical spinal origin.

RESUME OF DEVELOPMENT

In the third week of embryonic life, the longitudinal axis of the embryo is formed by the growth of the notochord between the ectoderm and the endoderm. The notochord is the precursor of the vertebral column. Paraxial mesoderm develops on each side of the notochord.

The notochord controls the further development of the mesodermal cells on each side of it, and has an important influence on the ectoderm, which lies immediately dorsal to it. First, it induces thickening of the dorsal ectoderm to form the neural plate, which folds to form the neural tube. Then the notochord and neural tube together cause the paraxial mesodermal cells to form a cylindrical mesodermal condensation around them, which is the primitive vertebral column. Before this mesodermal vertebral column is formed, the paraxial mesoderm segments into a large number of blocks of mesoderm called *somites*. These

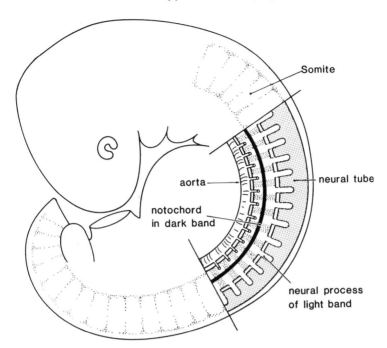

Fig. 1-1. Diagrammatic reconstruction of 7-mm embryo with external features removed from central part to show the notochord enclosed in the primitive vertebral column; the light bands (primitive vertebrae), whose neural processes partly enclose the neural tube; and the dorsal aorta, whose intersegmental branches supply the centres of the light bands. Compare with Fig. 1-2. (From Taylor and Twomey,[11] with permission.)

somites are ranged along each side of the notochord and neural tube, and their medial parts (sclerotomes) are the raw material from which the original vertebral column is made. The dorsal aorta lies anterior to the original, unsegmented condensation of mesoderm around the notochord and neural tube, and its regular intersegmental branches supply this mesodermal vertebral column. Vertebral column development is usually described in three stages[10,11] (Fig. 1-1).

Mesodermal Stage

The original column is formed around the notochord by the mesoderm from the ventromedial portions of the somites. Although formed from segmented mesoderm, this mesodermal column is continuous and unsegmented. It resegments into alternate light and dark bands all the way along its length. Neural processes grow around the neural tube from each light band. The aorta sends

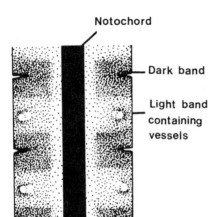

Notochord

Dark band

Light band containing vessels

Fig. 1-2. Coronal section of 7-mm embryo. Note the paired intersegmental vessels in the light bands (vertebrae). Fissures in the dark bands (discs) are a transient feature. (From Taylor and Twomey,[11] with permission.)

intersegmental branches around the middle of each light band. The light bands grow in height more rapidly than the adjacent dark bands[12] (Fig. 1-2).

Cartilaginous Stage

Each light band with its neural processes differentiates into a cartilaginous model of a vertebra at about 2 months gestation. The differentiation and rapid growth of the light bands into fetal cartilage models of vertebral bodies is accompanied by notochordal segmentation. The cylindrical notochord swells within each dark band or primitive intervertebral disc and constricts and disappears from each cartilaginous vertebra. Each notochordal segment will form a nucleus pulposus at the center of a disc. At the periphery of the primitive intervertebral disc, fibroblasts lay down collagen fibers in outwardly convex lamellae. The cartilaginous stage of vertebral development is a short one, and blood vessels grow into the cartilaginous vertebra, heralding the appearance of the primary centers of ossification.

Osseous Stage

Three primary centers of ossification are formed in each vertebra. Bilateral centers for the vertebral arch appear first, then one center for each vertebral body. The earliest vertebral arch centers in the cervicothoracic region, so that cervical arches ossify relatively early and the most caudal centers appear last. The single ossification center for each vertebral body forms the centrum. The first centra appear in the thoracolumbar region and the cervical centra appear relatively late.

Ossification extends transversely through the cartilage model of each vertebra, replacing cartilage with bone, except for three cartilage growth plates. The bilateral neurocentral growth plates and the single growth plate between the laminae persist in the ring around the spinal canal to ensure continuing growth in girth of the canal to accommodate growth of the spinal cord. When the required growth in girth of the spinal canal is almost complete, the three growth plates around it fuse. The two halves of the vertebral arch fuse at about 1 year postnatally. The bilateral neurocentral growth plates between the arch and the centrum on each side fuse at 3 years in cervical vertebrae. These growth plates are within the vertebral body, so that the lateral quarter of each cervical vertebra is ossified from the vertebral arch.

Growth plates and cartilage plates also persist at the upper and lower margins of the vertebral body, next to the discs, to ensure growth in height. Each cartilage plate remains cartilaginous throughout life, except at its circumference, where a ring apophysis appears. This bony "ring apophysis" appears between 9 and 12 years of age and fuses with the vertebral body at 16 to 18 years, 2 years earlier in girls than in boys.

GROWTH IN LENGTH OF THE VERTEBRAL COLUMN

Growth is most rapid before birth, and the rate decreases progressively in infancy and childhood, with a final growth spurt at adolescence. The spine contributes 60 percent of sitting height. Sitting-height measurements are used to chart postnatal growth in length of the spine. Sitting height increases by 5 cm in the second year of life. The rate of increase declines to 2.5 cm per annum from 4 years to 7 years, then declines further to 1.5 cm per annum by 9 or 10 years. The adolescent growth spurt between 10 and 14 years in girls peaks at 12 years with a growth velocity of 4 cm per annum. In boys the growth spurt lasts from 12 to 17 years with a peak growth velocity of 4 cm per annum at 14 years. Sitting height reaches 99 percent of its maximum by 15 years in girls and 17 years in boys.[13]

NOTOCHORDAL, NEURAL, VASCULAR, AND MECHANICAL INFLUENCES ON DEVELOPMENT

The notochord and neural tube induce formation of the mesodermal vertebral column around them from the medial parts of the somites. Regular segmentation of the mesodermal column is influenced by the regular arrangement of intersegmental arteries within it. The notochord makes a small contribution to the original nucleus pulposus in cervical discs, and forms the greater part of the nucleus in other discs, but notochordal tissue atrophies and disappears during childhood. The small notochordal contribution to the cervical nucleus and the correspondingly greater contribution to the cervical nucleus from surrounding fibroblastic cells means that from an early stage there is more collagen in the cervical nucleus than in other regions.

Persistence of live notochord cells in vertebrae may lead to the formation of chordomas in adults. These rare malignant tumors are usually seen in high retropharyngeal or sacrococcygeal situations. Congenital fusion of vertebrae, butterfly vertebra, or hemivertebra may result from abnormal development of the notochord or the segmental blood vessels. Congenital fusion of vertebrae is quite common in the cervical spine.

Growth of the spinal cord influences growth of the vertebral arches and canal, just as brain growth influences skull-vault growth. An enlarged spinal cord results in an enlarged canal. Spina bifida is a developmental anomaly that varies from a simple cleft in the vertebral arch (spina bifida occulta), which is common and innocuous, to complete splitting of skin, the vertebral arch, and the underlying neural tube with associated neurologic deficits. In meningomyelocele, abnormal development of the neural tube is the primary event, and the skeletal defects are secondary. This abnormality occurs most often in the lumbosacral spine, but also occurs in the cervical region.

Following birth, the cervical spine forms a secondary lordotic curve during the first 6 months of postnatal life. When the infant assumes erect posture, a lumbar lordosis appears. These postural changes produce changes in the shape of the intervertebral discs and slow changes in the position of the nucleus pulposus. They also produce changes in the shape of the vertebral end-plates.

Uncinate processes grow upward from the posterolateral margins of each cervical vertebra during childhood, and uncovertebral clefts begin to appear in the lateral parts of each intervertebral disc just before adolescence. The appearance of these uncovertebral clefts or joints is unique to the cervical spine, and is favored by its greater mobility and the narrowing of the lateral parts of the interbody space.

SEGMENTATION AND VERTEBRAL ANOMALIES

Normal Segmentation

The mesodermal column is formed from the medial parts of the somites (sclerotomes), which are segmented blocks of mesoderm, but it is itself continuous and unsegmented. It resegments into its own sequence of alternate light and dark bands in such a way that the vertebrae develop between the myotomes, the segmental blocks of muscle derived from the middle parts of the somites. Thus the muscles will bridge over from vertebra to vertebra. This alternation of muscle and bone is essential to the proper function of the locomotor system.

Regularly spaced intersegmental branches of the dorsal aorta pass around each developing vertebra and provide nutrition for rapid growth. Vascular anomalies may result in anomalies of segmentation.[14]

Segmental Anomalies

A hemivertebra develops if one side of the vertebral body fails to grow. Absence of an intersegmental vessel on one side may result in failure to grow on that side; only one side grows and a hemivertebra appears. Absence of a notochordal segment may cause centra to fuse, forming congenital fusion between vertebrae. The relatively high frequency of this in the cervical spine may relate to the smaller contribution made by the notochord to the nucleus in the cervical region.

Chordoma

Notochordal cells produce substances that loosen and digest the inner margins of the surrounding envelope; this "invasive" characteristic contributes to the growth of the expanding nucleus in fetuses and infants.[15] Notochordal cells do not normally survive beyond early childhood, except perhaps deeply buried in the developing sacrum or at the craniocervical junctional region. If notochordal cells survive, they may be "released" by trauma to the containing tissues and begin to multiply again, causing a malignant chordoma. Fortunately this is a rare tumor.

"Butterfly Vertebra"

The mucoid streak persists for a while in the cartilage models of fetal and a few infant vertebrae as an acellular notochordal track. Ossification of the centrum usually obliterates it. If the notochordal track persists through the centrum, it locally inhibits ossification and a butterfly vertebra will result.

NORMAL ADULT ANATOMY OF THE CERVICAL SPINE

Atlas and Axis Vertebrae

The *atlas* or first cervical vertebra (C1) has a ring structure around a wide vertebral foramen. The ring is formed by two lateral masses joined by anterior and posterior arches. The atlas develops without a centrum; its centrum joins the axis (C2) to form its dens. The atlas has no articular facets corresponding to those on the cervical vertebrate below C2 (Fig. 1-3).

The Atlanto-Occipital Joint

The lateral masses of the atlas articulate with the occiput above and with the axis below. The concave upper articular surfaces articulate with the convex occipital condyles, which project downward on each side of the foramen magnum. The upper articular facets of C1 are elongated from front to back, and kidney shaped in outline, with their anterior ends closer together than their posterior ends. Their anterior ends project upward in a curved fashion to a greater extent than their posterior ends. This provides for much more extension

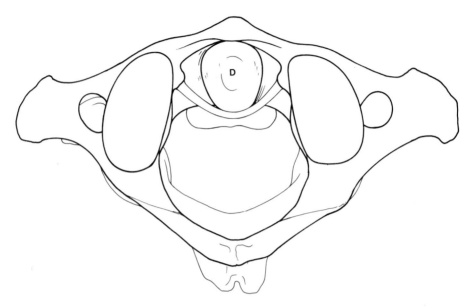

Fig. 1-3.   Atlas from above, with dens *(D)* of C2 and transverse ligament. The diagram of C1 shows the concave articular facets for the occipital condyles and the articulation of the anterior arch, with the odontoid process (dens) of C2. The transverse ligament, which holds the dens in place, is attached to two tubercles on the medial aspects of the articular masses. The foramina transversaria and the long transverse processes are seen lateral to the articular masses.

than flexion in the atlanto-occipital joint.[16] Atlanto-occipital dislocation, or fracture dislocation, can occur in severe injuries in motor vehicle accidents. It is usually fatal, because the junction of the brain stem and spinal cord is injured; in our current studies, we have seven examples of this injury in 90 cases of fatal trauma. The lateral margins of the upper facets of C1 are higher than the medial margins, and functionally, the lateral atlantoaxial joints can be considered as two parts of a single ellipsoid joint. This allows about 10° of lateral bending to each side.[16] This configuration also means than in axial compression injuries the lateral masses may be forced apart, with fracture of the slender anterior and posterior arches (Jefferson fracture).

Each joint is enclosed by a fibrous capsule, lined on its inner aspect by synovial membrane. Like the atlanto-occipital joint the atlantoaxial joint is usually well preserved in many elderly people whose lower cervical joints have become stiff.[17]

Medial to each articular facet is a prominent tubercle for the attachment of the vitally important transverse ligament, which holds the dens of the axis in position against the small facet on the central part of the posterior surface of the anterior arch (Fig. 1-3). This is part of the atlantoaxial joint complex.

The Transverse Processes and Arches of the Atlas

The atlas has long transverse processes that are palpable, but has no spinous process.[18] The long transverse processes project laterally, anteroinferior to the mastoid processes. In the medial part of each process is an outwardly angled foramen for the vertebral artery. The lateral masses are joined by two slender arches. There are small anterior and posterior tubercles on the outer aspect of each arch in the midline. The posterior tubercle is for the attachment of the nuchal ligament and the rectus capitis posterior minor. The anterior tubercle is for the upper end of the anterior longitudinal ligament and the longus cervicis. A vertebral artery grooves the upper surface of each posterior arch and the posterior aspect of each lateral mass. As the artery courses medially, to the foramen magnum from the foramen transversarium, the small 1st cervical nerve passes out between the artery and the arch on each side, under cover of the posterior atlanto-occipital membrane. This membrane passes from the posterior arch to the posterior margin of the foramen magnum. The posterior arch and the vertebral artery lie at the floor of the suboccipital triangle, deeply located under the overhanging posterior skull, between the rectus capitis posterior major and the superior and inferior oblique muscles. These muscles are supplied by the dorsal ramus of C1, and though quite small they are important in cervicocapital postural control. This region contains a plexus of suboccipital veins, easily bruised in injuries to the region. A thicker anterior atlanto-occipital membrane attaches the anterior arch to the base of the skull just in front of the anterior margin of the foramen magnum. This membrane is covered medially by the longus capitis and laterally by the rectus capitis anterior.

The Axis Vertebra (C2)

The central part of this vertebra is formed from the centra of both C1 and C2, giving it a normal sized lower vertebral body plus an upwardly projecting, toothlike dens or odontoid process.[19] Its lateral masses project laterally from this central part, midway between its lower margin and the tip of the dens, and to these masses are attached transverse processes and a vertebral arch with a thick, prominent spinous process in the form of an inverted "V." The lateral masses have upper flat facets for the atlantoaxial joint, and the laminae have downward and forward facing facets in line with the zygapophyseal facets of the lower cervical spine.[20] An upwardly projected line from the articular columns formed by these lower facets would pass posterior to the atlantoaxial and atlanto-occipital joints.

The transverse processes of C2 are much shorter than those of C1. The obliquely directed foramina transversaria, which gouge out deep grooves in the lower lateral parts of the lateral masses near the atlantoaxial joints, reflect the 45° outward and upward course of the vertebral arteries through C2 as they pass onto the posterolateral capsules of the joints.

The anterior longitudinal ligament narrows to a point as it attaches to the anterior tubercle of the atlas, and this is reflected by the projecting triangular outline on the anterior surface of the body of C2, where the ligament gains some attachment.[21] The posterior longitudinal is continuous with the membrana tectoria, which covers the cruciate ligamentous complex behind the dens, where it articulates with the anterior arch of the atlas and the transverse ligament. The membrana tectoria attaches to the basiocciput inside the foramen magnum.

The Atlantoaxial Joint

This interesting joint complex has three parts, two symmetrical lateral parts between the lateral masses of the atlas and axis and a central part formed by the enclosure of the upwardly projecting dens between the anterior arch of the atlas and the strong transverse ligament. These joints provide the largest component of cervical axial rotation, which is required for both voluntary and reflex turning of the head to direct the gaze to right or left. The stability of the joint depends on the integrity of the transverse ligament, which holds the dens in place[22] (Fig. 1-3). The dens acts as the "axis" around which rotation takes place.

The lateral joints are described as planar, but while flat in the coronal plane, both articular surfaces are convex in the sagittal plane, making them incongruous (Fig. 1-4). When viewed in sagittal section the articular surfaces are covered by articular cartilage that is thick centrally and thin peripherally, with a white, glistening, smooth surface in young subjects. These surfaces are often well preserved in older subjects. The anterior and posterior articular margins are separated by large triangular gaps, containing large, vascular, fat-filled synovial folds. These triangular meniscoid inclusions are attached at their bases to the inner aspect of the fibrous capsule, and their inner surfaces are lined by synovial membrane (Fig. 1-4). In young subjects they are soft and change shape readily on joint movement; they are filled by fat containing a plentiful vascular network. In older subjects they are fibro-fatty and stiffer, but generally remain vascular. These triangular meniscoid inclusions are often bruised in flexion–extension injuries.[17]

A well-defined but fairly loose fibrous capsule, about 1 to 2 mm thick, is attached around the articular margins of the joints. The roots of the second cervical nerve leave the spinal canal close to the medial capsule. They join as the spinal nerve passes transversely behind the posterior fibrous capsule, where the large dorsal-root ganglion dwarfs the small anterior root. The larger dorsal ramus forms the greater occipital nerve, which hooks under the inferior oblique muscle to ascend through the semispinalis capitis into the posterior scalp.[23,24]

The inferior oblique muscle passes transversely close behind the atlantoaxial joint, enclosing a space containing the C2 nerve and a plexus of thin-walled veins medial to and around the vertebral artery. The vertebral artery is loosely attached to the lateral capsule of the joint, its tortuous vertical course allowing

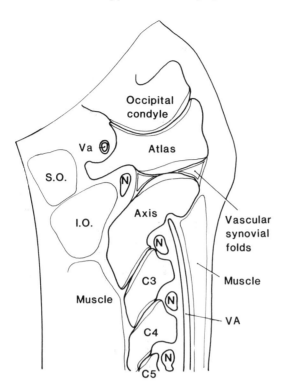

Fig. 1-4. This sagittal section from a young adult shows the zygapophyseal joints, whose facets are oriented at 45° to the long axis of the spine. The biconvex atlantoaxial facets are incongruous; triangular, vascular, synovial folds occupy the anterior and posterior parts of the joint. The convex occipital condyle fits neatly into the concave facet of the atlas. The vertebral artery *(Va)* is seen in transverse section on the posterior arch of the atlas and in sagittal section, ascending through the foramina transversaria of the cervical vertebrae. The dorsal root ganglion of C2 lies behind the atlantoaxial joint, covered by the inferior oblique *(IO)* and the superior oblique *(SO)* muscles. Anterior to the articular masses of C3 to C5, the dorsal root ganglia of C3, C4, and C5 *(N)* lie behind the vertebral artery.

for movements of the joint. Bleeding from the thin-walled veins may form a large hematoma around the C2 nerve in nonpenetrating injuries to this region.

The centra part of the joint complex is formed by the articulation of the dens with the anterior arch of the atlas and the enclosure of the dens by the strong transverse ligament which passes between large tubercles on the medial aspects of the lateral masses of the atlas. Articular cartilage covers the articulation between the dens and the arch of the atlas. There are separate synovial cavities in this articulation and between the transverse ligament and the dens. From near the tip of the dens on each side, strong alar or "check" ligaments pass upward and outward to the medial margins of the occipital condyles.[25] A much finer apical ligament passes from the tip of the dens to the anterior margin of the foramen magnum, and an inferior longitudinal bundle passes from the transverse ligament to the back of the body of C2, completing a cruciate ligamentous complex that is covered behind by the membrana tectoria and the anterior dura mater. The skull and atlas rotate around the axis of the dens, excessive movement being checked by the alar ligaments, which may be injured in rotational strains.

It is also of interest that the incongruity between the lateral masses of C1 and C2 allows rocking with flexion and extension in this joint. Panjabi[16] recorded 20° of sagittal plane movement here, compared to 30° in the atlanto-occipital joint.

The Lower Cervical Spine (C3 to T1)

The Vertebrae

Cervical vertebrae have the smallest bodies and the largest spinal foramina of the vertebral column. The third to sixth cervical vertebrae are described as being typical cervical vertebrae, but the sixth is atypical in some respects, having a longer spinous process than C3 to C5 and prominent, palpable, anterior tubercles, called the *carotid tubercles,* on its transverse processes. A typical cervical vertebra has a small vertebral body whose upper surface is flat centrally but is shaped like a seat with side supports (uncinate processes), and whose lower surface is concave in the sagittal plane (Fig. 1-5). From the posterolateral "corners" of this vertebral body the thin pedicles project posterolaterally. From the pedicles, thin laminae are sharply angled posteromedially to enclose a large triangular spinal foramen. Short bifid spinous processes extend back from C3 to C5. The spinous process of C7 is long and pointed, and C7 is called the *vertebra prominens.* The spinous process of C6 is usually not bifid and is intermediate in length between those of C5 and C7. It has often been taught that between C2 and C7 the spinous process are not readily palpable, but this is false; with a patient supine and muscles relaxed, C6 is easily palpable and with care, all the spinous processes can usually be identified by palpation.[26]

Lateral to the junction of the pedicles and laminae are the articular masses, with articular facets on their upper and lower surfaces. The upper facets are directed upward and backward and the lower facets are directed forward and downward. These facets are flat and form synovial, zygapophyseal joints with the facets of the adjacent vertebrae. The articular masses from C3 to T1 form articular columns, which bear a significant proportion of axial loading.[22]

Facet Angles. The cervical zygapophyseal facets are described as lying in an oblique coronal plane.[18] Milne (1993, unpublished data) has measured the angle between the facets and the superior surface of the corresponding vertebral body in 67 human skeletons. He found this to range from an average of 127° in C5 to 116° in C7 and 112° in T1. Considering that the superior surface of each

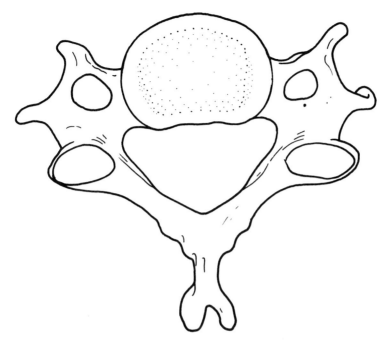

Fig. 1-5. Typical cervical vertebra from above. The C3 to C5 vertebrae each show a small vertebral body, bifid transverse and spinous processes, a large triangular spinal canal, and zygapophyseal facets that lie in an oblique coronal plane at 45° to the long axis of the spine.

cervical vertebral body slopes downward and forward, this would correspond to angles varying from about 45° to the long axis of the spine in the mid-cervical spine to just over 30° to the long axis of the spine at T1. In sagittal sections of adult cervical vertebrae, we found these angles to vary considerably, but we agree that 45° is close to the average in the mid-cervical spine and that 30° is close to the average for T1.

The transverse processes project anterolaterally from the articular masses and the vertebral bodies as two elements enclosing foramina transversaria for the vertebral arteries (Fig. 1-5). The anterior or costal element of this transverse process projects from the vertebral body. The posterior or true transverse element projects from the articular mass. Each element has a small tubercle at its tip in the C3 to C6 vertebrae for attachment of the scalene muscles, with the scalenus anterior attaching to the anterior tubercles and the scalenus medius to the posterior tubercles. The transverse processes are concave or gutter shaped on their superior aspects, especially from C5 down, corresponding to the large size of the nerves forming the brachial plexus, which passes out behind the vertebral artery into the inter-scalene plane in the root of the neck.

The atlas, axis, and C7 are described as atypical cervical vertebrae. The atlas and axis have already been described. The C7 vertebra differs from the others in having a very long spinous process and more vertically oriented zyga-pophyseal facets. There is in fact a gradual transition from the 45° angle of typical cervical facets to the 20° to 30° angle of thoracic facets. Though C7 has a small foramen transversarium, it does not transmit the vertebral arteries but only some vertebral veins.

Vertebral Arteries. The vertebral artery arises from the first part of the subclavian artery and passes upward on the longus colli to enter the foramen transversarium of C6, and then ascends through C6 to C1 inclusive, accompanied by the vertebral veins and a plexus of small sympathetic nerves before piercing the dura and arachnoid to enter the foramen magnum.[27,28] Within the cranial cavity, the two arteries ascend between the base of the skull and the medulla in the subarachnoid space, and join to form the basilar artery at the level of the pontomedullary junction. They are usually asymmetrical to some degree. In a study of 150 cadavers, Stopford,[29] claimed that 51 percent showed the left artery to be larger than the right, 41 percent showed the right to be larger than the left, and only 8 percent were equal in size. In an unpublished study based on measurements of the arterial images in magnetic resonance imaging (MRI) scans of 267 patients, Kearney[30] found the left vertebral artery to be larger in 49%, the right artery to be larger in 29 percent, and approximate equality in 22 percent. This has relevance in passive movement and manipulative studies. When there is gross asymmetry there may be a greater risk of depriving the hindbrain of its blood supply from maneuvers that obstruct a single vertebral artery.[31] We have observed a small number of instances of intimal damage with dissection and the formation of loose inner flaps in traumatized arteries, following motion-segment subluxation in motor vehicle accidents. In survivors of such accidents, vertebral artery thrombosis would be likely.

The vertebral arteries within the cervical spine give off small branches to supply the vertebrae and deep muscles and a few small feeders to the arteries of the spinal cord, the main arteries to the cord (one anterior and two posterior spinal arteries) being derived from the terminal portions of the vertebral arteries within the cranial cavity. Each vertebral artery is said to supply small branches at the level of C2, which form spiral arteriolar "glomeruli" to enter ampullary veins below the base of the skull in the suboccipital region.[32] These small arteries have a rich autonomic nerve supply. Injuries to these arteries could have the effect of causing arteriovenous fistulae. The vertebral veins have plentiful connections with the body-wall veins and with the internal vertebral venous plexus in the epidural space. Since these veins are valveless, blood can flow in either direction, and these veins act as routes for the spread of cancer cells, usually to thoracic or lumbar vertebrae.

The Motion Segments

Each lower cervical motion segment consists of "interbody joints" (an intervertebral disc and two uncovertebral joints) and two zygapophyseal (facet) joints. The lower cervical motion segments have an average of about 15° of

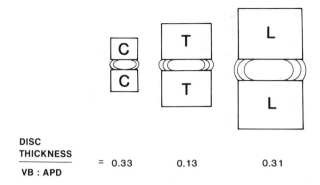

DISC
THICKNESS
――――――― = 0.33   0.13   0.31
VB : APD

Fig. 1-6. Factors controlling movement range. The slenderness of cervical vertebrae and the relative thickness of the discs favor mobility. An index of disc thickness over the anteroposterior diameter of the vertebral body is highest in the cervical spine *(C)*, next highest in the lumbar spine *(L)*, and lowest in the thoracic spine *(T)*.

sagittal range per segment, compared to an average of about 10° per motion segment in the lumbar spine.[3,33] These ranges of movement depend on the thickness of the intervertebral discs relative to the horizontal dimensions of the vertebral bodies (Fig. 1-6). The dimensions and compliance of the intervertebral disc determine the amount of movement possible; the extent and orientation of the zygapophyseal articular surfaces control the types of movement possible and make an essential contribution to stability by restraining excessive movement.

Van Mameren et al.[34] showed than in living subjects, the range of active cervical motion in the sagittal plane could vary considerably depending on variation in the instructions given to the subjects. The complex interplay of soft-tissue restraints and other factors resulted in the same subjects moving through different ranges in successive attempts to perform essentially the same movement.

Special features of lower cervical motion segments are (1) the development and natural history of the nucleus pulposus; (2) the growth of uncinate processes and formation of unco-vertebral joints; (3) the orientation of zygapophyseal facets at 45° to the long axis of the spine; and (4) the age-related formation of uncovertebral osteophytes encroaching on the intervertebral canals, together with bar-like posterior disc protrusions into the spinal canal.

The Development and Natural History of the Nucleus Pulposus. The notochord segments in cervical discs are much smaller than those in thoracic or lumbar discs. The rapid growth of notochordal segments and their interaction with the surrounding disc tissues forms a large, soft, gelatinous mass at the center of each lumbar intervertebral disc. In cervical discs the notochordal segment often remains small and rudimentary at birth, and its appearance is variable in infant cervical discs. Thus the cervical nucleus of infants and young children owes less to the notochord than the nucleus of the lumbar disc, and is often made of soft fibrocartilage.[15] From an early stage there is more collagen in the cervical than in the lumbar nucleus. Moreover, horizontal fissuring of the cervical annulus fibrosus develops from adolescence onward, and the nucleus pulposus of cervical discs has only a brief existence, in childhood and young adulthood, as an "encapsulated nucleus" enclosed by an intact fibrous and cartilaginous envelope. With the advent of fissuring in early adulthood, nuclear material may escape slowly from its annular envelope, or it becomes enmeshed in a collagenous network.

Therefore, the cervical disc should not be regarded as a smaller version of a lumbar disc. It is different in many respects. It has less soft nuclear material in the first place, and what remains is enmeshed in collagen in adults, so that nuclear prolapse is less likely, except in severe traumatic incidents, when herniated disc material is more likely to pass backward into the wide spinal canal than to pass laterally through the uncovertebral joints into the intervertebral canals. The cervical disc bears less axial load than the lumbar disc. Since proteoglycan and water content relate to load bearing, it is interesting that measurements of relative proteoglycan content confirm that it is lower in cervical than in lumbar discs.[29] As a degenerative phenomenon, lumbar discs herniate posterolaterally, but it is more usual for the fissured cervical annulus to show a generalized, bar-like, posterior bulge as a transverse, annular, and osteophytic protrusion into the spinal canal.

Growth of the Uncinate Processes: the Uncovertebral Joints of Luschka. The lateral parts of a cervical vertebral body are formed from the neural arch centers of ossification and not from the centrum. The width of the infant intervertebral disc does not extend to the whole transverse extent of the vertebral body. The outer edge of the annulus reaches just lateral to the line of fusion of the centrum and vertebral arches. From the upper lateral borders of each vertebral body, processes grow upward toward the vertebral body above (Fig. 1-7) in the loose vascular fibrous tissue at the lateral margins of the annulus.[6] Each process or uncus has grown enough by about 8 years of age to form a kind of adventitious joint called the uncovertebral joint on each side of the disc. There is some doubt about whether this "joint" or pseudoarthrosis develops within true disc tissue or whether it appears as a cleft in the looser connective tissue immediately lateral to the annulus.[5,7,33,35] The tip of the uncus and the groove in the lateral margin of the vertebra above are lined by a fibrocartilage that is probably derived from the horizontally cleft outer annulus, whose lamellae are bent outward and compacted together; a thin fibrous "capsule" limits each "joint" cleft laterally. The formation of the uncovertebral "joints" effectively narrows the horizontal band within which the translatory movements accompanying flexion take place (Fig. 1-7). It "concentrates" the plane of shear to a narrow horizontal band within the annulus because of the gliding movements in the adjacent uncovertebral "joints."[36] This appears to result in medial extension of horizontal fissures into the annulus from the uncovertebral clefts (Fig. 1-8). These fissures

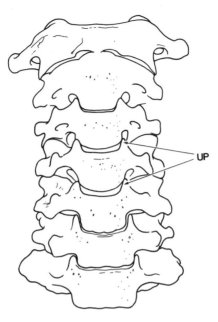

Fig. 1-7. Anterior view of cervical spine shows the unique shape of cervical vertebral bodies, which have uncinate processes *(UP)* projecting upward from their lateral edges to form uncovertebral joints with the vertebra above.

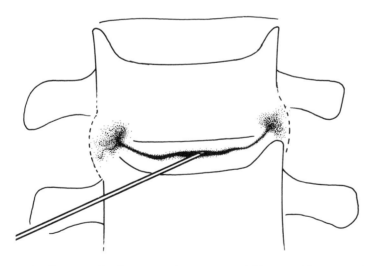

Fig. 1-8. This diagram of a discogram from a normal 36-year-old woman shows how contrast medium injected centrally typically spreads transversely through linear fissures in the normal disc into both uncovertebral joints, where an expanded cavity allows diffuse spread of the contrast medium.

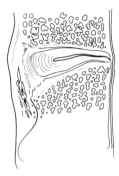

Fig. 1-9. This diagram of a sagittal section of an elderly cervical disc near the midline shows how the posterior half of the disc is completely fissured, except for the posterior longitudinal ligament, while the anterior annulus remains intact.

frequently extend right through the posterior part of the adult intervertebral disc between two uncovertebral joints, leaving only the anterior annulus and the longitudinal ligaments relatively intact (Fig. 1-9). Such extensive fissuring changes the disc, in middle life, form a structure that deforms around a central nucleus on movement, to yield a bipartite disc with a "gliding joint" between its upper and lower parts, which allows translation of several millimeters forward and backward in full flexion and extension. This arrangement is related to the wide range of mobility of the cervical spine, which entails much less stability than in the thoracolumbar spine. Thus, the cervical spine is heavily dependent, for its stability, on the integrity of the zygapophyseal joints and posterior musculature and ligaments. The additional loading of the uncovertebral joints that accompanies disc fissuring, loss of nuclear material, and "disc collapse" leads to lateral osteophytosis from the uncinate processes into the intervertebral canals. In some individuals the osteophytes are very large; they severely limit the space available to the spinal nerves and may compress the anterior part of the spinal cord.[37,38]

The Zygapophyseal Joints.   These joints, by their structure and the orientation of their articular facets, determine the directions of intervertebral movements. Their articular surfaces are oriented at about 45° to the long axis of the spine, with a range of 30° to 60°.[33] The cranial facets are directed upward and backward; the caudal facets are directed downward and forward. The facet orientation facilitates sagittal-plane movements and requires that axial rotation and lateral bending always be coupled.

The joint capsules are described as lax, permitting great mobility.[33,39] In our studies of sagittal sections of over 100 cervical spines of all ages, we have found that the lateral joint capsule is lax and fibrous and is partly formed by the ligamentum flavum anteriorly, but that the posterior capsule is very thin, especially medially, where the large triangular fat pad at the lower posterior joint margin is simply enclosed by the insertions of the deep cervical muscles. Where the upper end of the joint adjoins the intervertebral canal anteromedially, the capsule contains very little fibrous tissue and is formed by the synovial fat pad that projects into the joint. Vascular, fat-filled synovial folds project between the articular surfaces from the upper and lower joint recesses as "meniscoid inclusions'' that are vulnerable to bruising or rupture in injuries, forming hemarthroses in the joints (Fig. 1-4).

In flexion, a cervical vertebra both tilts and slides forward on the subjacent vertebra, with ventral compression and dorsal distraction of the disc, ''spreading the spinous processes like a fan.''[39] The forward rotation and translation probably occur together, but Jones[40] maintains that the forward slide is most evident in the later stages of flexion. In full flexion, there may only be about 5 mm of facetal contact remaining. Lateral radiographs of the flexed cervical spine show a ''stepped'' arrangement of the vertebral bodies because of the forward slide, an appearance that might be associated with instability if observed in the lumbar spine but is regarded as normal in the flexed cervical spine. With the 15° or more of rotation, there are about 2 mm of translation. Therefore, the centers of motion for sagittal plane movements are located in the subjacent vertebra. These centroids are relatively low in the vertebral body in upper segments and relatively high in the vertebral body in cervicothoracic sements.[33]

Both the orientation of the cervical facets and the presence of uncovertebral joints contributes to the process that leads to shearing and fissuring in adult cervical intervertebral discs. These changes would appear to be the price paid in reduced stability for the required range of cervical mobility. The reduced stability in full flexion, which depends on maintenance of a few millimeters of facet contact, obviously requires the strength and integrity of the posterior muscles and ligaments.

Degenerative Pathology. The disc fissuring already described involves the posterior parts of the disc and extends between the two uncovertebral joints on each side, though the posterior longitudinal ligament usually remains largely intact.[6] Isolated disc thinning is quite common as a degenerative phenomenon, when the uncus comes to bear more directly and firmly on the lower lateral margin of the vertebra above. When the ''articular surfaces'' of these pseudarthroses become weightbearing, the uncinate processes grow posterolateral osteophytes. Osteophytes projecting into the intervertebral canals are common in middle-aged and elderly cervical spines. Anteriorly directed osteophytes from the zygapophyseal superior articular facets are also quite common.[37]

Meanwhile, the disc bulges posteriorly as a bar into the anterior epidural space. The structures vulnerable to compression or distortion as a result of this degenerative spondylosis are the cervical nerve roots, the vertebral arteries, and the spinal cord.

Cervical Nerve Roots. The lateral recesses of the spinal canal are wider in the cervical spine than in the lumbar spine, but the intervertebral canals are almost filled by the large cervical dorsal root ganglia, which are at or below the level of the uncovertebral and zygapophyseal joint lines. The lumbar dorsal root ganglia, by contrast, occupy only the upper parts of large intervertebral canals, so that nerve roots are less at risk of entrapment in cervical than in

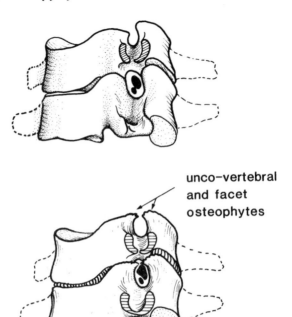

unco–vertebral
and facet
osteophytes

Fig. 1-10. Oblique views of normal and arthritic vertebrae. These anterior oblique views along the intervertebral foramina show the large dorsal and small ventral roots of the cervical nerves emerging between the zygapophyseal and uncovertebral joints. Note the reduced space for the nerves when uncovertebral and facet osteophytes appear.

lumbar lateral recesses but more at risk of close confinement in the intervertebral canals, through a combination of uncovertebral and facet osteophytes (Fig. 1-10). They are liable to be squeezed in pincer fashion between the zygapophyseal and uncovertebral osteophytes, or squeezed down by the encroaching osteophytes into the lower part of the intervertebral canal.

The Spinal Cord. As described above, posterior bars made of disc protrusions, flanked by posterior vertebral osteophytes, project backward into the anterior epidural space. The cervical spinal canal is fortunately relatively large in its anteroposterior dimensions, ranging from 13 to 22 mm in mid-sagittal diameter between C3 and C7, with a mean value of about 17 mm.[26] The spinal cord normally occupies only about 60 percent of this anteroposterior space.[33] However, in the extended position, particularly with degenerative changes in the lower cervical region, anterior bars and posterior infolding or buckling of the dura and ligamenta flava may imperil the cord. In some elderly people with thoracic osteoporosis, the thoracic kyphosis requires a considerable compensatory cervical lordosis.

In performing postmortem examinations on the cervical spines of elderly subjects, we often find the anterior surface of the spinal cord to be indented by disc and osteophytic bars. It appears that these may exist in many subjects without producing recognized symptoms. However, in cervical injuries to such subjects, the likelihood of spinal cord damage is much greater than in young subjects.[41]

Laterally directed osteophytes from the uncus can also encroach on the course of the vertebral vessels between the foramina transversaria of two successive cervical vertebrae, making forceful cervical manipulation in elderly subjects potentially hazardous.

ANATOMY OF INJURIES

In flexion, the posterior elements of the spine are distracted and the anterior elements are compressed. In extension, the anterior elements (discs) are distracted and the posterior elements are compressed. In the cervical spine, the facet orientation means that translation accompanies these anterior and posterior rotations, so that shearing forces occur in the tissues of the motion segments. Extension injury frequently causes splits to occur in the anterior discs at the disc–vertebra interface, owing to shear, without rupture of the anterior longitudinal ligament. This may and frequently does occur in several different discs as a result of a single injury. At the same time, compression of the facets with one another bruises the vascular, intra-articular synovial folds or fractures the tip of a facet where it is forced against an adjacent vertebral arch.

The cervical spine is inadequately protected from extension injuries by anterior muscles. The longus colli et cervicis with the prevertebral fascia are very small in bulk compared to the posterior muscles and their fasciae. We have observed in many fatally injured persons subjected to violent movements in both flexion and extension, that the main injuries have been sustained in extension. This relates to the inadequate protection given by seat belts in head-on collisions, where the majority of drivers and front-seat occupants of cars involved in high-speed collisions, strike their heads on the steering wheel or some other part of the car and sustain craniofacial trauma with a neck-extension injury. Well over 90 percent of these individuals show disc injuries, and about 80 percent also show soft-tissue injuries to the facet joints. About 15 percent also show intraneural bruises in the dorsal root ganglia.[42–44] Our heads and necks have built-in protection to sudden flexion but inadequate provision for sudden extension. When flexion injuries do occur they require a greater violence, which is enough to overcome the restraint offered by the posterior muscles and fasciae. In this case, one or both facets, usually at one specific level, may be dislocated, with grave risk of damage to the spinal cord.

INNERVATION OF CERVICAL MOTION SEGMENTS

The Intervertebral Disc

The longitudinal ligaments and the annulus of cervical intervertebral discs are innervated from the ventral rami, sinuvertebral nerves, and vertebral nerves (around the vertebral arteries). According to Bogduk,[45] only the outer annulus is innervated, but Mendel[46] demonstrated nerves through the whole thickness of the annulus. Nerves are not found in the cartilage plates or in the nucleus pulposus of normal discs.

The Zygapophyseal Joints

The medial branch of each dorsal ramus contributes to the innervation of two zygapophyseal joints.[24,47] The medial branches of the C4 to C8 dorsal rami curve dorsally around the waists of the articular pillars. There are often two of these branches on each articular pillar. They supply the zygapophyseal joint capsules above and below, and innervate the corresponding segments of the multifidus and semispinalis muscles. The fibrous capsule and joint recesses are innervated, but the ligamentum flavum does not appear to have any nociceptive nerves.[48–50] The synovial folds projecting into the joints from the polar recesses are probably innervated. Innervation has been demonstrated in these structures in the lumbar spine.[49,50]

Pain may arise from injury to any innervated part of the motion segment. It may also arise from injury to spinal nerves or dorsal root ganglia where they are closely related to these joints. For example, the dorsal rami of C2 and C3, which form the greater occipital nerve and the third occipital nerve, can be affected by injury. They supply the skin of the medial upper neck and the occipital scalp as far as the vertex. They also supply rostral segments of postvertebral muscles and the posterior capsules of the lateral atlantoaxial joints and the C2-3 and C3-4 zygapophyseal joints. We have observed both perineural and intraneural bruising in our postmortem studies of neck injuries.

PAIN REFERRAL PATTERNS

Pain is often referred to the skin, but pain is also referred through the sensory nerves of muscles. The trapezius, sternomastoid, and levator scapulae are innervated by C3 and C4, the rhomboids by C5, the short scapulohumeral muscles by C5 and C6, and the longer trunk-humeral muscles have multisegmental innervation (C5 to T1). When these muscles are injured or involved in reflex spasm, they may generate patterns of referred pain similar to those of the underlying spinal joints.[28] Explaining cervical headache, Bogduk[47] points to the convergence of afferents from C1 to C3 with the spinal tract of the trigeminal nerve in the grey matter of the upper cervical cord, in the "trigeminocervical nucleus." The ophthalmic and maxillary divisions of the trigeminal nerve are best represented in this "nucleus."

Two neck-sprain syndromes are described: a "cervico-encephalic syndrome" in which trauma to upper cervical motion segments (discs, facets, muscles, or dura) causes neck pain and headaches; and a "lower cervical syndrome" from traumatic lesions to lower cervical motion segments, in which pain radiates from the neck to the upper limb, shoulder, or scapular region.[51-53]

SUMMARY

In summary, the unique anatomy of lower cervical mobile segments gives the cervical spine a wide range of mobility but carries the risk of less stability in these mobile joints. The orientation of the cervical zygapophyseal joints at 45° to the long axis of the spine, and the childhood development of uncovertebral joints, both contribute to early fissuring of cervical intervertebral discs, with loss of the "encapsulated nucleus found in lumbar intervertebral discs. This is associated with loss of cervical disc height and degenerative spondylitic changes that pose threats to the cervical spinal nerves. The relative instability of cervical mobile segments as compared to thoracolumbar segments increases the importance of the posterior ligaments and muscles of the neck. If these structures are injured in sudden deceleration injuries, the mobility of the cervical triad may prove a grave disadvantage; while unilateral dislocation of a zygapophyseal joint facet may leave enough room for the cord in the spinal canal, bilateral dislocation often results in severe cord damage.

REFERENCES

1. Huelke DF, Nusholz GS: Cervical spine biomechanics: a review of the literature. J Orthop 109:42, 1986
2. Penning L, Wilmink JT: Rotation of the cervical spine: a CT study in normal subjects. Spine 12:732, 1987
3. Taylor JR, Twomey L: Sagittal and horizontal plane movement of the lumbar vertebral column in cadavers and in the living. Rheum Rehab 19:223, 1980
4. White AA, Panjabi MM: Clinical Biomechanics of the Spine. 2nd Ed. JB Lippincott, Philadelphia, 1990
5. Hayashi K, Yakubi T: The origin of the uncus and of Luschka's joint in the cervical spine. J Bone Joint Surg 67A:788, 1985
6. Kramer J: Intervertebral Disc Lesions: Causes, Diagnosis, Treatment and Prophylaxis. Georg Thieme Verlag, Stuttgart, 1981
7. Tondury G: Anatomie fonctionelle des petites articulations du rachis. Ann Med Phys 15:173, 1972
8. Brunnstrom S: Clinical Kinesiology. 1st Ed. FA Davis, Philadelphia, 1962
9. Kakulas BA, Taylor JR: Pathology of injuries of the vertebral column. pp. 21–54. In Frankel HL (ed): Handbook of Clinical Neurology. Vol 61. Elsevier, Amsterdam, 1992

10. Bardeen CR: Early development of cervical vertebrae in man. Am J Anat 8:181, 1908
11. Taylor JR, Twomey L: The role of the notochord and blood vessels in development of the vertebral column and in the aetiology of Schmorl's nodes. p. 21. In Grieve GP (ed): Modern Manual Therapy of the Vertebral Column. Churchill Livingstone, Edinburgh, 1986
12. Verbout AJ: The Development of the Vertebral Column. Vol. 90. In Beck F, Hild W, Ortmann R (eds): Advances in Anatomy, Embryology, and Cell Biology. Springer Verlag, Berlin, 1985
13. Taylor JR, Twomey L: Factors influencing growth of the vertebral column. pp. 30–36. In Grieve G (ed): Modern Manual Therapy. Churchill Livingstone, Edinburgh, 1986
14. Tanaka T, Uhthoff HK: The pathogenesis of congenital vertebral malformations. Acta Orthop Scand 52:413, 1981
15. Taylor JR: Growth and development of the human intervertebral disc. Ph.D. thesis, Edinburgh, 1973
16. Panjabi M, Dvorak J, Duranceau J et al: Three dimensional movement of the upper cervical spine. Spine 13:727, 1988
17. Schonstrom N, Twomey L, Taylor J: Lateral atlanto-axial joint injuries. J Trauma 35:886, 1993
18. Williams PL, Warwick R, Dyson M, Bannister LH: Grays Anatomy. 37th Ed. Churchill Livingstone, Edinburgh, 1989
19. Schaffler MB, Alkson MD, Heller JG, Garfin SR: Morphology of the dens: a quantitative study. Spine 17:738, 1992
20. Ellis JH, Martel W, Lillie JH, Aisen AM: Magnetic resonance imaging of the normal craniovertebral junction. Spine 16:105, 1991
21. Yoganandan N, Pintar F, Butler J et al: Dynamic response of human cervical spine ligaments. Spine 14:1102, 1989
22. Pal GP, Sherk HH: The vertical stability of the cervical spine. Spine 13:447, 1988
23. Bogduk N: The rationale for patterns of neck and back pain. Patient Management 8:13, 1984
24. Bogduk N, Marsland A: The cervical zygapophysial joint as a source of neck pain. Spine 13:610, 1988
25. Dvorak J, Panjabi MM: Functional anatomy of the alar ligaments. Spine 12:183, 1987
26. Panjabi MM, Duranceau J, Geol V et al: Cervical human vertebrae: quantitative three dimensional anatomy of the middle and lower regions. Spine 16:861, 1991
27. Dommisse GF: Blood supply of spinal cord. J Bone Joint Surg 56B:225, 1974
28. Travell J, Simons D: Myofascial Pain and Dysfunction: The Trigger Point Manual. Williams & Wilkins, Baltimore, 1983
29. Scott JE, Bosworth T, Cribb A, Taylor JR: A biochemical and ultrastructural study of the age related changes in human intervertebral disc glycosaminoglycans from the cervical, thoracic and lumbar nucleus pulposus and annulus fibrosus. J Anat (In press)
30. Kearney D: Asymmetry of the human vertebral arteries: an unpublished research project. Department of Anatomy and Human Biology, University of Western Australia, 1993
31. Fast A, Zincola DF, Marin EL: Vertebral artery damage complicating cervical manipulation. Spine 12:840, 1987
32. Parke WW: The vascular relations of the upper cervical vertebrae. Orthop Clin North Am 9:879, 1978

33. Penning L: Functional Pathology of the Cervical Spine. Excerpta Medica Foundation. Williams & Wilkins, Baltimore, 1968
34. Van Mameren H, Drukker J, Sanches H, Beurgsgens J: Cervical spine motions in the sagittal plane. I: Ranges of motion of actually performed movements, an x-ray cine study. Eur J Morphol 28:47, 1990
35. Hirsch C, Schajowicz F, Galante J: Structural Changes in the Cervical Spine. Monograph. Orstadius Boktryckeri Aktiebolag, Gothenberg, 1967
36. Taylor JR, Milne N: The cervical mobile segments. p. 21. In Whiplash Symposium, Australian Physiotherapy Association Symposium, Adelaide, 1988
37. Bohlman HH, Emory SE: The pathophysiology of cervical spondylosis and myelopathy. Spine 13:843, 1988
38. Clark CC: Cervical spondylitic myelopathy: history and physical findings. Spine 13:847, 1988
39. Lysell E: Motion in the cervical spine: an experimental study on autopsy specimens. Acta Orthop Scand, suppl. 123:1, 1969
40. Jones MD: Cited by Penning L: In Functional Pathology of the Cervical Spine. Williams & Wilkins, Baltimore, 1968
41. Scher AT: Hyperextension trauma in the elderly: an easily overlooked spinal injury. J Trauma 23:1066, 1983
42. Taylor JR: Whiplash Injury: the cause and the lesion. In Proceedings of the National Conference of the Australian Association of Musculo-Skeletal Medicine, Adelaide, 1991
43. Taylor JR: Injuries to cervical motion segments. In Proceedings of the 20th Scientific Meeting of the Australian Orthopaedic Association, Perth, 1992, Abstract 11.
44. Taylor JR, Kakulas BA: Neck Injuries. Lancet 338:1343, 1991
45. Bogduk N, Windsor M, Inglis A et al: The innervation of the cervical intervertebral discs. Spine 13:2, 1988
46. Mendel T, Wink CS, Zimny ML: Neural elements in human cervical intervertebral discs. Spine 17:132, 1992
47. Bogduk N: Cervical causes of headache and dizziness. pp. 289–302. In Grieve G (ed): Modern Manual Therapy of the Vertebral Column. Churchill Livingstone, Edinburgh, 1986
48. Ashton IK, Ashton BA, Gibson SJ et al: Morphological basis for back pain: the demonstration of nerve fibres and neuropeptides in the lumbar facet joint but not in ligamentum flavum. J Orthop Res 10:72, 1992
49. Giles L, Taylor J: Innervation of human lumbar zygapophyseal joint synovial folds. Acta Orthop Scand 58:43, 1987
50. Giles LG, Taylor JR, Cockson A: Hyman zygapophyseal joint synovial folds. Acta Anat 126:110, 1986
51. Cloward RB: Cervical discography: a contribution to the etiology and mechanism of neck, shoulder and arm pain. Ann Surg 150:1052, 1959
52. Dwyer AC, Bogduk N, Aprill C: Cervical zygapophyseal joint pain patterns. I: A study in normal volunteers. Spine 15:453, 1990
53. Radanov BP, Dvorak J, Valac L: Cognitive deficits in patients after soft tissue injury of the cervical spine.'' Spine 17:127, 1992

2 | Biomechanics of the Cervical Spine

Nikolai Bogduk

Fundamental to the understanding of disorders of an organ is a knowledge of its normal physiology. Such a body of knowledge exists for organs such as the heart, the kidneys, and the lungs. Consequently, the causes and results of cardiac failure, renal failure, and respiratory failure can be understood in terms of the normal function of these organs, and subsequently, treatment can be instituted on a rational and valid basis.

Such a body of knowledge does not exist for the musculoskeletal system. Some appreciation has emerged of the physiology of the lower limbs through gait analysis, but there is no information of a comparable standard for the vertebral column.

Biomechanics is the first step to determining the physiology of the musculo-skeletal system. By applying the principles of engineering and by using mathe-matical analyses, the way in which a mechanical system operates can be deter-mined. However, the more complicated the system, the more laborious and difficult is its analysis and the more complicated seems the result.

The first stage of biomechanical analysis is the study of *kinematics*—ob-serving and measuring how the system moves. The second stage is *kinet-ics*—determining the forces that operate on the system (to produce the observed or observable movements). Initially, this latter stage involves analyses of the forces in various, static (equilibrium) states: different postures in which no movement is actually occurring. Subsequently, the dynamics of the system can be studied, determining how forces vary as movement occurs.

For a system like the vertebral column, biomechanical studies are barely beyond their infancy. With respect to the cervical spine, little progress has been made beyond studying elementary kinematics. The study of the cervical spine lags woefully behind that even of the lumbar spine, whose physiology is

27

barely understood. It is little wonder, then, that disorders of the cervical spine are poorly understood and often poorly treated, if not maltreated.

The rate of progress of biomechanical study has differed for different regions of the neck. Only an elementary, descriptive understanding is available for the atlanto-occipital joints; somewhat more is available for the atlantoaxial joints, largely through the advent and application of computed tomographic (CT) scanning. In terms of sophistication, the greatest advances have so far been made with respect to the lower cervical spine.

ATLANTO-OCCIPITAL KINEMATICS

The atlanto-occipital joints are designed to allow flexion–extension but to preclude other movements. During flexion, the condyles of the occiput roll forward and glide backward in their atlanteal facets; in extension, the converse combination of movement occurs. Axial rotation and lateral flexion of the occiput are precluded because each movement requires one or both occipital condyles to rise out of their atlanteal sockets, essentially distracting the joint.

Studies of the ranges of these movements in cadavers have found the range of flexion–extension to be about 13°; that of axial rotation was 0°; but about 8° was possible.[1] A detailed radiographic study of cadaveric specimens[2] found the mean ranges (±SD) to be flexion–extension: 18.6° (±0.6), axial rotation 3.4° (±0.4°), and lateral flexion 3.9° (±0.6°). It also revealed that when flexion–extension was executed it was accompanied by negligible movements in the other planes, but that when axial rotation was executed as the primary movement, 1.5° of extension and 2.7° of lateral flexion occurred. Thus, axial rotation was achieved artificially through a combination of these other movements.

Radiographic studies of the atlanto-occipital joints in vivo have addressed only the range of flexion–extension because axial rotation and lateral flexion are impossible to determine accurately from plain radiographs. Most studies agree that the average range of motion is 14° to 15° (Table 2-1); for some reason, the values reported by Fielding[6] are distinctly out of character. What is conspic-

Table 2-1. Summary of Reported Results of Studies of Normal Ranges of Motion of the Atlanto-Occipital Joint

	Range of Motion (Degrees)		
Source	Mean	Range	SD
Brocher[3]	14.3	0–25	
Lewit and Krausova[4]	15		
Markuske[5]	14.5		
Fielding[6]	35		
Kottke and Mundale[7]		0–22	
Lind et al.[8]	14		15

uous from Table 2-1 is the enormous variation in range of motion exhibited by normal individuals, which indeed led one group of investigators[7] to refrain from offering either an average or representative range. This variation is reflected formally by the results of Lind et al.,[8] in which the coefficient of variation is over 100 percent.

ATLANTOAXIAL KINEMATICS

The atlantoaxial joints are designed to accommodate axial rotation of the head and atlas as a single unit on the remainder of the cervical spine. Consequently, the atlas exhibits a large range of axial rotation. However, the atlas is also quite mobile in other respects; it is not bound directly to the axis by any substantive ligaments, and few muscles act directly on it to control its position or movements. Consequently, the atlas essentially lies like a passive washer between the skull and C2, and is subject to passive movements in planes other than that of axial rotation. This underlies some of the paradoxical movements exhibited by the atlas.

Paradoxical movements arise because of the location of the joints of the atlas with respect to the line of gravity and the line of action of the flexor and extensor muscles acting on the head. No extensor muscles insert into the atlas; consequently, its extension movements are purely passive and dependent on the forces acting on the skull. Whether the atlas flexes or extends during flexion–extension of the head depends on where the occiput rests on the atlas. If, during flexion of the head, the chin is first protruded, the center of gravity of the head will come to lie relatively anterior to the atlantoaxial joints. Consequently, the atlas will be tilted into flexion by the weight of the head, irrespective of any action by the longus cervicis on its anterior tubercle. However, if the chin is tucked backward, the center of gravity of the head tends to lie behind the atlantoaxial joints and, paradoxically, the atlas will be squeezed into extension by the weight of the head, even though the head and the rest of the neck move into flexion.

In cadavers, the atlantoaxial joints exhibit about 47° of axial rotation and some 10° of flexion–extension.[1] Such lateral flexion as does occur is brought about by the atlas sliding sideways; an apparent tilt occurs because the facets of the axis slope downward and laterally; therefore, as the atlas slides laterally, it slides down the ipsilateral facet of the axis and up the contralateral facet, thereby incurring an apparent rotation that measures about 5°.[9]

Plain radiography cannot be used to determine accurately the range of axial rotation of the atlas, for direct, top views of the moving vertebra cannot be obtained. Consequently, the range of axial rotation can only be inferred from plain films. For this reason, few investigators have hazarded an estimate of the range of axial rotation of the atlas; most have reported only its range of flexion-extension (Table 2-2).

One approach to obtaining values of the range of axial rotation of the atlas has been to use biplanar radiography.[11] The results of such studies reveal that

Table 2-2. Ranges of Motion of the Atlantoaxial Joints

Source	Ranges of Motion (Degrees)		
	Axial Rotation		
	One Side	Total	Flexion-extension
Brocher*[3]			18 (2–16)
Kottke and Mundale[7]			11
Lewit and Krausova[4]			16
Markuske[5]			21
Lind et al.[8]			13 (±5)
Fielding[6]		90	15
Hohl and Baker[10]	30		(10–15)

the total range of rotation (between both sides) of the occiput versus C2 is 75.2° (±11.8°) (mean ± SD). Moreover, axial rotation is accompanied by 14° (±6°) of extension and 2.4° (±6°) of contralateral lateral flexion. Axial rotation of the atlas is therefore not a pure movement; it is coupled with a substantial degree of extension, and in some cases flexion. The coupling arises because of the passive behavior of the atlas under axial loads from the head; whether it flexes or extends during axial rotation depends on the shape of the atlantoaxial joints and the exact orientation of any longitudinal forces acting through the atlas from the head.

Another approach to studying the range of axial rotation of the atlas has been to use computed tomography (CT) scanning. This facility was not available to early investigators of cervical kinematics, and data stemming from its application have appeared only in recent years.

In a rigorous series of studies, Dvorak and colleagues examined first the anatomy of the atlantoaxial ligaments,[12] the movements of the atlas in cadavers,[13–15] and how these could be demonstrated using CT.[16] Subsequently, they applied the same scanning technique to normal subjects and to patients with neck symptoms following motor vehicle trauma in whom atlantoaxial instability was suspected clinically.[17,18]

Dvorak and associates[18] confirmed earlier demonstrations[19] that the transverse ligament of the atlas was critical in controlling flexion of the atlas and its anterior displacement.[14] They showed that the alar ligaments are the cardinal structures that limit axial rotation of the atlas,[13,14] although the capsules of the lateral atlantoaxial joints contribute to a small extent.[14] In cadavers, 32° (±10°) (mean ± SD) of axial rotation to either side could be obtained; but if the contralateral alar ligament was transected, the range increased by some 30% (i.e., by about 11°).[16]

In normal individuals, the range of axial rotation, as evident in CT scans, is 43° ± 5.5° (mean ± SD) with an asymmetry of 2.7° ± 2.0° (mean ± SD).[17] These figures establish 56° as a reliable upper limit of rotation, above which pathologic hypermobility can be suspected, with rupture of the contralateral alar ligament being the most likely basis for this.[17]

In studying a group of patients with suspected hypermobility, Dvorak et al.[17,18] found their mean range of rotation to be 58°. Although the number of patients so afflicted as perhaps small, the use of functional CT to identify them constitutes a significant breakthrough. Functional CT is the only available means of reliably diagnosing damage to the alar ligament. Without the application of CT, patients with such damage would continue to remain unrecognized, and their complaint ascribed to unknown or psychogenic causes.

LOWER CERVICAL KINEMATICS

Many studies have been devoted to the movements of the lower cervical spine. In the literature it has been almost traditional for yet another group each year to add another contribution to issues such as the range of movement of the neck.[20–42]

Early studies examined the range of movement of the entire neck, typically by applying goniometers to the head.[20–24] Fundamentally, however, such studies describe the range of movement of the head. Although they provide implicit data on the global function of the neck, they do not reveal what actually is happening inside the neck.

Some investigators examined neck movements by studying cadavers.[25,26,27] Such studies are an important first iteration, for they establish what might be expected when individual segments come to be studied in vivo, and how it might best be measured. However, cadaver studies are relatively artificial; the movement of skeletons without muscles does not accurately reflect how intact, living individuals move.

Investigators recognized that for a proper comprehension of cervical kinematics, radiographic studies of normal individuals were required,[28–42] and a large number of investigators produced what might be construed as normative data on the range of motion of individual cervical segments and the neck as a whole (Table 2-3).

What is conspicuous about these data, however, is that while ranges of values were sometimes reported, standard deviations were not. It seems that most of these studies were undertaken in an era before the advent of statistical and epidemiologic rigor.

Two early studies[31,35] provided raw data from which means and standard deviations could be calculated, and two recent studies[8,40] provided data properly described in statistical terms[8,40] (Table 2-4).

However, the early studies of cervical motion are marred by lack of attention to the reliability of the technique used; inter- and intraobserver errors were not reported. This leaves unknown the extent to which observer errors and technical errors compromise the accuracy of the data reported. Only those studies conducted in recent years specify the accuracy of their techniques,[8,40] and only the data from these studies can therefore be considered acceptable.

The implication of collecting normative data is that somehow they might be used diagnostically to determine abnormality. Unfortunately, without means

Table 2-3. Summary of Reported Results of Studies of Normal Ranges of Motion of Cervical Spine in Flexion and Extension

Source	Number	Total Average Range of Motion in Degrees (with Ranges, if Reported)				
		C2–3	C3–4	C4–5	C5–6	C6–7
Bakke[28]	15	13 (3–22)	16 (8–23)	17 (11–24	20 (12–29)	18 (11–26)
de Seze[29]	9	13	16	19	28	18
Buetti-Bauml[30]	30	11 (5–18)	17 (13–23)	21 (16–28)	23 (18–28)	17 (13–15)
Kottke and Mundale[7]	78	11	16	18	21	18
Penning[32]	20	13 (5–16)	18 (13–26)	20 (15–29)	22 (16–29)	16 (6–25)
Zeitler and Markuske[33]	48	16 (4–23)	23 (13–38)	26 (10–39)	25 (10–34)	22 (13–29)
Mestdagh[36]	33	11	12	18	20	16
Johnson et al.[37]	44	12	18	20	22	21
Dunsker et al.[38]	25	10 (7–16)	13 (8–18)	13 (10–16)	20 (10–30)	12 (6–15)

and standard deviations, and without values for observer errors, normative data are at best illustrative and cannot be adopted for diagnostic purposes. To declare an individual or a segment to be abnormal, an investigator must clearly be able to calculate the probability of a given observation constituting a normal value, and must determine whether or not technical errors have biased the observation.

The one study that has pursued this application using reliable and well-described data appeared only relatively recently.[40] For the quantification of active and passive cervical flexion, mean values and standard deviations were determined for the range of motion of every cervical segment, using a method of stated reliability. Furthermore, it was claimed that symptomatic patients could be identified on the basis of hypermobility or hypomobility.[40] However, the normal range adopted in this study was one standard deviation on either side of the mean.[40] This is irregular and illusory.

It is more conventional to adopt the two-standard-deviation range as the normal range. This convention establishes a range within which 96% of the asymptomatic population lies; only 2 percent of the normal population will have

Table 2-4. Summary of Results of Studies of Cervical Flexion and Extension that Reported Both Mean Values and Standard Deviations

Source	Number	Mean Range and Standard Deviation of Motion in Degrees				
		C2–3	C3–4	C4–5	C5–6	C6–7
Aho et al.[31]	15	12 ± 5	15 ± 7	22 ± 4	28 ± 4	15 ± 4
Bhalla and Simmons[35]	20	9 ± 1	15 ± 2	23 ± 1	19 ± 1	18 ± 3
Lind et al.[8]	70	10 ± 4	14 ± 6	16 ± 6	15 ± 8	11 ± 7
Dvorak et al.[40]	28	10 ± 4	15 ± 3	19 ± 4	20 ± 4	19 ± 4

flexion values that fall above these limits, and only 2 percent will have values that fall below. Adopting a one-standard-deviation range classifies only 67 percent of the normal population within the limits, leaving 33% of normal individuals outside the range. This means that any population of putatively abnormal individuals will be "contaminated" with 33 percent of the normal population. This reduces the specificity of the test and increases its false-positive rate.

Axial Rotation

The majority of studies of lower cervical kinematics have focused on movements in the sagittal plane. Axial rotation and other movements have only begun to be studied. The reasons for this are twofold. First, the radiographic study of cervical motion requires that the movement in question remain in a single plane, since the images acquired are two-dimensional. If aberrant movement out of the plane occurs (such as axial rotation coupled with flexion), the images of a given vertebra in two separate positions of the subject are not identical; landmark recognition becomes fallacious and unreliable, and measurements and the calculations and results based on them become unreliable.

The second limitation was the availability of technique. Anteroposterior and lateral cervical spine radiographs do not directly depict axial rotation. This can only be seen in a top view. One approach to this problem was the application of biplanar radiography. In this technique, simultaneous anteroposterior and lateral radiographs are taken during a movement, and the three-dimensional motion is calculated trigonometrically by plotting the movement of several points on the proband vertebrae. From such calculations the inferred axial rotation can be determined. Such studies have provided normative data on axial rotation of the cervical spine (Table 2-5). The data, however, are derived, and depend on the accuracy of identifying like points on four separate views of the same vertebra (an anteroposterior view and a lateral view in each of two positions). Accuracy in this process is not easy to achieve.[43]

Table 2-5. Normal Ranges of Motion of Cervical Spine in Axial Rotation and Ranges of Coupled Motions, as Determined by Biplanar Radiography

Segment	Axial Rotation Mean Degrees (SD)	Coupled Movement	
		Flexion/Extension Mean Degrees (SD)	Lateral Flexion Mean Degrees (SD)
Occ–C2	75 (12)	− 14 (6)	− 2 (6)
C2–3	7 (6)	0 (3)	− 2 (8)
C3–4	6 (5)	− 3 (5)	6 (7)
C4–5	4 (6)	− 2 (4)	6 (7)
C5–6	5 (4)	2 (3)	4 (8)
C6–7	6 (3)	3 (3)	3 (7)

(Data from Mimura et al.[11])

Table 2-6. Mean Values and Ranges of Axial
Rotation of Cervical Motion Segments as
Determined by CT Scanning

Segment	Range of Motion (Degrees)	
	Mean	Range
Occ–C1	1.0	–2–5
C1–2	40.5	29–46
C2–3	3.0	0–10
C3–4	6.5	3–10
C4–5	6.8	1–12
C5–6	6.9	2–12
C6–7	2.1	2–10
C7–T1	2.1	–2–7

(Data from Penning and Wilmink.[44])

The advent of CT scanning was required before axial rotation could be studied directly. One such study has provided normative data[44] (Table 2-6). However, while attractive as a first iteration, and while attractive as the only available normative data base to date, these data are questionable. Axial rotation of a cervical vertebra is coupled with lateral flexion. This results in movement occurring out of the plane of view, and the image of the vertebra is altered. Consequently, identical landmarks cannot be identified, and calculations of the observed range of motion must be in error. These errors could be eliminated if CT scanning were undertaken for each vertebra across its plane of axial rotation, which requires tilting and adjusting the gantry of the CT machine for each and every segment to coincide exactly with its plane of motion. Such studies have not yet been undertaken.

Uncinate Processes

One of the long-standing mysteries of the cervical spine has been the function of the uncinate processes. In some interpretations their role has been trivialized to that of "guide rails" for flexion and extension.[26] However, Penning[44,45] has been enunciated a fascinating and compelling theory for these structures.

By taking CT scans, first parallel to the plane of the cervical zygapophyseal joints and then perpendicular to this plane, Penning[44,45] revealed that the uncinate processes form a concave cup under the reciprocally curved convex vertebral body above (Fig. 2-1). This invites the interpretation that the cervical interbody joints are in fact saddle joints.

In the sagittal plane, the upper surface of a vertebral body is gently convex and the inferior surface of the vertebra above it is gently concave. This permits the movements of flexion and extension in the sagittal plane. Meanwhile, in the plane of the zygapophyseal joints, the upper surface of the vertebral body

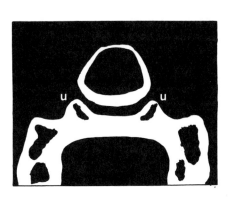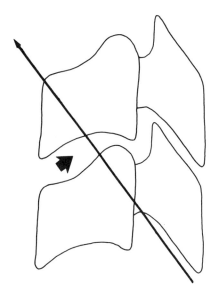

Fig. 2-1. Appearance of the uncovertebral region as revealed by CT scans parallel to the plane of the zygapophyseal joints. The long arrow depicts the plane of scan; the short arrow depicts the direction in which the segment is viewed. Note how the uncinate processes *(u)* present a concave cup to the reciprocally curved vertebral body above, thereby constituting the transverse component of a saddle joint between the cervical vertebral bodies.

is concave between the uncinate processes, and the reciprocal surface of the superior vertebra is convex. This permits side-to-side rotation in the saddle of the joint; but this freedom of motion is not in the conventional, coronal plane; it occurs in the plane of the zygapophyseal joints (i.e., some 40° ventrad to the coronal plane).

When viewed in this way, the cervical interbody joints permit only two forms of movement: sagittal rotation and axial rotation in the plane of the zyga-pophyseal joints (Fig. 2-2). This latter movement is tantamount to a modified form of what has been called axial rotation. Side-bending of the cervical verte-brae is not possible; movement perpendicular to the plane of the zygapophyseal joints is precluded by impaction of the joints (Fig. 2-3).

This model of cervical motion is attractive not only because it explains the function of the uncinate processes, but also because it explains the development of the clefts in the posterior annulus fibrosus. These are normal features of the cervical intervertebral discs from an early age,[46] and are essential to allowing the posterior half of the vertebral body to move about the modified axis of axial rotation. Without the clefts, the intact annulus fibrosus would preclude any axial rotation. In essence, the clefts are the joint spaces of the saddle joints of the cervical spine.

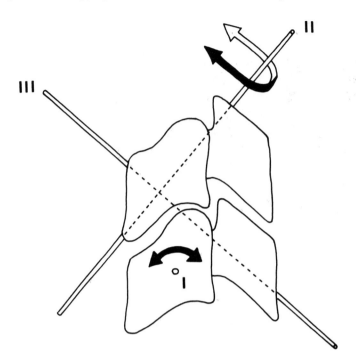

Fig. 2-2.   Planes of motion of a cervical motion segment. Flexion and extension occur around a transverse axis *(axis I)*. Axial rotation occurs around a modified axis *(axis II)* passing perpendicular to the plane of the zygapophyseal joints, and this motion is cradled by the uncinate processes. The third axis *(axis III)* lies perpendicular to both of the first two axes but no motion can occur about this axis (see Fig. 2-3).

Range of Motion

Regardless of how fashionable it may have been to study ranges of motion of the neck, and regardless of how genuine may have been the intent and desire of early investigators to derive data that could be used to detect abnormalities, a definitive study has now superseded all previous studies, and renders irrelevant any further studies of cervical motion using conventional radiographic techniques. No longer are any of the tabulated, earlier data (see Tables 2-3 and 2-4) of any use.

Van Mameren and colleagues[47] used an exquisite technique to study cervical motion in flexion and extension in normal volunteers. High-speed cineradiographs were taken, in which top-quality images were produced on each frame, allowing accurate biomechanical analyses to be undertaken on a frame-by-frame basis. The subjects undertook flexion from full extension, and also extension from full flexion. Twenty-five exposures were obtained during each sequence. The experiments were repeated 2 weeks and 10 weeks after the first observation. These studies allowed the ranges of motion of individual cervical segments

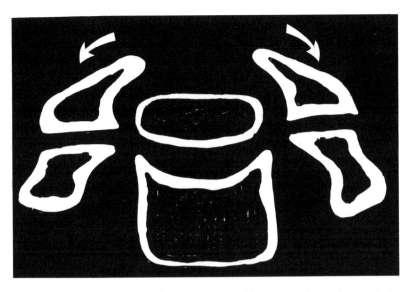

Fig. 2-3. View of a cervical motion segment looking upward and forward along axis III (see Fig. 2-2) to demonstrate how rotation around this axis is precluded by impaction of the facets of the zygapophyseal joints.

to be studied and correlated both against total range of motion of the neck and against the direction in which movement was undertaken. Moreover, the stability of the observations over time could be determined. The results are astonishing.

The maximum range of motion of a given cervical segment is not necessarily reflected by the range that is apparent when the position of the vertebra in full flexion is compared to its position in full extension. Often, the maximum range of motion is exhibited at some stage during the excursion but prior to the neck reaching its final position. In other words, a vertebra may reach its maximum range of flexion, but as the neck continues toward ''full flexion'' that vertebra actually reverses its motion and extends slightly. This behavior is particularly apparent in upper cervical segments (Occ-C1, C1-2).

A consequence of this behavior is that the total range of motion of the neck is not the arithmetic sum of its intersegmental ranges of motion. Therefore, what others have observed and quantified as the range of total cervical motion is not even directly related to intersegmental motion. For clinical purposes it is imperative that the range of intersegmental motion be studied explicitly, lest abnormal movements be masked within the range of total neck movements; but a further point is that a single flexion film and a single extension film is not enough to reveal maximum intersegmental motion; that can only be revealed cineradiographically.

A second result is that intersegmental range of motion differs according to whether the motion is executed from flexion to extension or from extension to flexion. At the same sitting, in the same individual, differences of 5° to 15°

can be recorded, particularly at Occ-C1 and C6-7. The collective effect of these differences, segment by segment, can result in differences of 10° to 30° in the total range of cervical motion.

There is no criterion for selecting which movement strategy should be preferred. It is not a question of standardizing a convention about which direction of movement should (arbitrarily) be recognized as standard. Rather, the behavior of cervical motion segments simply raises a caveat that no single observation defines a unique range of motion. Since the strategy used can influence the observed range, an uncertainty arises; depending on the segment involved, an observer may record a range of motion that may be 5° or even 15° less or more than the range of which the segment is actually capable. By the same token, claims of therapeutic success in restoring a range of motion must be based on ranges in excess of this range of uncertainty.

The third result is that ranges of motion are not stable with time. A difference in excess of 5° for the same segment in the same individual can be recorded in a study employing the same technique but on another occasion, particularly at segments Occ-C1, C5-6, and C6-7. Rhetorically, the question becomes: Which observation was the true normal? The answer is that normal ranges, within an individual, do not come in discrete quanta; they vary, and it is this variation and the range of variation that constitute the normal behavior of the cervical vertebrae, and not a single value. The implication is that a single observation of a range must be interpreted, and can be used for clinical purposes only with this variation in mind. A lower range of motion today, a higher range tomorrow, or vice versa, could be only the normal, diurnal variation in the range and not something attributable to a disease or therapeutic intervention.

Quality of Motion

Having noted the lack of utility of range-of-motion studies, and spurred even more by the findings of van Mameren et al.,[47] some investigators have explored the notion of quality of motion of the cervical vertebrae. They have contended that although perhaps not revealed by abnormal ranges of motion, abnormalities of the cervical spine might be revealed by abnormal patterns of motion.

One approach has been to examine the way in which various movements of a given vertebra are coupled to one another. Normative data were collected, and it was subsequently demonstrated that patients with neck pain following whiplash injury exhibited significantly different coupling patterns of the C1 vertebra.[43] Unfortunately, this work has not been further pursued, and the mechanical basis and clinical significance of disturbed coupling has not so far been elucidated.

Otherwise, investigators have pursued the phenomenon of instantaneous axes of rotation in the sagittal plane. The conjecture has been that abnormal segments exhibit abnormal locations of their axes of movement.

Instantaneous Axes of Rotation

When a cervical vertebra moves from full extension to full flexion, its path appears to lie along an arc whose center lies somewhere below the moving vertebra. This center is called the instantaneous axis of rotation (IAR), and its location can be determined using simple geometry. If tracings are obtained from lateral radiographs of the cervical spine in flexion and in extension, the pattern of motion of a given vertebra can be revealed by superimposing upon it the corresponding tracings of the vertebra below it. This reveals the extension and flexion positions of the moving vertebra in relation to the one below it (Fig. 2-4). The location of the IAR is determined by drawing the perpendicular bisectors of intervals connecting like points on the two positions of the moving vertebra. The point of intersection of the perpendicular bisectors marks the location of the IAR (Fig. 2-4).

The first normative data on the IARs of the cervical spine were provided by Penning.[32,34,45] He found them to be located in different positions for different cervical segments. At lower cervical levels the IARs were located close to the intervertebral disc of the segment in question, but at higher segmental levels the IAR was located substantially lower than this position.

A problem emerged, however, with Penning's data.[32,34,45] Although he displayed the data graphically, he did not provide any statistical parameters,

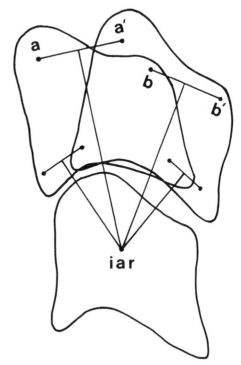

Fig. 2-4. Sketch of a cervical motion segment, illustrating how the location of its instantaneous axis of rotation (*iar*) can be determined by geometry.

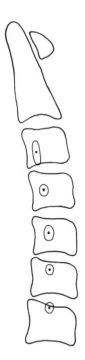

Fig. 2-5. Sketch of an idealized cervical vertebral column illustrating the mean location and two-standard-deviation range of distribution of the instantaneous axes of rotation of the typical cervical motion segments.

such as the mean location and variance; nor did he explain how IARs from different individuals with vertebra of different sizes were plotted onto a single, common silhouette of the cervical spine. This process requires some form of normalization, but Penning did not describe this.[32,34,45]

Subsequent studies pursued the accurate determination of the location of the IARs of the cervical spine. First, it was found that the technique used by Penning[32,34,39,45] to plot IARs was insufficiently accurate; the basic flaw lay in how well the images of the cervical vertebrae could be traced.[48] Subsequently, an improved technique, with smaller interobserver error, was developed[49] and used to determine the location of IARs in a sample of 40 normal individuals.[50]

Accurate maps were developed of the mean location and distribution of the IARs of the cervical motion segments (Fig. 2-5), based on raw data normalized for vertebral size and coupled with measures of interobserver error. The locations and distributions were concordant with those described by Penning,[32,34,45] but because the new data were described statistically, they offered the advantage of being able to be used to accurately test hypotheses about the normal or abnormal locations of IARs.

Some writers have protested against the validity and reliability of IARs, but the techniques they have used to determine the location of these axes have been poorly described and not calibrated for error and accuracy.[51] In contrast, van Mameren et al.[52] have rigorously defended IARs. They have shown that a given IAR can be reliably and consistently calculated within a small margin of technical error. Moreover, in contrast to the case for the range of motion of the cervical vertebrae, the location of the IAR is independent of whether it is calculated on the basis of anteflexion or retroflexion films. Moreover, and strikingly, the IAR is stable over time; no significant differences in location occur if the IAR is recalculated 2 weeks or 10 weeks after the initial observation.[52] Thus, the IAR stands as a reliable, stable parameter of the quality of vertebral motion through which abnormalities of motion can be explored.

Abnormal IARs

The first exploration of abnormal quality of cervical motion was undertaken by Dimnet and colleagues.[53] They proposed that abnormal quality of motion would be exhibited by abnormal locations of the IARs of the cervical motion segments. In a small study of six symptomatic patients, they found that in patients with neck pain the IARs exhibited a wider scatter than in normal individuals. However, they compared samples of patients and not individual patients; their data did not reveal which and how many IARs in a given patient were normal or abnormal, or to what extent.

A similar study was pursued by Mayer et al.[54] They claimed that patients with cervical headache exhibited abnormal IARs of the upper cervical segments. However, their normative data were poorly described with respect to ranges of distribution, nor did they describe the accuracy of the technique they used to determine both normal and abnormal axes.

Nevertheless, these two studies indicated that if reliable and accurate techniques were used, it was likely that abnormal patterns of motion could be identified in patients with neck pain in the form of abnormal locations of their IARs. This contention was formally investigated.

Amevo and colleagues[55] studied 109 patients with post-traumatic neck pain. Flexion–extension radiographs were obtained and wherever possible, IARs were determined for all segments from C2-3 to C6-7. These locations were subsequently compared with previously determined normative data.[50]

It emerged that 77 percent of the patients with neck pain exhibited an abnormally located axis at at least one segmental level. This relationship between axis location and pain was highly significant statistically (Table 2-7); there was clearly a relationship between pain and abnormal patterns of motion.

Table 2-7. Chi-squared Analysis of Relationship Between Presence of Pain and Location of Instantaneous Axes of Rotation

	Instantaneous Axis of Rotation[a]		
	Normal	Abnormal	
Pain	31	78	109
No pain[b]	44	2	46
	75	80	155

[a] $\chi^2 = 58.5$; df $= 1$; $p < 0.001$
[b] For patients with no pain, n $= 46$, and by definition 96% of these (44) exhibit normal IARs.[51,55]

Further analysis revealed that most abnormal axes were at upper cervical levels, notably at C2-3 and C3-4. However, there was no evident relationship between the segmental level of an abnormally located IAR and the segment found to be symptomatic on the basis of provocation discography or cervical zygapophyseal joint blocks.[55] This suggested that perhaps abnormal IARs were not caused by intrinsic abnormalities of a painful segment, but were secondary to some factor such as muscle spasm. However, this contention could not be explored, because insufficient numbers of patients had undergone investigation of upper cervical segments with discography or joint blocks.

STATE OF THE ART

Elementary data are available on the range of motion of the atlanto-occipital joints; biomechanical studies of abnormalities of these joints are still lacking.

More data are available on the atlantoaxial joints. Whereas these joints defied study in the past, the advent and application of CT scanning has enabled their range of motion to be determined accurately. States of hypermobility of these joints can now be reliably diagnosed using functional CT.

Because of the peculiar orientation of the plane of motion for axial rotation of the cervical vertebrae, few data are available about the patterns of motion in vivo of the cervical vertebrae in axial rotation. This movement still needs to be studied with modified CT scanning techniques.

Detailed data are available on the ranges of motion of the cervical vertebrae in the sagittal plane, but such data have not proved useful for identifying whether or not a patient has neck pain or for determining which particular segment is the source of the pain. Computerized cineradiography is the only available means of accurately and reliably determining segmental ranges of motion. Simple, static radiographs do not accurately reflect the actual range of motion of a segment, and normative data on plain radiography are obsolete.

However, ranges of motion are not stable parameters of cervical function. They differ with time and according to the movement executed. They have not proved to be of diagnostic value.

Accurate data are available on the normal locations of the IARs of the typical cervical vertebrae. In normal individuals these axes are tightly clustered around mean locations, which indicates that most normal necks operate in very similar ways. In normal individuals, IARs are stable with time and are independent of the direction in which movement in the sagittal plane is undertaken.

Abnormal IARs correlate strongly with the presence of neck pain, but do not seem to correlate with segmental location of the source of the pain. At present, it seems most likely that abnormal IARs represent a secondary disturbance of the cervical spine in response to pain. Nonetheless, it is evident that patients with neck pain exhibit objectively detectable abnormalities of the quality of motion of their vertebrae, even though the actual range of motion may not be abnormal.

Studies of the biomechanics of the cervical spine are emerging from their infancy. Normative data on the patterns of motion and the location of IARs pave the way for studying the kinetics of the neck by permitting the development of models that incorporate the cervical muscles and those of the shoulder that act on the cervical spine to control or disturb its normal motion. Such studies, however, cannot yet be pursued, since they required accurate and detailed descriptions of the cervical musculature, and the descriptions available in textbooks of anatomy are insufficient for biomechanical purposes. Once appropriately detailed data are available on the segmental attachments and disposition of every fascicle of the neck muscles, the next step can be taken in exploring and determining the normal physiology of the neck.

REFERENCES

1. Werne S: The possibilities of movement in the craniovertebral joints. Acta Orthop Scand 28:165, 1958
2. Worth DR, Selvik G: Movements of the craniovertebral joints. p. 53. In Grieve G (ed): Modern Manual Therapy of the Vertebral Column. Churchill Livingstone, Edinburgh, 1986
3. Brocher JEW: Die Occipito-Cervical-Gegend. Eine diagnostische pathogenetische Studie. Georg Thieme Verlag, Stuttgart, 1955
4. Lewit K, Krausova L: Messungen von Vor- and Ruckbeuge in den Kopfgelenken. Fortschr Rontgenstr 99:538, 1963
5. Markuske H: Untersuchungen zur Statik und Dynamik der kindlichen Halswirbelsaule: Der Aussagewert seitlicher Rontgenaufnahmen. p. 50. Die Wirbelsaule in Forschung und Praxis Hippokrates, Stuttgart, 1971
6. Fielding JW: Cineroentgenography of the normal cervical spine. J Bone Joint Surg 39A:1280, 1957
7. Kottke FJ, Mundale MO: Range of mobility of the cervical spine. Arch Phys Med Rehab 40:379, 1959
8. Lind B, Shilbom H, Nordwall A, Malchau H: Normal ranges of motion of the cervical spine. Arch Phys Med Rehab 70:629, 1989
9. Dankmeijer J, Rethmeier BJ: The lateral movement in the atlanto-axial joints and its clinical significance. Acta Radiol 24:55, 1943
10. Hohl M, Baker HR: The atlanto-axial joint. J Bone Joint Surg 46A:1739, 1964
11. Mimura M, Moriya H, Watanabe T, et al: Three-dimensional motion analysis of the cervical spine with special reference to the axial rotation. Spine 14:1135, 1989
12. Saldinger P, Dvorak J, Rahn BA, Perren SM: Histology of the alar and transverse ligaments. Spine 15:257, 1990
13. Dvorak J, Panjabi MM: Functional anatomy of the alar ligaments. Spine 12:183, 1987
14. Dvorak J, Scheider E, Saldinger P, Rahn B: Biomechanics of the craniocervical region: the alar and transverse ligaments. J Orthop Res 6:452, 1988
15. Crisco JJ, Oda T, Panjabi MM et al: Transections of the C1–C2 joint capsular ligaments in the cadaveric spine. Spine 16:S474, 1991
16. Dvorak J, Panjabi M, Gerber M, Wichmann W: CT-functional diagnostics of the rotatory instability of the upper cervical spine. I: An experimental study on cadavers. Spine 12:197, 1987

17. Dvorak J, Hayek J, Zehnder R: CT-functional diagnostics of the rotatory instability of the upper cervical spine. II: An evaluation on healthy adults and patients with suspected instability. Spine 12:725, 1987
18. Dvorak J, Penning L, Hayek J et al: Functional diagnostics of the cervical spine using computer tomography. Neuroradiology 30:132, 1988
19. Fielding JW, Cochran GVB, Lawsing JF, Hohl M: Tears of the transverse ligament of the atlas. J Bone Joint Surg 56A:1683, 1974
20. Schoening HA, Hanna V: Factors related to cervical spine mobility. I. Arch Phys Med Rehab 45:602, 1964
21. Ferlic D: The range of motion of the "normal" cervical spine. Bull Johns Hopkins Hosp 110:59, 1962
22. Bennett JG, Bergmanis LE, Carpenter JK, Skowund HV: Range of motion of the neck. J Am Phys Ther Assoc 43:45, 1963
23. O'Driscoll SL, Tomenson J: The cervical spine. Clin Rheum Dis 8:617, 1982
24. Colachis SC, Strohm BR: Radiographic studies of cervical spine motion in normal subjects. Flexion and hyperextension. Arch Phys Med Rehab 46:753, 1965
25. Ball J, Meihers KAE: On cervical mobility. Ann Rheum Dis 23:429, 1964
26. Lysell E: Motion in the cervical spine: an experimental study on autopsy specimens. Acta Orthop Scand, suppl. 123:4, 1969
27. Ten Have HAMJ, Eulerllink F: Degenerative changes in the cervical spine and their relationship to mobility. J Pathol 132:133, 1980
28. Bakke SN: Rontgenololgischen Beobachtungen uber die Bewegungen der Wirbelsaule. Acta Radiol, suppl. 13, 1931
29. de Seze S: Etude radiologique de la dynamique cervicale dans la plan sagittale. Rev Rhum Mal Osteoartic 3:111–116, 1951
30. Buetti-Bauml C: Funcktionelle Rontgendiagnsotik der Halswirbelsaule. Georg Thieme Verlag, Stuttgart, 1954
31. Aho A, Vartianen, Salo O: Segmentary antero-posterior mobility of the cervical spine. Annales Medicinae Internae Fenniae 44:287, 1955
32. Penning L: Funktioneel rontgenonderzoek bij degeneratieve en traumatische afwijikingen der laag-cervicale bewingssegmenten. Thesis, Reijuniversiteit Groningen, Groningen, The Netherlands, 1960
33. Zeitler E, Markuske H: Rontegenologische Bewegungsanalyse der Halswirbelsaule bei gesunden Kinden. Forstschr Rontgestr 96:87, 1962
34. Penning L: Nonpathologic and pathologic relationships between the lower cervical vertebrae. AJR 91:1036, 1964
35. Bhalla SK, Simmons EH: Normal ranges of intervertebral joint motion of the cervical spine. Can J Surg 12:181, 1969
36. Mestdagh H: Morphological aspects and biomechanical properties of the vertebroaxial joint (C2-C3). Acta Morphol Neerl-Scand 14:19, 1976
37. Johnson RM, Hart DL, Simmons EH, et al: Cervical orthoses. J Bone Joint Surg 59A:332, 1977
38. Dunsker SB, Coley DP, Mayfield FH: Kinematics of the cervical spine. Clin Neurosurg 25:174, 1978
39. Penning L: Normal movement in the cervical spine. AJR 130:317, 1978
40. Dvorak J, Froehlich D, Penning L et al: Functional radiographic diagnosis of the cervical spine: flexion/extension. Spine 13:748, 1988
41. Dvorak J, Panjabi MM, Grob D et al: Clinical validation of functional flexion/extension radiographs of the cervical spine. Spine 18:120, 1993
42. Dvorak J, Panjabi MM, Novotny JE, Antinnes JA: In vivo flexion/extension of the normal cervical spine. J Orthop Res 9:828, 1991

43. Worth D: Cervical Spine Kinematics. PhD Thesis, Flinders University of South Australia, 1985
44. Penning L, Wilmink JT: Rotation of the cervical spine. A CT study in normal subjects. Spine 12:732, 1987
45. Penning L: Differences in anatomy, motion, development and aging of the upper and lower cervical disk segments. Clin Biomech 3:37, 1988
46. Oda J, Tanaka H, Tsuzuki N: Intervertebral disc changes with aging of human cervical vertebra from the neonate to the eighties. Spine 13:1205, 1988
47. Van Mameren H, Drukker J, Sanches H, Beursgens J: Cervical spine motion in the sagittal plane. I: Range of motion of actually performed movements, an X-ray cinematographic study. Eur J Morphol 28:47, 1990
48. Amevo B, Macintosh J, Worth D, Bogduk N: Instantaneous axes of rotation of the typical cervical motion segments. I: an empirical study of errors. Clin Biomech 6: 31, 1991
49. Amevo B, Worth D, Bogduk N: Instantaneous axes of rotation of the typical cervical motion segments. II: optimisation of technical errors. Clin Biomech 6:38, 1991
50. Amevo B, Worth D, Bogduk N: Instantaneous axes of rotation of the typical cervical motion segments: a study in normal volunteers. Clin Biomech 6:111, 1991
51. Fuss FK: Sagittal kinematics of the cervical spine—how constant are the motor aaxes? Acta Anat 141:93, 1991
52. van Mameren H, Sanches H, Beurgsgens J, Drukker J: Cervical spine motion in the sagittal plane. II: Position of segmental averaged instantaneous centers of rotation—a cineradiographic study. Spine 17:467, 1992
53. Dimnet J, Pasquet A, Krag MH, Panjabi MM: Cervical spine motion in the sagittal plane: kinematic and geometric parameters. J Biomech 15:959, 1982
54. Mayer ET, Hermann G, Pfaffenrath V et al: Functional radiographs of the craniovertebral region and the cervical spine. Cephalalgia 5:237, 1985
55. Amevo B, Aprill C, Bogduk N: Abnormal instantaneous axes of rotation in patients with neck pain. Spine 17:748, 1992

3 | Biomechanics of the Thorax

Diane Lee

A biomechanical approach to the assessment and treatment of musculo-skeletal dysfunction of the thorax requires an understanding of its normal behavior. Without a working model, the clinician is limited to using often unreliable signs and symptoms for direction and treatment planning. If we understand how the osteoarticular system behaves normally, we can apply this knowledge when examining the deviant movement patterns of the thorax behaving abnormally. A systematic examination of mobility/stability of the associated bones and joints can then be done. The intent of this chapter is to present a model of in vivo biomechanics of the thorax that has been used clinically as the basis for assessing and treating mechanical dysfunctions of both the spinal and costal joints. Some parts of this model have been substantiated through scientific research,[1] while others remain empirical.

LITERATURE REVIEW

Reference to the literature reveals very little that is known about the in vivo biomechanics of the thoracic region. Four studies of the human thorax[2-5] were based on three-dimensional mathematical models and are difficult to apply clinically. Andriacchi[4] noted that the rib cage increased the bending stiffness of the spine by a factor of two in extension. He found that when the rib cage was left intact, the spine could support three times the load in compression before lateral instability occurred. The clinical implication of this is that any loss of integrity of the segmental "thoracic ring" would impair the ability of the entire cage to sustain a vertical load.

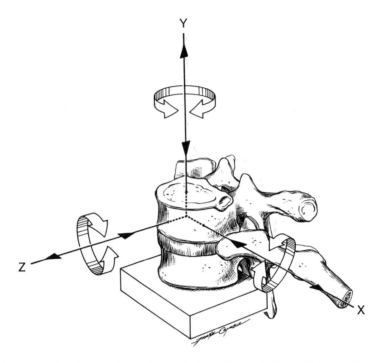

Fig. 3-1. In an in vitro study by Panjabi, Brand, and White,[1] 396 load-displacement curves were obtained for six degrees of motion at each thoracic segment. The amplitude of the induced motion as well as the amplitude and direction of any consequential coupled motion was recorded. (From Lee,[14] with permission.)

Saumarez[2] noted that there can be considerable independent movement of the sternum and the spine, "thus allowing mobility of the spine without forcing concomitant movements of (the) rib cage." Neither study[2,4] proposed a kinematic model of the in vivo biomechanics of the thorax.

Panjabi, Brand, and White[1] investigated the mechanical properties of the thoracic spine through an in vitro study. Three hundred and ninety six load-displacement curves were obtained for six degrees of motion, comprising three translations and three rotations along and about the *x, y,* and *z* axes (Fig. 3-1) for each of the eleven motion segments of the thoracic spine. The specimens tested ranged in age from 19 to 59 years. The motion segment tested included the anterior interbody joint, the posterior zygapophyseal joints, and the costovertebral and costotransverse joints. The ribs were cut 3 cm lateral to the costotransverse joints and the front of the chest was removed. The functional spinal unit was left intact, but the functional costal unit was not. The results of this study will be discussed later.

DEFINITION OF TERMINOLOGY

To facilitate the subsequent discussion, the terminology used requires definition. Table 3-1 outlines the terms used and their definition.

Table 3-1. Definition of Terminology

Term	Definition
Osteokinematics[6]	Study of the motion of bones regardless of the motion of the joints
	Angular motions are named according to the axis about which they rotate
	Coronal axis: flexion/extension
	Paracoronal axis: anterior/posterior rotation
	Sagittal axis: side-flexion
	Vertical axis: axial rotation
	Linear motions are named according to the axis along which they translate
	Coronal axis: mediolateral translation
	Paracoronal axis: anteromedial/posterolateral translation
	Vertical axis: traction/compression
	Sagittal axis: anteroposterior translation
Arthrokinematics[6]	Study of the motion of joints regardless of the motion of the bones that form them
	Named according to the direction in which the joint surfaces glide
Coupled motion	The combination of movements that occur as a consequence of an induced motion

HABITUAL MOVEMENTS

The thorax is capable of six degrees of motion (Fig. 3-1) along and about the three cardinal axes of the body; however, no movement occurs in isolation.[1] In other words, all angular motion is coupled with a linear motion and vice versa. The habitual movements of the thorax include forward and backward bending, lateral bending, and axial rotation of the trunk. Simultaneously, the chest moves to accommodate inspiration and expiration. The biomechanics of the thorax varies according to the region considered. Two regions will be discussed in this chapter; the midthorax and the lower thorax. The midthorax is defined as the region between T3 and T9 and includes the associated vertebral, costal, and sternal components. The lower thorax is defined as the region between T10 and L1 and includes the associated vertebral and costal components.

THE MIDTHORACIC REGION

Flexion

Flexion of the thoracic vertebrae occurs during forward bending of the trunk. Panjabi, Brand, and White[1] found that forward sagittal rotation (flexion) around the x axis was coupled with anterior translation along the z axis (0.5 mm) and very slight distraction (Fig. 3-2). When anterior translation along the z axis (1 mm) was induced in the experimental model, forward sagittal rotation around the x axis and very slight compression also occurred.[1]

The osteokinematic motion of the ribs that occurs during forward sagittal rotation of the thoracic vertebrae was not noted in the study by Panjabi et al.[1] Clinically, three movement patterns are apparent and are dependant upon the relative flexibility between the spinal column and the rib cage. In the very young (less than 12 years of age), the head of the rib does not fully articulate

Flexion   Anterior Translation

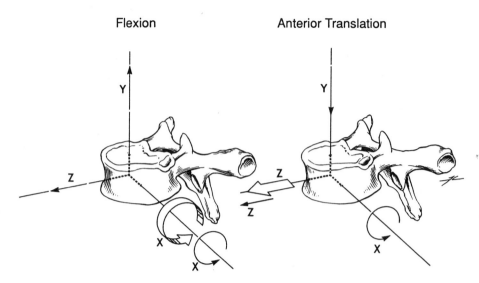

Fig. 3-2.   Forward sagittal rotation around the *x* axis induced anterior translation along the *z* axis and slight distraction along the *y* axis. Anterior translation along the *z* axis induced forward sagittal rotation around the *x* axis and slight compression along the *y* axis. (Modified by Lee,[14] from Panjabi et al.,[1] with permission.)

with the inferior aspect of the superior vertebra.[7] In other words, the superior costovertebral joint is not completely developed before puberty. The secondary ossification centers for the head of the rib do not develop until puberty, and the young chest is therefore much more mobile. In the skeletally mature, the superior costovertebral joints limit the degree of rotation possible in all three planes. In old age the costal cartilages tend to ossify superficially,[7] thereby further decreasing the pliability and relative flexibility of the thorax. This change in relative flexibility is apparent when examining the specific costal osteokinematics during forward and backward bending of the trunk.

1. During flexion of the *young mobile thorax,* forward sagittal rotation of the superior vertebra couples with anterior translation. This anterior translation appears to "pull" the superior aspect of the head of the rib forward at the costovertebral joint, inducing an anterior rotation of the rib. The rib rotates about a paracoronal axis along the line of the neck of the rib such that the anterior aspect travels inferiorly while the posterior aspect travels superiorly (Fig. 3-3).

Arthrokinematically, the inferior facets of the superior thoracic vertebrae glide superoanteriorly at the zygapophyseal joints during flexion of the thoracic vertebrae. The superior articular processes of the inferior thoracic vertebrae present a gentle curve that is convex posteriorly in both the sagittal and transverse plane. The superior motion of the inferior articular processes follows the curve of this convexity and the result is a superoanterior glide. Thus, the

Flexion

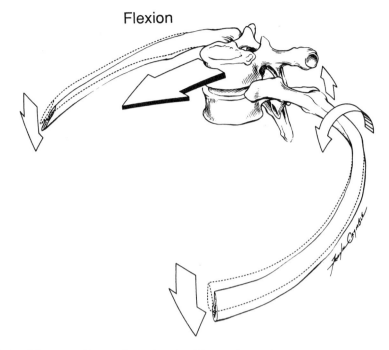

Fig. 3-3. The osteokinematic and arthrokinematic motion proposed to occur in the young, mobile thorax during flexion. (From Lee,[14] with permission.)

arthrokinematic motion of the joint surfaces supports the osteokinematic motion of the vertebrae, anterior translation being coupled with forward sagittal rotation.

The anterior rotation of the neck of the rib results in a *superior glide* of the tubercle at the costotransverse joint (Fig. 3-3). Since the costotransverse joints of the midthoracic vertebrae are concavoconvex (the facet on the transverse process is concave) in both a sagittal and transverse plane,[7] the superior glide of the tubercle results in an anterior rotation of the neck of the rib. Once again, the arthrokinematic motion at the costotransverse joint supports the osteokinematic motion of the rib during forward bending of the trunk.

In the *skeletally mature thorax* the ribs appear to be less flexible than the spinal column. During flexion of the thorax the anterior aspect of the rib travels inferiorly while the posterior aspect travels superiorly. Once the range of motion of the rib cage is exhausted, the thoracic vertebrae continue to forward flex on the now stationary ribs. The arthrokinematics of the zygapophyseal joints remain the same as in the first movement pattern described, but the degree of anterior translation is less. At the costotransverse joints, the arthrokinematics are different. As the thoracic vertebrae continue to forward flex, the concave facets on the transverse processes travel superiorly relative to the tubercle of the ribs. The result is a relative *inferior glide* of the tubercle of the rib at the costotransverse joint.

The third movement pattern occurs when the relative flexibility between the spinal column and the rib cage is the same. During flexion of the thorax, the extent of movement is reduced and there is no apparent movement between the thoracic vertebrae and the ribs. Some superoanterior gliding occurs at the zygapophyseal joints, but very little if any posteroanterior translation occurs.

The limiting factors to flexion of the thoracic functional spinal unit (FSU) include all of the ligaments posterior to and including the posterior half of the intervertebral disc. In an interesting study by Panjabi, Hausfeld, and White,[8,9] the thoracic FSU was loaded to failure in both flexion and extension. Failure was defined as a complete separation of the two vertebrae of the FSU or more than 10 mm of translation or 45° of rotation. The ligaments were transected sequentially and the contribution of the various ligaments to stability of the FSU was noted. They found that the FSU remained stable in flexion until the costovertebral joint was transected (Fig. 3-4). The integrity of the posterior one-third of the disc and the costovertebral joints is critical to the stability of anterior translation in the thorax.

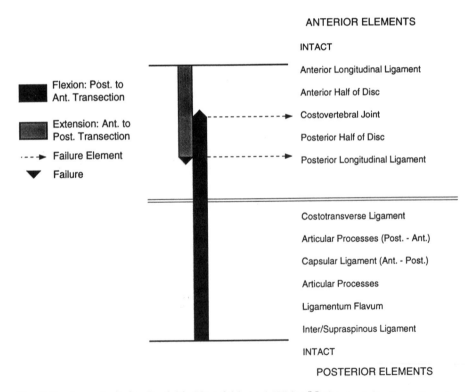

Fig. 3-4. In a study by Panjabi, Hausfeld, and White,[8,9] the contribution of various structures to stability of the thoracic segment was determined for both flexion and extension. Failure in flexion occurred when the costovertebral joint was transected. Failure in extension occurred when the posterior longitudinal ligament was transected. (Modified by Lee,[14] from Panjabi et al.,[9] with permission.)

Extension

Extension of the thoracic vertebrae occurs during backward bending of the trunk and during bilateral elevation of the arms. Panjabi, Brand, and White[1] found that backward sagittal rotation (extension) around the x axis was coupled with posterior translation along the z axis (1 mm) and very slight distraction (Fig. 3-5). When backward translation along the z axis (2.5 mm) was induced in the experimental model, posterior sagittal rotation around the x axis and very slight compression also occurred.[1]

The osteokinematic motion of the ribs that occurs during backward sagittal rotation of the thoracic vertebrae was not noted in the study by Panjabi et al.[1] Clinically, the movement patterns observed appear to depend on relative flexibility between the spinal column and the rib cage. Three patterns have been noted, as follows:

During extension of the *young mobile thorax*, the clinical hypothesis is that the backward sagittal rotation of the superior vertebra couples with the posterior translation and "pushes" the superior aspect of the head of the rib backward at the costovertebral joint, inducing a posterior rotation of the rib (Fig. 3-6). The rib rotates about a paracoronal axis along the line of the neck of the rib, such that the anterior aspect travels superiorly while the posterior aspect travels inferiorly.

Arthrokinematically, the inferior facets of the superior thoracic vertebrae glide inferoposteriorly at the zygapophyseal joints during extension of the thoracic vertebrae. The superior articular processes present a gentle curve that is

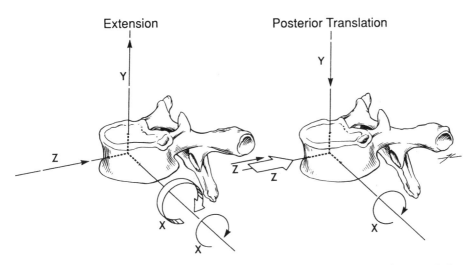

Fig. 3-5. Backward sagittal rotation around the x axis induced posterior translation along the z axis and slight distraction along the y axis. Posterior translation along the z axis induced backward sagittal rotation around the x axis and slight compression along the y axis. (Modified by Lee,[14] from Panjabi et al.,[1] with permission.)

Extension

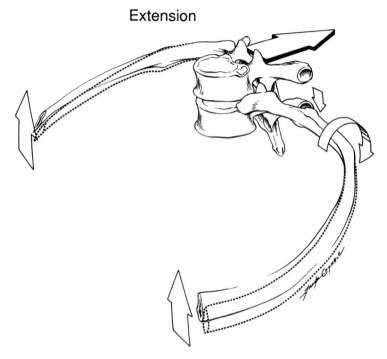

Fig. 3-6.   The osteokinematic and arthrokinematic motion proposed to occur in the thorax during extension. (From Lee,[14] with permission).

convex posteriorly in both the sagittal and transverse planes. The inferior motion of the inferior articular processes follows the curve of this convexity, and the result is an inferoposterior glide. Thus the arthrokinematic motion of the joint surfaces supports the osteokinematic motion of the vertebrae, posterior translation being coupled with backward sagittal rotation.

The posterior rotation of the neck of the rib results in an *inferior glide* of the tubercle at the costotransverse joint (Fig. 3-6). Since the costotransverse joints of the midthoracic vertebrae (T2 to T8) are concavoconvex in both the sagittal and transverse planes, the inferior glide of the tubercle results in a posterior rotation of the neck of the rib. Once again, the arthrokinematic motion supports the osteokinematic motion of the rib during backward sagittal rotation.

During extension of the *skeletally mature thorax,* the ribs are less flexible than the spinal column. Initially, the anterior aspect of the rib travels superiorly while the posterior aspect travels inferiorly. Once the range of motion of the rib cage is exhausted, the thoracic vertebrae continue to extend on the now stationary ribs. The arthrokinematics of the zygapophyseal joints remain the same as in the first movement pattern described, but the degree of posterior translation is less. At the costotransverse joints, the arthrokinematics are different. As the thoracic vertebrae continue to extend, the concave facets on the transverse processes travel inferiorly relative to the tubercle of the ribs. The result is a relative *superior glide* of the tubercle of the rib at the costotransverse joint.

The third movement pattern occurs with the relative flexibility between the spinal column and the rib cage is the same. During extension of the thorax, the extent of movement is reduced and there is no apparent movement between the thoracic vertebrae and the ribs. Some inferoposterior gliding occurs at the zygapophyseal joints only, but very little if any anteroposterior translation occurs.

The limiting factors to extension of the thoracic FSU include all of the ligaments anterior to and including the posterior longitudinal ligament. Panjabi et al.[8,9] sequentially transected the anterior longitudinal ligament, the anterior half of the intervertebral disc, the costovertebral joints, and the posterior half of the intervertebral disc and noted the contribution of each to the stability of the FSU in extension. It was found that the FSU remained stable in extension until the posterior longitudinal ligament was transected (Fig. 3-4).

Lateral Bending

Side-flexion of the thoracic vertebrae occurs during lateral bending of the trunk. Panjabi et al.[1] found that side-flexion, or rotation around the z axis, was coupled with contralateral rotation around the y axis and ipsilateral translation along the x axis. Translation along the x axis was coupled with ipsilateral side-flexion around the z axis and contralateral rotation around the y axis (Fig. 3-7).

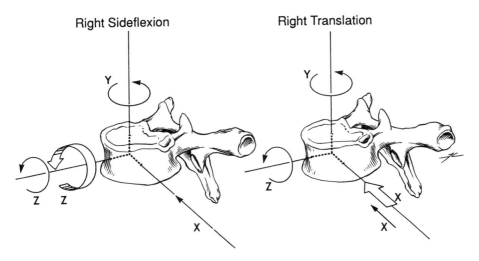

Fig. 3-7.   Right side-flexion around the z axis induced left rotation around the y axis and right translation along the x axis. Right lateral translation along the x axis induced right side-flexion around the z axis and left rotation around the y axis. (Modified by Lee,[14] from Panjabi et al.,[1] with permission.)

It is interesting to postulate about what produces this coupled motion in the thorax. It is thought[10,11] that in the mid-cervical spine, the oblique orientation of the zygapophyseal joints together with the uncinate processes directs the ipsilateral rotation and side-flexion that occurs. In the lumbar spine, the zygapophyseal joints also are known[12] to influence the direction of motion coupling during rotation. However, the facets of the zygapophyseal joints in the thoracic spine lie in a somewhat coronal plane and would not limit pure side-flexion during lateral bending of the trunk. It is difficult to see how they could be responsible for the contralateral rotation found to occur during side-flexion.[1]

Clinical Hypothesis

As the trunk bends laterally to the right, a left convex curve is produced. The thoracic vertebrae side-flex to the right, the ribs on the right approximate and the ribs on the left separate at their lateral margins (Fig. 3-8). In both the young mobile thorax and the skeletally mature thorax the ribs appear to stop moving before the thoracic vertebrae. The thoracic vertebrae then continue to side-flex to the right. This motion can be palpated at the costotransverse joint.

This slight increase in right side-flexion of the thoracic vertebrae against the fixed ribs is believed to cause a relative superior glide of the tubercle of the right rib and a relative inferior glide of the tubercle of the left rib at the

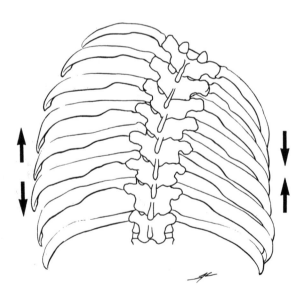

Fig. 3-8.   As the thorax side-flexes to the right, the ribs on the right approximate and the ribs on the left separate at their lateral margins. The costal motion appears to stop first; the thoracic vertebrae then continue to side-flex slightly to the right. (From Lee,[14] with permission.)

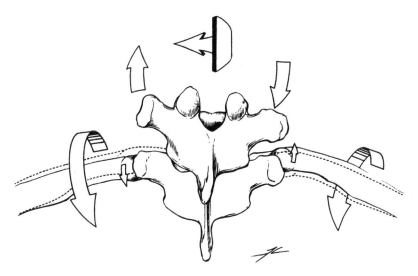

Fig. 3-9. The superior glide of the right rib at the costotransverse joint induces anterior rotation of the same rib due to the convexoconcavity of the joint surfaces. The inferior glide of the left rib at the costotransverse joint induces posterior rotation of the same rib. This relative costal rotation is proposed to "drive" the superior vertebra into left rotation such that the coupling of vertebral motion that occurs during right lateral bending of the trunk is right side-flexion and left rotation. (From Lee,[14] with permission.)

costotransverse joints, as the vertebra side-flexes against the fixed ribs. Since the costotransverse joint is concavoconvex in a sagittal plane, the superior glide of the right rib produces a relative anterior rotation of the neck of the rib with respect to the transverse process. The inferior glide of the left rib produces a posterior rotation of the neck of the rib relative to the transverse process. It is important to note that the moving bone is the thoracic vertebra, not the rib; however, the relative motion is described as though the rib was moving. Bilaterally, the effect of this rotation is to rotate the superior vertebral body to the left (contralateral to the direction of the side-flexion) (Fig. 3-9).

Panjabi, Brand, and White[1] found that the right lateral translation along the x axis (0.5 to 1 mm) occurred during right side-flexion (Fig. 3-7). The effect of this right lateral translation is negated by the left lateral translation that occurs as the superior vertebra rotates to the left. The net effect is minimal, if any, mediolateral translation of the ribs along the line of the neck of the rib at the costotranverse joints. The clinical impression is that no anteromedial or posterolateral slide of the ribs occurs during lateral bending of the trunk.

At the zygapophyseal joints, the left inferior articular process of the superior thoracic vertebra glides superomedially and the right process glides inferolaterally to facilitate right side-flexion and left rotation of the superior vertebra. The arthrokinematic motion of the joint surfaces supports the osteokinematic motion of the vertebrae and ribs.

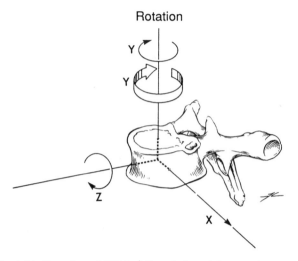

Fig. 3-10. Panjabi, Brand, and White[1] found that right rotation around the *y* axis induced left side-flexion around the *z* axis and left translation along the *x* axis. (Modified from Panjabi et al.,[1] with permission.)

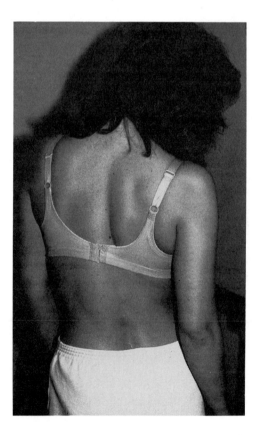

Fig. 3-11. Right side-flexion couples with right rotation during right axial rotation of the trunk.

Rotation

Panjabi, Brand, and White[1] found that rotation around the *y* axis was coupled with *contralateral* rotation around the *z* axis and contralateral translation along the *x* axis (Fig. 3-10). This is not consistent with clinical observation (Fig. 3-11). In the midthoracic spine, rotation around the *y* axis has been found to be coupled with *ipsilateral* rotation around the *z* axis and contralateral translation along the *x* axis. In other words, when axial rotation is the first motion induced, rotation and side-flexion appear to occur to the same side in the midthoracic spine (Fig. 3-11). It may be that the thorax must be intact and stable both anteriorly and posteriorly for this in vivo coupling of motion to occur. The anterior elements of the thorax were removed 3 cm lateral to the costotransverse joints in the study by Panjabi et al.[1]

When the anterior elements of the thorax are removed surgically, ipsilateral side-flexion and rotation cannot occur in the midthorax. The 17-year-old youth illustrated in Figures 3-12 and 3-13 had had the costocartilage of his left sixth rib removed for cosmetic reasons 4 years earlier. He presented with persistent

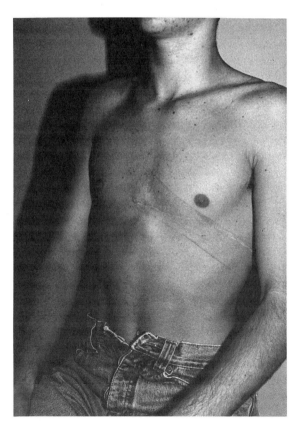

Fig. 3-12. This 17-year-old had the costal cartilage of his left 6th rib removed (note the incision).

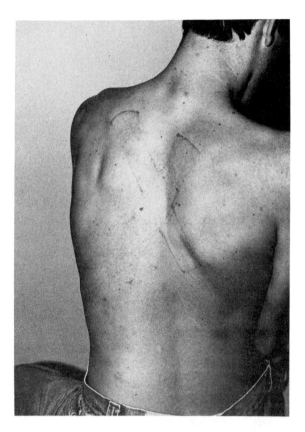

Fig. 3-13. Right rotation of the midthorax couples with left side-flexion when the anterior aspect of the chest is unstable.

pain in the midthorax, and on examination of axial rotation he could not produce ipsilateral rotation/side-flexion of the midthoracic region.

Clinical Hypothesis

During right rotation of the trunk, the following biomechanics appear to occur in the midthorax: The superior vertebra rotates to the right and translates to the left (Fig. 3-14). Right rotation of the superior vertebral body "pulls" the superior aspect of the head of the left rib forward at the costovertebral joint, inducing anterior rotation of the neck of the left rib, and "pushes" the superior aspect of the head of the right rib backward, inducing posterior rotation of the neck of the right rib. The left lateral translation of the superior vertebral body "pushes" the left rib posterolaterally along the line of the neck of the rib and causes a posterolateral translation of the rib at the left costotransverse joint. Simultaneously, the left lateral translation "pulls" the right rib anteromedially

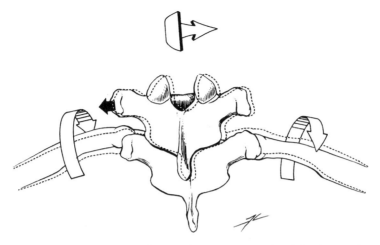

Fig. 3-14. As the superior thoracic vertebra rotates to the right, it translates to the left. The right rib posteriorly rotates and the left rib anteriorly rotates as a consequence of the vertebral rotation. The left lateral translation pushes the left rib in a posterolateral direction and pulls the right rib anteromedially. (From Lee,[14] with permission.)

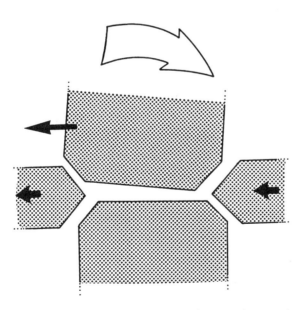

Fig. 3-15. At the limit of left lateral translation, the superior vertebra side-flexes to the right along the plane of the pseudo ''U'' joint (analogous to the uncovertebral joint of the midcervical spine) formed by the intervertebral disc and the superior costovertebral joints. (From Lee,[14] with permission.)

along the line of the neck of the rib and causes an anteromedial translation of the rib at the right costotransverse joint. An anteromedial/posterolateral slide of the ribs relative to the transverse processes to which they attach is thought to occur during axial rotation.

When the limit of this horizontal translation is reached, both the costovertebral and the costotransverse ligaments are tensed. Stability of the ribs both anteriorly and posteriorly is required for the following motion to occur. Further right rotation of the superior vertebra occurs as the superior vertebral body tilts to the right (glides superiorly along the left superior costovertebral joint and inferiorly along the right superior costovertebral joint). This tilt causes right side-flexion of the superior vertebra during right rotation of the midthoracic segment (Fig. 3-15).

At the zygapophyseal joints, the left inferior articular process of the superior vertebra glides superolaterally and the right inferior articular process glides inferomedially to facilitate right rotation and right side-flexion of the thoracic vertebrae. The arthrokinematic motion of the joint surfaces supports the osteokinematic motion of the vertebrae and ribs.

THE LOWER THORACIC REGION

Significant differences in the anatomy of the lower thorax influence its biomechanics. The facets on the transverse processes of the lower midthoracic vertebrae are more planar than those of the upper midthoracic vertebrae and tend to be oriented in a superolateral direction.[7] A superoinferior glide of the rib will therefore not necessarily be associated with the same degree of anteroposterior rotation as is found in the upper midthoracic region. The costocartilages of ribs 7 to 10 are less firmly attached to the sternum.[7] The costocartilages of the 11th and 12th ribs do not articulate with the anterior chest. The inferior demi-facet on the body of T9 for the 10th rib is small and often absent. The 10th rib articulates with one facet on the body of T10, and often does not attach to the transverse process at all. The 11th and 12th ribs do not have a costotransverse joint, and articulate only with T11 and T12, respectively.

Flexion/Extension

Flexion of the thoracic vertebrae in the lower thoracic region is also accompanied by anterior translation of the superior vertebra.[1] Extension of the lower thorax is accompanied by posterior translation of the superior vertebra.[1] Clinically, it appears that the associated ribs follow the sagittal motion, although minimal articular motion is necessary at the costovertebral joints of ribs 10, 11, and 12, since they do not attach to the respective superior vertebrae. The zygapophyseal joints glide superiorly during flexion and inferiorly in extension.

Lateral Bending

The biomechanics of the lower thorax during lateral bending of the trunk depends upon the apex of the curve produced in side-flexion. For example, if during right lateral bending of the trunk the apex of the side-flexion curve is at the level of the greater trochanter on the left, then all of the thoracic vertebrae will side-flex to the right and the ribs will approximate on the right and separate on the left. As the rib cage is compressed on the right and stops moving, further right side-flexion of the lower thoracic vertebrae will result in a superior slide of the ribs at the costotransverse joints on the right. Given the orientation of the articular surfaces, the glide that occurs is posteromediosuperior on the right and anterolateroinferior on the left, with minimal if any rotation of the neck of the rib. The ribs to not appear to direct the superior vertebrae into contralateral rotation, as they do in the midthorax. The vertebrae are then free to follow the rotation that is congruent with the levels above and below them.

If, however, the apex of the side-flexion curve is within the thorax (i.e., at T8), then the osteokinematics of the lower thoracic vertebrae appear to be very different. The rib cage remains compressed on the right and separated on the left, but the thoracic vertebrae side-flex *to the left* below the apex of the right side-flexion curve (i.e., T9 to T12). Given the orientation of the articular surfaces of the costotransverse joints, the glide that occurs on the right is in an anterolateroinferior direction (posteromediosuperior on the left), with minimal if any rotation of the neck of the rib. Once again, the ribs do not appear to direct the superior vertebrae to rotate in a sense incongruent with the levels above and below them.

Rotation

The same flexibility in the coupling of motion is apparent in the lower thorax when rotation is considered. In fact, the lower thoracic levels appear to be designed to rotate with minimal restriction from the costal elements. The coupled movement pattern for rotation in this region can be ipsilateral side-flexion or contralateral side-flexion. The coronally oriented facets of the zygapophyseal joints do not dictate a coupling of side-flexion when rotation is induced. The absence of a costotransverse joint and the lack of a direct anterior attachment of the associated ribs facilitates this flexibility in motion patterning.

CONCLUSION

The known biomechanics of the intact thorax is far from complete. Nevertheless, clinicians in the field of manual medicine who follow a biomechanical approach to the assessment and treatment of musculoskeletal dysfunction require a model from which to work. Recently, the quantitative three-dimensional surface anatomy of the thoracic vertebrae has been studied[13] with the intent of constructing an accurate mathematical model of the spine. It is hoped that further research will validate or dispute the hypotheses presented in this chapter.

REFERENCES

1. Panjabi MM, Brand RA, White AA: Mechanical properties of the human thoracic spine. J Bone Joint Surg 58A:642, 1976
2. Saumarez RC: An analysis of possible movements of human upper rib cage. J Appl Physiol 60:678, 1986
3. Saumarez RC: An analysis of action of intercostal muscles in human upper rib cage. J Appl Physiol 60:690, 1986
4. Andriacchi T, Schultz A, Belytschko T, Galante J: A model for studies of mechanical interactions between the human spine and rib cage. J Biomech 7:497, 1974
5. Ben-Haim SA, Saidel GM: Mathematical model of chest wall mechanics: a phenomenological approach. Ann Biomed Eng 18:37, 1990
6. MacConaill MA, Basmajian JV: Muscles and Movements; a Basis for Human Kinesiology. 2nd Ed. Kreiger, New York, 1977
7. Williams P, Warwick R, Dyson M, Bannister LH: Gray's Anatomy. 37th Ed. Churchill Livingstone, Edinburgh, 1989
8. Panjabi MM, Hausfeld JN, White AA: A biomechanical study of the ligamentous stability of the thoracic spine in man. Acta Orthop Scand 52:315, 1981
9. Panjabi MM, Thibodeau LL, Crisco JJ, White AA: What constitutes spinal instability? Clin Neurosurg 34:313, 1988
10. Penning L, Wilmink JT: Rotation of the cervical spine—a CT study in normal subjects. Spine 12:732, 1987
11. Bogduk N: Contemporary biomechanics of the cervical spine. pp. 1–7. In: Manipulative Physiotherapists Association of Australia 7th Biennial Conference Proceedings, Blue Mountains, New South Wales, Australia, November 27–30, 1991
12. Bogduk N, Twomey LT: Clinical anatomy of the lumbar spine. 2nd Ed. Churchill Livingstone, Melbourne, 1991
13. Panjabi MM, Takata K, Goel V et al: Thoracic human vertebrae: quantitative three-dimensional anatomy. Spine 16:888, 1991
14. Lee DG: Biomechanics of the thorax: a clinical model of in vivo function. J Manual Manipulative Ther 1:13, 1993

4 | Innervation and Pain Patterns of the Cervical Spine

Nikolai Bogduk

Since publication of the first edition of this book, major advances have been made in understanding the innervation and pain patterns of the cervical spine. Data on the innervation of cervical intervertebral discs that was only foreshadowed in the first edition of this chapter have since been formally published and subsequently confirmed and elaborated by other groups. Rules on the patterns of referred pain that previously were reserved and nihilistic have now been transformed into guidelines with firm, positive, predictive values.

CERVICAL PAIN SYNDROMES

Neck pain may occur as an isolated symptom or in association with pain in the upper limb girdle, pain in the upper limb itself, pain in the chest, or headache. However, these various combinations can be classified into two basic pathophysiologic forms: somatic pain syndromes and radicular pain syndromes.

Somatic pain syndromes are those in which the source of pain lies in one or another of the musculoskeletal elements of the cervical spine. These syndromes are not associated with neurologic abnormalities and do not involve nerve root compression. Radicular pain syndromes are those in which compression or irritation of spinal nerves or nerve roots is the cause of pain, and objective neurologic signs are a cardinal compartment of these syndromes.

Somatic Pain

Neck pain can arise from any structure in the cervical spine that receives a nerve supply. Consequently, an appreciation of the innervation of the cervical spine forms a foundation for interpreting the differential diagnosis of cervical pain syndromes.

The posterior elements of the neck are those structures that lie behind the intervertebral foramina and nerve roots. These are all innervated by the dorsal rami of the cervical spinal nerves.[1] The lateral branches of the cervical dorsal rami supply the more superficial posterior neck muscles such as the iliocostalis cervicis, longissimus cervicis and capitis, and splenius cervicis and capitis.[1] The medial branches of the cervical dorsal rami supply the deeper and more medial muscles of the neck, such as the semispinalis cervicis, capitis, and multifidus, and the interspinalis.[1] These nerves also innervate the cervical zygapophyseal joints[1,2] (Fig. 4-1). The suboccipital muscles are innervated by the C1 and C2 dorsal rami.[1]

The anterior elements of the neck are those in front of the cervical spinal nerves and include the cervical intervertebral discs, the anterior and posterior longitudinal ligaments, the prevertebral muscles, and the atlanto-occipital and atlantoaxial joints and their ligaments. The prevertebral muscles of the neck (longus cervicis and capitis) are innervated by the ventral rami of the C1 to C6 spinal nerves.[3,4] Other muscles in the neck also innervated by cervical ventral

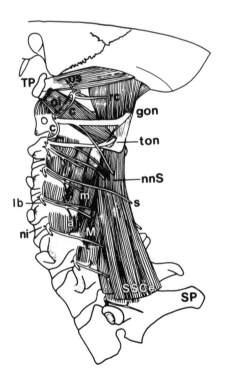

Fig. 4-1. Deep dissection of the left cervical dorsal rami. The superficial posterior neck muscles have been resected. The lateral branches *(lb)* of the dorsal rami and the nerves to the intertransversarii *(ni)* have been transected, leaving only the medial branches *(m)* intact. The C1 dorsal ramus supplies the obliquus superior *(os)*, obliquus inferior *(oi)*, and rectus capitis *(rc)* muscles. The medial branches of the C2 and C3 dorsal rami, respectively, form the greater occipital *(gon)* and third occipital *(ton)* nerves. Communicating loops *(c)* connect the C1, C2, and C3 dorsal rami. Three medial branches *(nnS)* of the C2 innervate the semispinalis capitis, while the C3 to C8 medial branches send articular branches *(a)* to the zygapophyseal joints before innervating the multifidus *(M)* and semispinalis cervicis *(SSCe)*, and those at C4 and C5 form superficial cutaneous branches *(s)*. TP, transverse process of atlas; SP, spinous process of T1. (From Bogduk,[1] with permission.)

Fig. 4-2. Distribution of the upper three cervical sinuvertebral nerves and the innervation of the atlanto-occipital and atlantoaxial joints. Articular branches *(arrowed)* to the atlanto-occipital and atlantoaxial joints arise from the C1 and C2 ventral rami, respectively. The C1 to C3 sinuvertebral nerves *(svn)* pass through the foramen magnum to innervate the dura mater over the clivus. En route, they cross and supply the transverse ligament of the atlas *(TL)*. The dura mater of the more lateral parts of the posterior cranial fossa is innervated by meningeal branches of the hypoglossal *(xii)* and vagus *(x)* nerves.

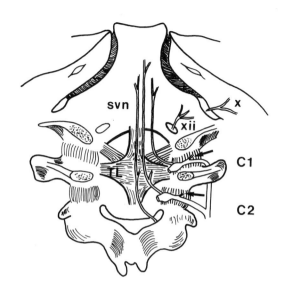

rami are the scalenes, the trapezius, and the sternocleidomastoid. Although the latter two muscles receive their motor innervation from the accessory nerve, their sensory supply is from the upper two or three cervical ventral rami.[3] The atlanto-occipital and lateral atlantoaxial joints are innervated respectively by the C1 and C2 ventral rami[2] (Fig. 4-2).

The ligaments of the atlantoaxial region are innervated by the C1 and C3 sinuvertebral nerves, and these same nerves also innervate the dura mater of the upper spinal cord and the posterior cranial fossa[5] (Fig. 4-2). At lower cervical levels (C3 to C8), the dura mater is innervated by an extensive plexus of nerves derived from the cervical sinuvertebral nerves.[6] Fibers within the plexus extend along the dural sac for several segments above and below their segment of origin.

The cervical intervertebral discs derive their nerve supply from a variety of sources (Fig. 4-3). Posteriorly, they are innervated by branches of a posterior longitudinal plexus that is derived from the cervical sinuvertebral nerves and which accompanies the posterior longitudinal ligament.[7] Anteriorly they are innervated by a similar plexus that is derived from the cervical sympathetic trunks and the vertebral nerves and that accompanies the anterior longitudinal ligament.[7] Laterally, the discs receive penetrating branches from the vertebral nerve.[7,8] Nerve fibers penetrate at least the outer third and up to the outer half of the annulus fibrosus of cervical discs.[7–9]

The demonstration of the extensive, microscopic plexus accompanying the posterior longitudinal ligament and from which the cervical intervertebral discs derive a nerve supply[7] supersedes previous descriptions in which the nerve supply to the posterior aspects of the cervical intervertebral discs was portrayed as stemming explicitly from the cervical sinuvertebral nerves.[8] The cervical

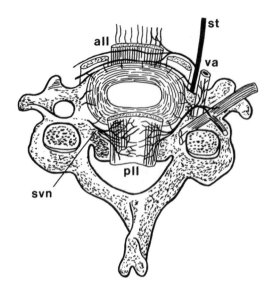

Fig. 4-3. The innervation of a cervical intervertebral disc. Nerve fibers enter the anterior and anterolateral aspect of the annulus fibrosus from branches of the cervical sympathetic trunk *(st)* that form a plexus accompanying the anterior longitudinal ligament *(all)*. Nerve fibers enter the posterolateral aspect of the annulus fibrosus from branches of the vertebral nerve, which accompanies the vertebral artery *(va)*. From this nerve arise the cervical sinuvertebral nerves *(svn)*, which form a plexus accompanying the posterior longitudinal ligament *(pll)*, and from which branches enter the posterior aspect of the annulus fibrosus.

sinuvertebral nerves constitute only the larger, dissectable elements of the posterior longitudinal plexus.

The structures that receive an innervation and which are therefore potential sources of cervical pain are the cervical zygapophyseal joints, the posterior, prevertebral, and anterolateral neck muscles, the atlanto-occipital and atlantoaxial joints and their ligaments, the cervical dura mater, and the cervical intervertebral discs and their ligaments.

Somatic Referred Pain

Referred pain is pain perceived in a region separate from the location of the primary source of the pain. Strictly and more explicitly, referred pain is pain perceived in a territory innervated by nerves other than the ones that innervate the actual source of pain, although as a rule, both sets of nerves usually stem from the same spinal segment. In the case of visceral referred pain, the source lies within a viscus but the pain is perceived in some part of the body wall that is itself unaffected by disease. Pain caused by a lesion in a somatic structure may similarly be perceived in a distant location, and the term *somatic referred pain* is used to highlight the somatic origin of this form of pain and to distinguish it from visceral referred pain. In the cervical region, neck pain arising from the zygapophyseal joints, ligaments, muscles, and intervertebral discs of the cervical spine may be accompanied by pain perceived in the head, shoulder girdle, upper limb, and/or posterior or anterior chest wall.

The mechanism of cervical somatic referred pain has not been demonstrated explicitly by physiologic experiments, but certain clinical studies indicate that the mechanism involves convergence of afferent pathways in the central nervous system, either in the spinal cord or at a more rostral level. Convergence is an anatomic and physiologic process in which neurons in the central nervous system receive afferent fibers from two distinctly separate peripheral sites, with signals from either site relayed by the common second-order neuron to the brain. Because of this arrangement, an afferent signal from one site may be interpreted as arising from either or both peripheral sites.

In the case of cervical somatic referred pain, afferents from the vertebral column converge on common neurons with afferents from peripheral regions such as the head, chest wall, or upper limb. Consequently, a nociceptive signal arising from the vertebral column may be perceived as arising from the head, chest wall, or upper limb.

Whether referred pain occurs as a result of a particular, spinal lesion depends on whether the afferents from the lesion relay to convergent pathways. In turn, the site to which pain is referred depends on the site of origin of any other afferents that converge on the common neuron in the central nervous system. If afferents from the vertebral column converge with afferents from the head, headache occurs. If they converge with afferents from the chest wall, chest pain occurs.

To date, there have been no attempts to demonstrate that anatomic convergence is the basis of cervical referred pain. However, the results of various clinical experiments imply that convergence is the mechanism involved.

Stimulation of the cervical, interspinous ligaments and muscles with noxious injections of hypertonic saline produces somatic referred pain in normal volunteers. Stimulation of upper cervical levels produces referred pain in the head.[10–12] Stimulation of lower cervical levels produces pain in the chest wall, shoulder girdle, and upper limb.[11–13] Electrical and mechanical stimulation of the cervical intervertebral discs produces pain in the posterior chest wall and scapular region,[14] and pressure on the posterior longitudinal ligament produces pain in the anterior chest.[15] Distention of the cervical zygapophyseal joints with contrast medium produces referred pain in normal volunteers that is perceived in the head or shoulder girdle, depending on which segmental level is stimulated.[16]

All of these experimental and clinical observations indicate that noxious stimuli from the cervical spine are capable of causing pain in the head, upper limb, or chest wall. None of the experiments in normal volunteers involved the spinal nerves or nerve roots. Therefore, nerve root irritation cannot have been the cause of pain. Convergence in the central nervous system is the only mechanism postulated, to date, that explains these phenomena.

The capacity of cervical pain to be referred to the head, upper limb, or chest wall can pose diagnostic difficulties. For instance, patients with pain referred to the head may present with the complaint of headache rather than neck pain, and this headache may be misinterpreted as tension headache if the cervical cause is not recognized.[17,18] Referred pain to the anterior chest wall may mimic angina, and the phenomenon of cervical angina, or pseudoangina, and methods for distinguishing it from cardiac angina, have been reviewed.[19,20]

Patterns of Referred Pain

The early experiments on somatic referred pain were undertaken to establish charts of referred pain patterns.[13] It had been noted that referred pain tended to follow a segmental pattern, in that stimuli to lower levels in the vertebral column resulted in the referral of pain to more caudal areas in the upper limb or chest wall. The apparent patterns of referred pain differed from those of dermatomes, and to distinguish this different pattern the concept of *sclerotomes* was introduced.[21]

It was expected that by charting the patterns of referred pain in normal volunteers, maps of the sclerotomes could be constructed, with the view that these could then be used clinically to deduce the segmental origin of spinal pain on the basis of the peripheral distribution of any referred pain experienced by these patients. This ambition, however, was thwarted.

The charts produced did not provide clinically useful information. In the first instance they were not based on studies of clinically relevant structures. Stimuli were delivered to the interspinous spaces rather than to structures that are plausible sources of pain in patients. Second, the published charts of sclerotomes demonstrated inconsistencies. Different individuals reported different distributions of referred pain, even when exactly the same structures and segmental levels were stimulated. Moreover, the distributions of referred pain reported in different studies differed markedly (Fig. 4-4). There was too much variation and overlap in the patterns of referred pain for the site of referred pain to be used as a precise clue in the diagnosis of its segmental level of origin.

Nevertheless, these early experiments enabled certain rules to be elaborated. Pain referred to the head occurred only when upper cervical segments were stimulated. Stimulation of lower segments resulted in pain referred to the upper limb or chest wall.

More recently, however, studies have been completed on the patterns of pain referred from the cervical zygapophyseal joints. Distinctive patterns emerged. Joints at particular segmental levels seemed to be consistently associated with characteristic patterns of referred pain[16] (Fig. 4-5), and these patterns have been found to be reliable in determining the segmental location of a symptomatic, cervical zygapophyseal joint.[22] One caveat applies, however. These pain patterns are not diagnostic of cervical zygapophyseal joint pain. All they allow is that *if* the patient has cervical zygapophyseal joint pain, the location of the responsible joint can be reasonably well deduced from the pain pattern itself. How to determine if the patient actually has cervical zygapophyseal joint pain is another matter.[22]

Radicular Pain Syndromes

Virtually all of the previous literature on cervical pain syndromes has focused on cervical spondylosis and nerve root compression, and there is no doubt that disc bulges and osteophytes in either the uncovertebral region or

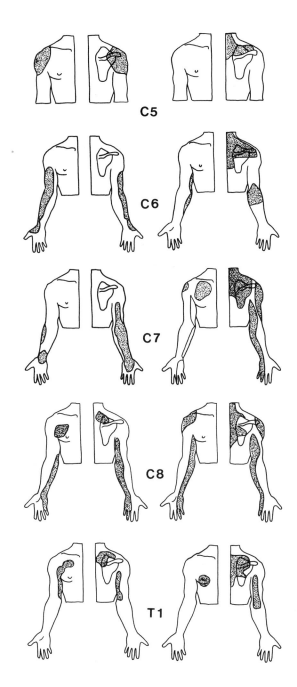

Fig. 4-4. Patterns of referred pain induced in normal volunteers by stimulation of the interspinous structures at the levels indicated. The left-hand figures are based on the studies of Kellgren.[13] The right-hand figures are based on the studies of Feinstein et al.[12] Comparison of the two sets of figures reveals the variation in patterns of referred pain from the same cervical structures and segmental levels.

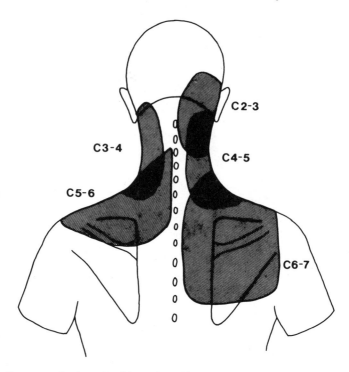

Fig. 4-5.   Patterns of referred pain produced by stimulating the cervical zygapophyseal joints in normal volunteers. (Modified from Dwyer et al.,[16] with permission.)

the cervical zygapophyseal joints can affect the cervical nerve roots.[23–31] However, the emphasis on nerve root compression has resulted in an inappropriate proclivity to interpret all cervical pain syndromes as due to nerve root compression.

Theories suggesting nerve root compression as a source of pain were developed to explain the association between low back pain and sciatica,[32,33] and these were extrapolated to the cervical region to explain the concurrence of neck pain and upper limb pain. However, these theories were formulated and the extrapolations made without regard to the contemporary experiments on somatic referred pain. Consequently, somatic mechanisms have remained largely overlooked as explanations for cervical pain syndromes, and nerve root compression has remained accepted as the principal (if not the only) mechanism for cervical pain. However, as a mechanism, nerve root compression is inconsistent with the clinical features of the majority of cervical pain syndromes, and in fact accounts for only a very specific proportion of cases.

Nerve root compression produces symptoms in two ways. First, objective neurologic signs can be produced if nerve root compression blocks conduction in the axons. The symptoms or signs that occur depend on exactly which axons are affected. If sensory fibers are compressed, sensory loss will be experienced. If motor fibers are affected, weakness will occur. The depth of any sensory loss or motor weakness will be proportional to the number of axons affected by the compression.

Paresthesia may be a feature of nerve root compression, but the mechanism is not compression of axons. Experiments on peripheral nerves have demonstrated that paresthesias occur as a result of ischemia of nerves.[34] Therefore, it can be deduced that paresthesia in the presence of nerve root compression is likely to be due to compression of radicular vessels, causing nerve root ischemia rather than frank compression of the root itself.

The second manifestation of nerve root compression may be pain, but the mechanism, quality, and distribution of this pain are different from those of somatic pain. Root pain, or radicular pain, is caused by the generation of ectopic impulses in nociceptive afferents in the affected root. These impulses can be generated by mechanical stimulation of the dorsal root ganglion or by mechanical stimulation of previously damaged dorsal nerve roots.[35–37]

Notwithstanding the capacity of nerve root compression to generate both objective neurologic signs and radicular pain, there are several anatomic and physiologic factors that limit nerve root compression as the explanation for most cervical pain syndromes, as follows:

1.   A cardinal feature of nerve root compression is that any symptom or sign must be in the territory innervated by the affected root. Thus, for example, compression of the C6 root should be associated with sensory symptoms in the C6 dermatome and/or motor weakness in the C6 myotome. Clinical features not in the appropriate distribution cannot legitimately be ascribed to root compression.

2.   There is no known mechanism whereby lesions causing nerve root compression can selectively affect only those axons that innervate the vertebral column, while sparing the other axons in the root that supply the upper limb or other, nonvertebral structures. Therefore, nerve root compression cannot be the responsible mechanism in patients presenting with neck pain unassociated with referred pain or peripheral neurologic signs.

3.   There is no known mechanism whereby nociceptive afferents can be selectively affected by lesions that cause root compression. Such lesions indiscriminately affect both large-diameter, afferent fibers (touch, vibration, and proprioceptive fibers) and small-diameter fibers (nociceptive fibers). Indeed, both compression and ischemia affect large-diameter sooner than small-diameter afferent fibers.[38] Therefore, nerve root compression cannot be the mechanism of symptoms if pain is the only feature. Any radicular pain must to some extent be associated with signs or symptoms of conduction block or ischemia of the large-diameter fibers in the affected root. Consequently, nerve root compression cannot legitimately be deemed to be the mechanism responsible for symptoms unless numbness, weakness, or paresthesia is present.

4.   Nerve root compression can be the mechanism of symptoms only at segmental levels at which roots are susceptible to compression. Because they run in the intervertebral foramina, the mid-cervical and lower cervical roots are susceptible to compression by disorders of the intervertebral discs, uncinate

processes, and zygapophyseal joints that form the boundaries of the interverte-bral foramina. However, the C1 and C2 roots do not run in intervertebral foram-ina and have no structural relations that render them liable to compression. Therefore, compression of the C1 or C2 roots cannot be held to be the mecha-nism of upper cervical pain.

    5. The quality and behavior of radicular pain are distinctive. Experiments on lumbar nerve roots have shown that mechanical or electrical stimulation of nerve roots produce pain that is quite distinct from somatic pain.[39,40] Lumbar radicular pain tends to be shooting or lancinating in quality, and travels into the lower limb along narrow bands. It is not dull, and aching and spread over diffuse areas where it is hard to localize, which are the characteristics of somatic pain and somatic referred pain.[41]

    Because of these several anatomic and physiologic factors, nerve root compression is a mechanism that must be restricted to levels C3 and below and to cases in which radicular pain is associated with objective neurologic signs or paresthesia in the appropriate segmental distribution. In the absence of these associated neurologic features, any pain is more likely to be some form of somatic pain and somatic referred pain stemming from one or another of the musculoskeletal elements of the cervical spine.

COMBINED STATES

    While it is important to highlight the differences between somatic pain states and root compression syndromes, and to redress the relative neglect of somatic referred pain in the differential diagnosis of cervical pain syndromes, it is equally important to recognize that the two conditions may coexist. Lesions that cause somatic pain and somatic referred pain also may secondarily cause nerve root compression, and the features of root compression syndrome may be superimposed on those of somatic pain syndrome.

    For example, disc disease may be intrinsically painful, causing local and referred somatic pain, but if the disc bulges, or if osteophytes develop, the adjacent nerve root may become compressed. Similarly, arthrotic zygapophy-seal joints may be intrinsically painful, but zygapophyseal osteophytes may concomitantly affect the nerve root in front of the joint. As a result of combina-tions such as these, patients may present with a combination of neck pain, somatic referred pain, objective neurologic signs, and radicular pain. It is imper-ative that such combinations and the multiplicity of mechanisms involved be recognized, lest the assessment and consequent treatment be incomplete or inappropriate. It would be erroneous to assume, in a patient with objective neurologic signs, that root compression was the only process operating. Root compression would certainly account for the objective neurologic signs, but the pain of which the patient complains could be somatic pain due to the lesion that only secondarily happens to be causing the root compression. Decompres-sion of the root might reverse the objective neurologic signs and relieve any associated radicular pain, but it will not necessarily relieve the somatic pain or any somatic referred pain unless the cause of the compressing lesion is inadvertently treated in the course of the decompression.

In the assessment of patients presenting with pain, each of the presenting symptoms and signs should be individually analyzed and the mechanism of each should be determined. Subsequently, treatment should be prescribed for each complaint in a manner consistent with its mechanism of causation. Because the mechanisms and sources of somatic referred pain and radicular pain are so different, they should be distinguished. Moreover, standard treatments for radicular pain may not be appropriate for somatic pain, and vice versa. Failure to distinguish the components of a patient's complaint in this way runs the risk of treatment being directed at only part of the problem, with the consequence of patient dissatisfaction and disillusionment with the therapist.

REFERENCES

1. Bogduk N: The clinical anatomy of the cervical dorsal rami. Spine 7:319, 1982
2. Lazorthes G, Gaubert J: L'innervation des articulations inter-apophysaire vertebrales. Comptes Rendues de l'Association des Anatomistes, 43 Reunion: 488, 1956
3. Williams PL, Warwick R, Dyson M, Bannister LH (eds): *Gray's Anatomy*. 37th Ed. pp. 584, 609, 1130. Churchill Livingstone, Edinburgh, 1989
4. Hovelacque A: Anatomie des nerfs craniens et rachidiens et du systeme grand sympathique. Doin, Paris, 1927
5. Kimmel DL: Innervation of the spinal dura mater and dura mater of the posterior cranial fossa. Neurology (NY) 10:800, 1960
6. Groen GJ, Baljet B, Drukker J: The innervation of the spinal dura mater: anatomy and clinical implications. Acta Neurochir 92:39, 1988
7. Groen GJ, Baljet B, Drukker J: Nerves and nerve plexuses of the human vertebral column. Am J Anat 188:282, 1990
8. Bogduk N, Windsor M, Inglis A: The innervation of the cervical intervertebral discs. Spine 13:2, 1989
9. Mendel T, Wink CS, Zimny ML: Neural elements in human cervical intervertebral discs. Spine 17:132, 1992
10. Cyriax J: Rheumatic headache. Br Med J 2:1367, 1938
11. Campbell DG, Parsons CM: Referred head pain and its concomitants. J Nerv Ment Dis 99:544, 1944
12. Feinstein B, Langton JBK, Jameson RM, Schiller F: Experiments on referred pain from deep somatic tissues. J Bone Joint Surg 36A:981, 1954
13. Kellgren JH: On the distribution of pain arising from deep somatic structures with charts of segmental pain areas. Clin Sci 4:35, 1939
14. Cloward RB: Cervical diskography. Ann Surg 150:1052, 1959
15. Murphey F: Sources and patterns of pain in disc disease. Clin Neurosurg 15:343, 1968
16. Dwyer A, Aprill C, Bogduk N: Cervical zygapophyseal joint pain patterns. I: A study in normal volunteers. Spine 15:453, 1990
17. Bogduk N, Marsland A: Third occipital headache. Cephalalgia 5, suppl. 3:310, 1985
18. Bogduk N, Marsland A: On the concept of third occipital headache. J Neurol Neurosurg Psychiatry 49:775, 1986

19. Booth RE, Rothman RH: Cervical angina. Spine 1:28, 1976
20. Brodsky AE: Cervical angina. A correlative study with emphasis on the use of coronary arteriography. Spine 10:699, 1985
21. Inman VT, Saunders JBCM: Referred pain from skeletal structures. J Nerv Ment Dis 99:660, 1944
22. Aprill C, Dwyer A, Bogduk N: Cervical zygapophyseal joint pain patterns. II: A clinical evaluation. Spine 15:458, 1990
23. MacNab I: Cervical spondylosis. Clin Orthop 109:69, 1975
24. Friedenberg ZB, Edeiken J, Spencer HN et al: Degenerative changes in the cervical spine. J Bone JOint Surg 41A:61, 1959
25. Friedenberg ZB, Broder HA, Edeiken JE, et al: Degenerative disk disease of the cervical spine. JAMA 174:375, 1960
26. Friedenberg ZB, Miller WT: Degenerative disc disease of the cervical spine. J Bone Joint Surg 27:248, 1945
27. Lyon E: Uncovertebral osteophytes and osteochondrosis of the cervical spine. J Bone Joint Surg 27:248, 1945
28. Horwitz T: Degenerative lesions in the cervical portion of the spine. Arch Intern Med 65:1178, 1940
29. Hirsch C, Schajowicz F, Galante J: Structural changes in the cervical spine. Acta Orthop Scand, suppl. 109:1, 1967
30. Pallis C, Jones AM, Spillane JD: Cervical spondylosis: incidence and implications. Brain 77:274, 1954
31. Holt S, Yates PO: Cervical spondylosis and nerve root lesions. J Bone Joint Surg 48B:407, 1966
32. Danforth MS, Wilson PD: The anatomy of the lumbosacral region in relation to sciatic pain. J Bone Joint Surg 7:109, 1925
33. Mixter WJ, Barr JS: Rupture of the intervertebral disc with involvement of the spinal canal. N Engl J Med 211:210, 1934
34. Ochoa JL, Torebjork HE: Paraesthesiae from ectopic impulse genration in human sensory nerves. Brain 103:835, 1980
35. Howe JF: A neurophysiological basis for the radicular pain of nerve root compression. p. 647. In Bonica JJ, Liebeskind JD, Albe-Fessard DG (eds): Advances in Pain Research and Therapy. Vol 3. Raven Press, New York, 1979
36. Howe JF, Loeser JD, Calvin WH: Mechanosensitivity of dorsal root ganglia and chronically injured axons: a physiological basis for the radicular pain of nerve root compression. Pain 3:25, 1977
37. Loeser JD: Pain due to nerve injury. Spine 10:232, 1985
38. Walton JN (ed): Brain's Diseases of the Nervous System. 8th Ed. Oxford University Press, Oxford, 1977
39. McCulloch JA, Waddell G: Variation of the lumbosacral myotomes with bony segmental anomalies. J Bone Joint Surg 62B:475, 1980
40. Smyth MJ, Wright V: Sciatica and the intervertebral disc. An experimental study. J Bone Joint Surg 40A:1401, 1959
41. Bogduk N, Twomey LT: Clinical Anatomy of the Lumbar Spine. 2nd Ed. p. 151. Churchill Livingstone, Melbourne, 1991

5 | Innervation and Pain Patterns of the Thoracic Spine

Nikolai Bogduk
Fernando Valencia

Since publication of the first edition of this book, few developments have occurred with regard to thoracic spinal pain. This issue remains as unserved as ever before by research studies and enlightening publications. Even basic information about the innervation of the thoracic spine remains incomplete. Such investigative methods as discography and zygapophyseal joint blockade, which have been so productive when applied to the cervical and lumbar spine, have only begun to be used on the thoracic spine, and little proper literature on their use has appeared.

The available literature on thoracic spinal pain focuses principally on fracture-dislocations and spinal cord compression in the thoracic region, and on thoracic outlet syndromes.[1] Deformities, fractures, tumors, and metabolic and rare diseases that affect the thoracic spine are well described in standard textbooks[2-4] but are not the cause of the majority of complaints of troublesome thoracic pain that are referred for physiotherapy. Clinical and experimental papers on what might be construed as idiopathic thoracic pain syndromes are rare. Consequently, there are few data on which one can base a comprehensive account of such pain syndromes. Any analysis must be based largely on hypotheses or suppositions and on extrapolated principles derived from studies of cervical and lumbar pain syndromes.

In this chapter, the neurologic anatomy of the thoracic spine is reviewed in order to establish a foundation for the theoretical differential diagnosis of thoracic pain, and the available evidence on the behavior of thoracic pain is reviewed. The principle followed is that any structure in the thoracic spine that receives a nerve supply must be a possible source of pain. Where available, clinical evidence is adduced to vindicate deductions made on the basis of anatomy. Otherwise, various putative sources of pain are described on theoretical grounds, with the suggestion that these sources be considered in the assessment of patients with undiagnosed thoracic pain.

INNERVATION

There have been no formal, comprehensive studies of the innervation of the thoracic spine. The available data relate only to certain aspects of this subject, such as the muscular[5] or cutaneous[6] distribution of the thoracic dorsal rami, and constitute incomplete accounts of these nerves. In order to provide as comprehensive a description as possible, one of us (F.V.) undertook dissections of two embalmed, human adult cadavers, and a combination of the data in the literature and the personal observations made during these dissections is the basis of the following description.

On the other hand, classical descriptions of the thoracic sinuvertebral nerves[5,7] have been elaborated by recent studies on the innervation of the thoracic intervertebral discs and bodies.[8]

Thoracic Dorsal Rami

The thoracic dorsal rami supply the posterior structures of the thoracic spine. Each dorsal ramus arises from a spinal nerve and passes directly posteriorly, entering the back through an osseoligamentus tunnel bounded by a transverse process, the neck of the rib below, the medial border of the superior costotransverse ligament, and the lateral border of a zygapophyseal joint (Fig. 5-1). The nerve then runs laterally through the space between the anterior lamella of the superior costotransverse ligament anteriorly and between the costolamellar ligament and posterior lamella of the superior costotransverse ligament posteriorly (Fig. 5-1). At the lateral end of this space it divides into a medial and a lateral branch.

The medial branch hooks around the lateral border of the posterior lamella of the superior costotransverse ligament, lying a short distance above the tip of the next lower transverse process. It crosses the back of the transverse process obliquely, running caudomedially between the fibers of the semispinalis and multifidus muscles, which arise from the back of the transverse process (Fig. 5-1). Along this part of its course, the medial branch divides into three branches. The shorter branches enter the fibers of the semispinalis and multifidus that arise from the transverse process, while a longer branch continues caudally and medially along the lateral surface of the multifidus muscle. At the upper thoracic levels (T1 to T6), these longer branches eventually penetrate

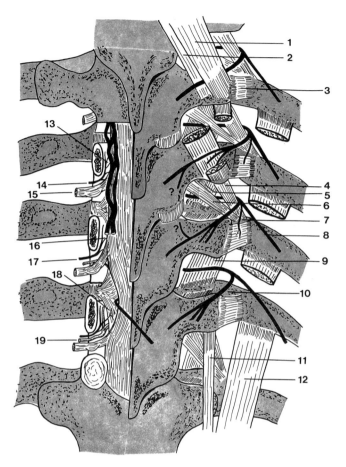

Fig. 5-1.   Innervation of the thoracic spine as viewed from the rear. On the left, the vertebral laminae have been resected to reveal the contents of the vertebral canal. The dural sac has been retracted to demonstrate the thoracic sinuvertebral nerves. On the right, the courses of the thoracic dorsal rami are shown. For clarity, muscles such as the levatores costarum and iliocostalis have not been depicted. *(1)* Semispinalis thoracis; *(2)* multifidus; *(3)* lateral costotransverse ligament covering costotransverse joint, *(4)* posterior lamella of the superior costotransverse ligament, *(5)* anterior lamella of the superior costotransverse ligament, *(6)* costolamellar ligament, *(7)* nerve to costotransverse joint, *(8)* lateral branch of dorsal ramus, *(9)* anterior lamella of superior costotransverse ligament, with dorsal ramus running across it posteriorly, *(10)* medial branch of dorsal ramus, *(11,12)* medial and lateral slips of longissimus thoracis, *(13)* branches of sinuvertebral nerves to epidural vessels, *(14)* sinuvertebral nerve, *(15)* spinal nerve, *(16)* branches of sinuvertebral nerve to dura mater, *(17)* sinuvertebral nerve, *(18)* branches to posterior longitudinal ligament, *(19)* radicular artery. Putative branches *(?)* are illustrated to the thoracic zygapophyseal joints.

the rhomboids, trapezius, and latissimus dorsi to become cutaneous. At lower thoracic levels the medial branches of the dorsal rami retain an exclusively muscular distribution.

The lateral branches of the thoracic dorsal rami descend caudally and laterally, weaving between the fascicles of the thoracic longissimus muscle (Fig. 5-1). As a rule, each nerve supplies the fascicles of the longissimus that attach to the transverse process and rib above the level of origin of the nerve, and sometimes the fascicle from the rib next above.[5] Continuing caudally and laterally, the lateral branches enter and supply the iliocostalis muscles. The lateral branches of the lower thoracic (T7 to T12) dorsal rami eventually emerge from the iliocostalis lumborum to become cutaneous. Those from higher levels have an entirely muscular distribution.

Articular branches to the costotransverse joints arise just above each joint where the dorsal ramus bifurcates.[9] They arise from the point of bifurcation or from the lateral branch of the dorsal ramus (Fig. 5-2). The pattern of innervation of the thoracic zygapophyseal joints has not been demonstrated, but it would be extraordinary if these synovial joints lacked an innervation. If their innervation is analogous to that of the lumbar and cervical joints,[10,11] articular branches would arise from the medial branches of the dorsal rami running above and below each joint (Fig. 5-1).

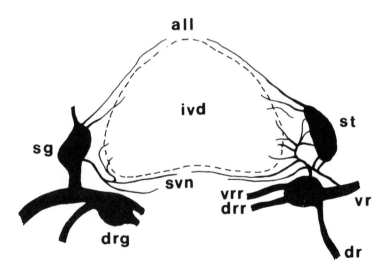

Fig. 5-2. The pattern of innervation of the thoracic vertebral bodies and intervertebral discs, as seen in human fetuses. Based on Groen et al.[8] **(A)** transverse section. Branches to the anterior longitudinal ligament *(all)* emanate from the sympathetic trunks *(st)* and sympathetic ganglia *(sg)*. Branches to the posterolateral and posterior aspects of the intervertebral disc *(ivd)* stem from the sympathetic trunk and from the sinuvertebral nerves *(svn)* that are directed to the posterior longitudinal ligament. *drg,* dorsal root ganglion; *dr,* dorsal ramus. *vr,* ventral ramus; *drr,* dorsal root; *vrr,* ventral root. (*Figure continues.*)

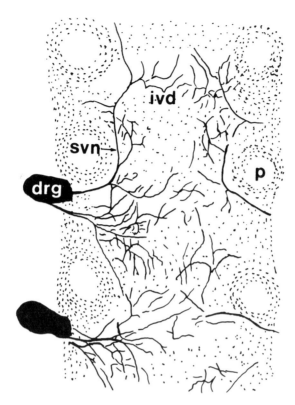

Fig. 5-2. *(Continued).* **(B)** Longitudinal view showing the posterior longitudinal plexus. The sinuvertebral nerves *(svn)* form a dense plexus that ramifies over the back of the intervertebral discs *(ivd)*. *p,* location of pedicles; *drg,* dorsal root ganglion.

Thoracic Sinuvertebral Nerves

The thoracic sinuvertebral nerves are recurrent branches of the thoracic spinal nerves. Each nerve arises from two roots: a somatic root and an autonomic root. The somatic root arises from the anterior surface or superior border of the spinal nerve just outside the intervertebral foramen. It passes into the intervertebral foramen, running in front of or sometimes above the spinal nerve, and joins with the autonomic root after a course of about 2 to 3 mm.[5,7] The autonomic root arises from the grey ramus communicans at each segmental level or, in some cases, from the sympathetic ganglion nearest the spinal nerve.[5,7] Having been formed, each sinuvertebral nerve passes through the intervertebral foramen and enters the vertebral canal, embedded amongst the branches of the segmental spinal artery and the tributaries of the spinal vein, anterior to the spinal nerve. In the intervertebral foramen the nerve gives rise to filaments that supply the vertebral lamina, and a branch that crosses the upper border of the neck of the nearby rib supplies the periosteum of the neck.[5,7]

Other branches are distributed to the vessels within the vertebral canal. Terminal branches ramify in the anterior surface of the vertebral laminae, the dural sac, and the posterior longitudinal ligament.[5,7]

The studies of Groen et al.[8] have clarified the innervation of the thoracic intervertebral discs and adjacent structures. As in the cervical and lumbar spine, the thoracic spine is innervated by dense microscopic plexuses that accompany the posterior and anterior longitudinal ligaments. The posterior plexus is derived from the thoracic sinuvertebral nerves and the anterior plexus from the thoracic sympathetic trunks and rami communicantes. Each plexus furnishes branches that supply the longitudinal ligaments and branches that penetrate the vertebral bodies and intervertebral discs. Branches from the posterior plexus innervate the ventral aspect of the dural sac.[8]

SOURCES OF PAIN

The structures that receive an innervation and are therefore possible sources of pain in the thoracic region are the thoracic vertebrae, dura mater, intervertebral discs, longitudinal ligaments, posterior thoracic muscles, and costotransverse joints. To this list should be added the thoracic zygapophyseal joints, although their source of innervation has not been explicitly demonstrated.

While conclusions about possible sources of thoracic pain may be made on the basis of anatomy, what is sorely missing are physiologic data supporting any deductions that might be made. Provocation discography and analgesic discography have shown that the intervertebral disc can be a source of pain in the cervical and lumbar regions,[12,13] but the use of discography has not been reported in the thoracic region. Thus, there is no published experimental evidence that pain can arise from thoracic discs.

There has been only one, brief report on the use of thoracic zygapophyseal joint blockade. Wilson[14] reported 17 patients with thoracic spinal pain who underwent intra-articular injections of bupivacaine and triamcinolone into their thoracic zygapophyseal joints. Thirteen of these patients obtained complete relief from their pain. This report constitutes preliminary evidence that thoracic zygapophyseal joints can be a source of pain.

Pathology

No pathologic data, not even circumstantial evidence, exists to explain why thoracic discs, muscles, zygapophyseal joints, or costovertebral joints might be sources of thoracic pain. It is only by analogy to the cervical and lumbar regions, which have been studied more extensively, that these structures can be believed to be sources of pain. In the absence of relevant pathologic studies or reports, it is difficult to state with certainty what disorders might afflict these various structures to produce pain.

Infectious and neoplastic diseases of bone can affect the thoracic vertebrae, but such conditions are usually evident on radiologic investigation and are not likely causes of idiopathic thoracic pain. Neoplastic disorders of the thoracic dura or epidural blood vessels typically manifest themselves by causing symptoms of spinal cord compression, and have not been described as causing pain without neurologic signs. Herniation of thoracic intervertebral discs is an uncommon disorder but is usually attended by signs of nerve root irritation or spinal cord compression.[15] Furthermore, thoracic disc herniations most commonly occur at lower thoracic levels (T9 and T10) and are associated with pain in the lumbar region and abdominal wall rather than in the chest.[15]

Very few pathologic conditions have been described as affecting the posterior thoracic muscles and synovial joints of the thoracic spine. The costotransverse and thoracic zygapophyseal joint can be involved in ankylosing spondylitis, but it would be unusual for this condition to be the source of thoracic pain in the absence of signs of concomitant involvement of the sacroiliac joints or other features of ankylosing spondylitis. Rheumatoid arthritis can affect the costotransverse joints[16,17] and may spread from these sites to involve the adjacent intervertebral discs.[17] Rheumatoid arthritis is also recognized as affecting the thoracic zygapophyseal joints, although not as severely as it affects the costotransverse joints.[17] The German literature[18] describes degenerative joint disease of the thoracic zygapophyseal and costotransverse joints, but there is no physiologic evidence of whether or not all joints so affected become painful.

A notion attractive to manipulative therapists is that either the thoracic zygapophyseal joints or the costotransverse joints can be affected by mechanical disorders that cause pain and are amenable to manipulative therapy. However, the pathology of these putative disorders is not known. Further study of these conditions depends critically on the development and implementation of diagnostic blockade of these joints.

The issue of muscular pain is even more speculative. The thoracic spine is abundantly covered by posterior muscles, and the thoracic transverse processes and ribs are virtually riddled with muscle attachments. Moreover, much of the posterior thoracic musculature is formed by lumbar muscles inserting at thoracic levels or cervical muscles arising from thoracic levels. This arrangement invites the suggestion that thoracic pain arising from muscles could be caused by cervical or lumbar disorders that disturb the normal function of these overlapping muscles. Spasm of these muscles as a result of cervical or lumbar pain, or excessive tension in them as a result of abnormal lumbar or cervical mechanics, could be perceived as straining their thoracic attachments and thereby causing pain. However, clinical or physiologic evidence substantiating any of these concepts is lacking. No studies have shown that anaesthetizing certain muscle insertions relieves thoracic pain caused by cervical or lumbar diseases, nor have any controlled studies verified that correction of abnormal cervical or lumbar postures relieves thoracic muscular pain.

These various reservations and seemingly negative conclusions should not be interpreted as denials of the possibility that idiopathic thoracic pain can be caused by disorders of the thoracic synovial joints or muscles. Indeed, the analogy with the lumbar and cervical regions makes it likely that at least the zygapophyseal and costotransverse joints would be potent sources of otherwise undiagnosed thoracic pain. However, what is emphasized is the absence, to date, of any definitive clinical, experimental, or pathologic data permitting endorsement of this notion.

PATTERNS OF PAIN

The phenomenon of referred pain in the thoracic region poses more diagnostic difficulties than are caused by such pain in any other region of the vertebral column. Of foremost importance is the diagnosis of visceral pain referred to the chest wall. Chest pain can be caused by cardiac, pulmonary, and pleural disease as well as by diseases of the mediastinum, esophagus, and diaphragm. Because many of these diseases are potentially life-threatening, they must be recognized and managed, or specifically excluded, and specialist consultation may be required for this purpose. However, preoccupation with visceral disease has led to the neglect and even denial of the possibility that chest wall pain may be somatic or skeletal in origin.

Pain in the chest wall (either posterior, anterior, or both) can arise from thoracic and even cervical vertebral structures. Experiments on normal volunteers have shown that noxious stimulation of the interspinous structures at thoracic and lower cervical levels can produce somatic pain referred to the chest wall.[19,20] It has also been shown that mechanical and electrical stimulation of the lower cervical intervertebral discs can produce pain over the scapula.[21] The capacity of cervical structures to produce referred pain in the chest, and the mechanism of this pain, are described in Chapter 1. The distribution of referred pain following the stimulation of thoracic structures is illustrated in Figure 5-3.

Figure 5-3 shows that somatic referred pain in the thoracic region follows a somewhat segmental pattern, in that stimulation of higher levels causes referred pain at higher levels in the chest wall. However, there is no consistent location for pain referred from a particular segment. The locations ascribed to different segments differ in different studies, and the segmental pattern is not always strictly sequential. Stimulation of a particular segment may cause referred pain at a higher level than stimulation of the segment below (Fig. 5-3). Because of these variations and irregularities, the location of any referred pain cannot be used to deduce the exact segmental location of its source.

Notwithstanding this limitation, the studies illustrated in Figure 5-3 demonstrate the principle that pain from posterior thoracic vertebral structures can be associated with referred pain in the anterior or posterior chest wall. Clinically, such referred pain may mimic the referred pain of visceral disease, and should be distinguished from it. Unfortunately, only the interspinous structures have been studied experimentally at thoracic levels, and only these structures have been shown to be capable of causing somatic referred pain. There are no data showing that any other thoracic structures also can produce such patterns

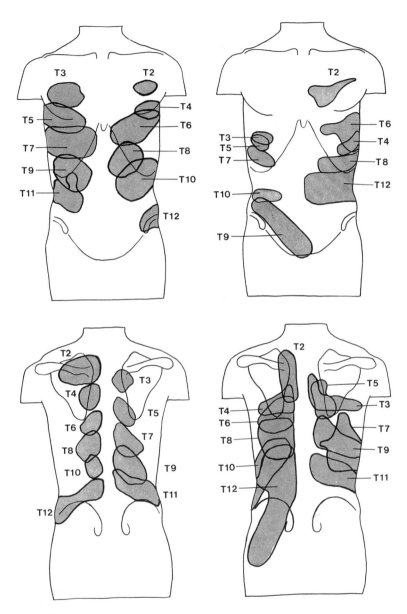

Fig. 5-3. Referred pain patterns in the chest. The shaded areas illustrate the distribution of referred pain reported by normal volunteers after stimulation of interspinous structures at the segmental levels indicated. The figures on the left are based on the data of Kellgren,[19] those on the right are based on the data of Feinstein et al.[20] Note the differences in the distribution of pain in the two sets of figures and the extensive overlap in distribution shown in the figures on the right.

of referred pain. However, the fact that interspinous structures can produce referred pain indicates that the appropriate circuitry for thoracic referred pain must exist in the central nervous system. The question that remains is whether or not other structures, such as the thoracic zygapophyseal joints or costotransverse joints, have access to this circuitry.

For many years this was the case at cervical and lumbar levels. Originally, only the cervical and lumbar interspinous structures were shown to be capable of producing referred pain. Zygapophyseal joints and other structures had not been studied. However, studies have now formally vindicated the extrapolation that because they had the same nerve supply as interspinous structures, the zygapophyseal joints could also produce referred pain[22] (see Ch. 1). It therefore seems highly likely that appropriate experiments in the future will demonstrate that thoracic zygapophyseal and costotransverse joints can cause referred pain to the chest wall.

DISCUSSION

In a sense, this chapter may not seem helpful for readers hoping to find explanations and answers to problems concerning thoracic pain since its conclusions are so diluted with reservations. However, this accurately reflects the state of the art with respect to idiopathic thoracic pain. In the absence of appropriate anatomic, experimental, and clinical data one cannot make legitimate conclusions, and there is a dire need for basic data in this field. Otherwise, thoracic pain can at best be interpreted only on the basis of extrapolations from the cervical and lumbar regions.

In this regard, however, the evidence is encouraging. Whereas the zygapophyseal joints were once disputed and disregarded as possible causes of lumbar and cervical pain, there is now abundant evidence for their having such a role. Similarly, it was disputed that lumbar and cervical discs had an innervation and that they could be sources of pain without affecting nerve roots, but contemporary evidence resolved this dispute in the affirmative. It seems only a matter of course that various structures in the thoracic spine will be shown to be possible sources of pain. All that is required are the appropriate anatomic and clinical studies. When the results of such studies become available, a stronger case may be mounted for resolving the differential diagnosis of idiopathic thoracic pain.

REFERENCES

1. Wyke B: A Back Pain Bibliography. p. 24. Lloyd-Luke, London, 1983
2. Epstein BS: The Spine. A Radiological Text and Atlas. 4th Ed. Lea & Febiger, Philadelphia, 1976
3. Rothman RH, Simeone FA (eds): The Spine. WB Saunders, Philadelphia, 1975

4. Schmorl G, Junghanns H: The Human Spine in Health and Disease. 2nd American Ed. Grune & Stratton, Orlando, FL, 1971
5. Hovelacque A: Anatomie des nerfs Craniens et Rachidiens et du System Grand Sympathique. Doin, Paris, 1927
6. Johnston HM: The cutaneous branches of the posterior primary divisions of the spinal nerves, and their distribution in the skin. J Anat Physiol 43:80, 1908
7. Hovelacque A: Le nerf sinu-vertebral. Ann Anat Pathol Medico-Chir 2:435, 1925
8. Groen GJ, Baljet B, Drukker J: Nerves and nerve plexuses of the human vertebral column. Am J Anat 188:282, 1990
9. Wyke BD: Morphological and functional features of the innervation of the costover-tebral joints. Folia Morphol Praha 23:286, 1975
10. Bogduk N, Wilson AS, Tynan W: The human lumbar dorsal rami. J Anat 134:383, 1982
11. Bogduk N: The clinical anatomy of the cervical dorsal rami. Spine 7:319, 1982
12. Bogduk N: The innervation of the lumbar intervertebral discs. In Grieve GP (ed): Modern Manual Therapy of the Vertebral Column. 2nd Ed. Churchill Livingstone, Edinburgh (In press)
13. Bogduk N: The innervation of intervertebral discs. p. 135. In Ghosh P (ed): The Biology of the Intervertebral Disc. CRC Press, Boca Raton, 1987
14. Wilson PR: Thoracic facet joint syndrome—clinical entity? Pain, suppl. 4:S87, 1987
15. Taylor TKF: Thoracic disc lesions. J Bone Joint Surg 46B:788, 1964
16. Weinberg H, Nathan H, Magora F et al: Arthritis of the first costrovertebral joint as a cause of thoracic outlet syndrome. Clin Orthop 86:159, 1972
17. Bywaters EGL: Rheumatoid discitis in the thoracic region due to spread from costo-vertebral joints. Ann Rheum Dis 33:408, 1974
18. Hohmann P: Degenerative changes in the costotransverse joints. Zeitschr Orthop 105:217, 1968
19. Kellgren JH: On the distribution of pain arising from deep somatic structures with charts of segmental pain areas. Clin Sci 4:35, 1939
20. Feinstein B, Langton JBK, Jameson RM et al: Experiments on referred pain from deep somatic tissues. J Bone Joint Surg 36A:981, 1954
21. Cloward RB: Cervical diskography. Ann Surg 150:1052, 1959
22. Bogduk N: Innervation, pain patterns, and mechanisms of pain production. p. 93. In Twomey LT, Taylor JR (eds): Physical Therapy of the Low Back. 2nd Ed. Churchill Livingstone, New York, 1994

6 | Clinical Reasoning in Orthopedic Manual Therapy

Mark Jones
Nicole Christensen
Judi Carr

Physical therapists daily address the evaluation and management of patient problems in varying ways and with varying levels of success. The distinguishing characteristics of successful and efficient clinical practice, typified by the performance of expert physical therapists, have been the focus of some of the more recent research in the field of physical therapy.[1-5] This has been partly a result of the ongoing struggle by physical therapists to advance the growth and validation of their profession. There is a recognized need to define and promote those characteristics that lead to superior clinical performance, in order to firmly establish physical therapists as autonomous, competent healthcare professionals capable of sound clinical decision-making and effective patient management.

Concern for the development of expert clinical performance by physical therapists has naturally led to a rapidly growing interest in the topic of clinical reasoning. Clinical reasoning can be defined as the cognitive processes, or thinking, used in the evaluation and management of patients.[6] This cognitive processing guides the clinician in the decision-making that dictates his or her course of action, and hence proficiency in clinical reasoning is likely to contribute to greater clinical success and efficiency in overall patient management. However, further research is required to substantiate this belief. Although cognitive processing and expert–novice differences have been studied extensively in the medical education field, under the heading of medical problem solving, there is still a relative lack of formal research into those aspects of clinical reasoning that might help to differentiate expert from less expert levels of performance among physical therapists.

This chapter attempts both to act as a reference point for related chapters and to assist readers in recognizing and analyzing their own clinical reasoning skills. As such, the chapter will briefly review relevant findings of research in the field of medical education in order to provide the background on which a model of clinical reasoning in physical therapy can reasonably be based. A structure for the organization of clinical knowledge in manual therapy is proposed, and the clinical reasoning processes facilitated by this type of organization of knowledge are then illustrated by a clinical example.

CLINICAL REASONING IN MEDICINE

Within the medical education literature dating back over more than 20 years, there exists an evolving debate about the nature of expertise in medical problem solving. Research in this area has undergone fundamental changes in methodology and focus since publication of the earliest reports of clinical problem solving.

Initially, research on clinical reasoning in the field of medical education was undertaken with the aim of identifying and understanding the process of problem solving used by expert physicians in order to facilitate the instruction of novice clinicians within the medical education curriculum.[7-9] This research was process-oriented: it focused on characterizing the actions or steps involved in the diagnosis of patient problems,[8] and was based on information-processing studies in areas such as chess.[10]

In 1978, Elstein et al. reported on 5 years of research, and their report has served as the basis for much of the investigation in the field. The core study described involved observation of two groups of physicians, consisting of peer-nominated experts and non-experts. Data were collected on the way in which the physicians sought information, on the information they obtained, and on the hypotheses they formed. These authors and others[7,9,11] concluded that clinical reasoning is a type of hypothetico-deductive reasoning, that is, one involving the generation and testing of hypotheses, followed by their modification as needed, depending on the outcome of testing.

Using the results of similar studies,[7] Barrows and Tamblyn (1980)[12] proposed a model of clinical reasoning based on the hypothetico-deductive process. They expanded slightly upon stages initially proposed by Elstein et al.[8] and described the steps in the clinical reasoning process as (1) information perception and interpretation; (2) hypothesis generation; (3) inquiry strategy and clinical skills; (4) problem formulation; and (5) diagnostic and/or therapeutic decisions.

The process is described as being cyclical and interactive rather than simply a linear series of steps. Barrows and Tamblyn[12] emphasized the relationship between memory and all stages of the process, and explained that the process of clinical reasoning itself enhances memory and adds to the existing knowledge base. Thus, this model proposed that the more experience a clinician has in going through the clinical reasoning process, the more his or her knowledge base is enriched because of it.[12]

General conclusions drawn from the early research on information processing in medical clinical reasoning included the nearly universal use of the hypothetico-deductive process of generating and testing hypotheses by clinicians, regardless of their specialty or level of experience.[8,9,11] However, Groen and Patel[13,14] have proposed that expert reasoning is more accurately described by a forward reasoning process involving the recognition of clinical patterns directly rather than the testing of hypotheses. It seems reasonable that this may indeed occur, since expert clinicians have vast knowledge bases of clinical patterns and variations on the basic patterns, so that a process of matching a patient problem to one already stored in memory might be a more efficient way of arriving at a diagnosis. However, as pointed out by Barrows and Feltovich,[15] the mechanisms by which these pattern-recognition systems were built probably included hypothesis testing at one time. In fact, experts seldom appear to miss subtle clues indicating that a patient's problem is not as it first appears, and must thus entertain alternate hypotheses as well.[15] In addition, many researchers in medical education have concluded that when faced with an unfamiliar problem, even experts revert to a hypothesis-testing process.[14–16]

Thus, it may be that the clinical reasoning process is best represented by a combination of pattern recognition and hypothesis testing. The determination of which of the two becomes primary in any clinical reasoning process depends on the extent of a clinician's prior experience with that particular type of patient presentation. The tendency of research in medical education to focus only on the diagnostic part of the clinical reasoning process may lead to overlooking of the other components of the reasoning process (i.e., management and reassessment). It is likely that for physical therapists, even if the initial diagnosis is based purely on pattern recognition, both the subsequent management and reassessment of a patient's condition will operate on a hypothesis-testing basis, since the clinician must prove that the diagnosis was accurate and the chosen treatment was effective.

Whether a hypothetico-deductive or pattern recognition process is utilized, the use of either alone appears insufficient to differentiate successful from unsuccessful clinical reasoning. Rather, the earliness with which hypotheses are generated and the quality of these early hypotheses seem to be central in determining outcome, since these hypotheses coordinate and guide all subsequent activity.[9,11,17] These conclusions suggested that the key to successful performance in diagnosis and patient management is a superior knowledge base from which to generate high-quality hypotheses. At this stage, research in medical problem solving turned its focus to the differences in the knowledge content and knowledge structure of experts as compared to novices.[14,17–26]

CLINICAL REASONING IN PHYSICAL THERAPY

Research specific to clinical reasoning among physical therapists suggests that the process they use is comparable to that used by medical clinicians.[2,4,5] Jones[6] has expanded upon the model of medical problem solving proposed by Barrows and Tamblyn[12] in developing a model of the clinical reasoning process in physical therapy. This model is illustrated in Figure 6-1.

The clinical reasoning model presented by Jones,[6] like that proposed by Barrows and Tamblyn,[12] emphasizes the cyclical and interactive nature of each step in the reasoning process. This model highlights the hypothesis generation, evaluation, and subsequent modification that take place not only in the subjective examination of the patient but throughout the physical examination, treatment, and reassessment of the patient as well.

The first step in the process as described by Jones[6] is the perception or observation of information and the interpretation of that initial information.

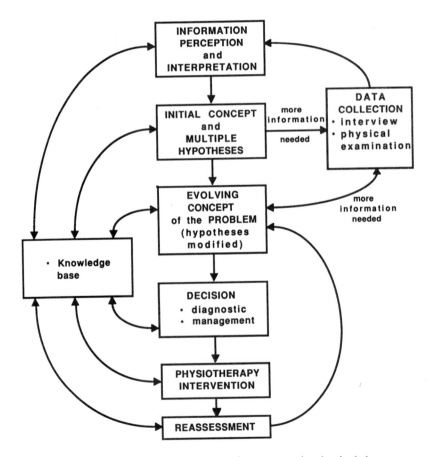

Fig. 6-1.   Model of the clinical reasoning process in physical therapy.

There is much valuable information to be gained by consciously taking a moment to process this available information before beginning formal interviewing of the patient. Even when greeting a patient a therapist can observe such specific cues as age, facial expression, appearance, resting posture, and movement patterns. Researchers in medical education have noted that experts make more extensive use than do novices of such initial information from patient encounters.[27] This fact seems to fit with the notion that expert clinicians use this information in identifying clinical patterns stored in memory.[28] Such information can be used in more effective development of an initial concept of the patient's problem and in the generation of early multiple hypotheses. These hypotheses then serve to guide the rest of the subjective and physical examination.

Data collection is tailored to the working hypotheses generated, and the therapist interprets the data by reference to his or her knowledge base in order to develop an evolving concept of the problem. That is, the collected data serve to prove or disprove hypotheses, refining, reranking, and narrowing the list of possibilities throughout the subjective and physical examination. Each new item of data that is obtained should be evaluated in light of the multiple hypotheses being considered. An important principle, as proposed by Maitland,[29] is described by the phrase "making the features fit." This implies that when information collected does not support current hypotheses, more information should be obtained to clarify the interpretation of the data. This process will also enable the clinician to build previously unrecognized variations into the existing knowledge of clinical patterns.

It is important to note that a superior performance in clinical reasoning alone is not enough to obtain good clinical results. The reasoning process itself and the decisions to which it leads are based on the data obtained through the subjective and physical examinations. It follows from this that if the data collected are faulty (e.g., incomplete, inaccurate, unreliable), clinical decisions are at risk. This raises the importance of communication skills, effective inquiry strategies, and physical examination and treatment procedures in the data-collection process. Means by which to enhance communication with patients include attention to nonverbal communication, provision of opportunity for the patient to offer spontaneous information related to his or her symptoms, using the patient's own words when communicating about the problem, and avoidance of assumptions by clarification of all information given. Examples of inquiry strategies include asking open-ended questions, forcing choices, repetition of a patient's story, and silence. While good communication is a key to quality data collection in the subjective and physical examination, superior manual skills are also invaluable in providing accurate data that will support or negate hypotheses about the structures at fault in a particular clinical disorder. The physical examination is not performed as a routine series of tests. Rather, it is a direct extension of the data-collection and hypothesis-testing performed throughout the subjective examination.

Both the subjective and physical examination benefit from the adoption of what Barrows and Tamblyn[12] referred to as "search and scan" strategies.

Search strategies are the main reasoning strategies in an examination, aimed at identifying the temporal features of a patient's symptoms, the factors that aggravate and improve them, and their relationship to other symptoms. Search strategies in physical therapy are those described above, which tend to provide information useful in supporting, refining, and reranking hypotheses. Scan inquiries, on the other hand, are routine data-gathering procedures unrelated to specific hypotheses. They provide background information, safety information, and quick checks of other areas less likely to be involved in a patient's condition.

When enough information has been gathered from both the subjective and physical examinations, the therapist is able to make a *diagnostic and management decision*. This decision includes whether to treat or not to treat the patient, whether to address initially the source(s) or contributing factor(s) in the patient's condition, or both, which type of treatment to try, and, for the treatment chosen, what specifications will be employed (i.e., with manual treatment will pain be avoided or provoked, and what grade and direction of mobilization will be employed). The treatment intervention that is chosen must be followed by continuous reassessment, for even treatment is viewed as a form of hypothesis testing. Results of treatment serve to modify or reform hypotheses, contributing further to the therapist's evolving concept of the patient's problem.

Unexpected or ineffective results of selected treatments may also lead to expansion of the knowledge base with regard to variations in the presentation and responses to treatment of various clinical patterns. It is easy to see that with accumulated experience in clinical reasoning, which includes reflecting on patient encounters and outcomes, a therapist's knowledge base has the potential to grow rapidly to a point at which pattern recognition becomes very rapid and the clinician can function intuitively in a large proportion of cases.

In addition to reflecting on clinical cases, the physical therapist can reflect on his or her own reasoning process throughout the subjective and physical examination of a patient. This awareness and monitoring of one's own thinking process is called *metacognition*. While cognitive skills such as data analysis and synthesis allow the clinical reasoning process to continue, the metacognitive skills provide a critical review of this cognitive performance. In essence, this requires the clinician to think, or process information, on two planes simultaneously. By reflecting on clinical cases, the therapist's knowledge of clinical presentations and their treatment will expand; by reflecting on his or her own performance, the therapist's knowledge of how to function efficiently and effectively will expand.

May and Dennis[30] provide an excellent discussion of factors that influence the clinical reasoning process, including the nature of the specific task at hand, the environment in which the task is set, and the decision maker. The focus in this chapter is on the process of clinical reasoning itself, and only those factors relating to the knowledge and cognitive skills of the decision maker will be discussed further.

KNOWLEDGE BASE CONTENT AND ORGANIZATION

It can be seen from the model proposed above that a physical therapist's knowledge base affects and is affected by every phase of the clinical reasoning process. Knowledge has been described in the literature of cognitive psychology as a record of the processing and reprocessing of information within human memory. This processing produces knowledge that is structured into networks of interrelationships.[31,32]

Problem-solving studies in areas such as chess and physics have demonstrated that experts in these fields are characterized by the possession of highly organized and interrelated patterns of meaningful information held in memory.[10,33,34] These patterns, or schemata, are modifiable information structures that represent generalized concepts underlying an object, situation, event, sequence of events, action, or sequence of actions.[32] They are prototypes in memory of frequently experienced situations that individuals use to recognize and interpret other situations. Within the more recent medical-education literature, researchers have emphasized that it is the organization, or structure, of a clinician's knowledge base more than the content of that knowledge that results in effective, accurate diagnosis.[17,19–23,35,36] When the knowledge is there but cannot be easily accessed by the clinician in a clinical situation because of a lack of organization, the clinical reasoning process suffers.

Physical therapists may call upon various types of knowledge in varying degrees when going through a process of clinical reasoning. These types of knowledge include basic science and biomedical knowledge, clinically acquired knowledge (often in the form of recognized clinical patterns and "If/Then" rules of action), everyday knowledge about life and social situations, and tacit knowledge, a term that connotes the habitual knowledge gained through experience, which is difficult to translate into words yet which greatly influences the way in which clinicians see and gather information from patients.[37]

A physical therapist's organization of knowledge may include schemata for facts, procedures, concepts, principles, and clinical pattern presentations. Relevant facts in the clinical reasoning process include anatomic information, pathophysiologic mechanisms, and the physical properties of modalities employed by physical therapists. Procedures might include examination and treatment strategies, manual techniques, and exercise progressions.

Examples of concepts represented by discrete schemata in memory are "adverse neural tension" and "irritability." Adverse neural tension signifies some form of alteration in the structure or mobility of the continuous tissue tract composing the nervous system. Involvement of adverse neural tension in a patient's symptoms necessitates attention to this aspect of the problem through the ongoing management and reassessment of the patient's condition. Irritability is a measure of how easily and to what extent the patient's symptoms are provoked by daily activities. Judgement about the irritability component of the patient's disorder is then used to guide the extent of the physical examination and treatment that can be performed at the first assessment without risk of aggravating the patient's disorder.

Principles represented in memory by schemata are the underlying rationales that guide the physical therapist in the application of specific knowledge from any other schema. Examples include the principles that guide the selection of techniques and grade of passive movement treatment appropriate for a particular combination of signs and symptoms[29,38] (see also Ch. 12).

A clinical pattern presentation is represented in memory by a schema that may contain information typical of that particular patient problem; data relating to predisposing or contributing factors, the sites and nature of symptoms, history, the behavior of symptoms, and physical signs that are present when such a pattern is seen clinically. These "subschemas" are linked, so that the identification of one item of data enables the clinician to easily recall other information related to that clinical pattern. A superficial representation of a schema for identifying the clinical pattern of an acutely locked cervical zygapophyseal joint is presented in Figure 6-2 and Table 6-1 to illustrate the subschema that might be activated in order to access this clinical pattern in memory. No attempt is made to illustrate the complete and multiple links that are likely to exist between subschemata.

It is evident that the content of knowledge varies among individuals. In addition, some medical-education literature suggests that there may be a different structure to the knowledge of clinicians at varying levels of expertise, (i.e., at different stages between novice and expert).[28,39–42] Boshuizen and Schmidt[42] have proposed that the development of expertise in medicine progresses through stages in which clinical reasoning and knowledge acquisition are interdependent. The first stage involves the accumulation of biomedical, basic scien-

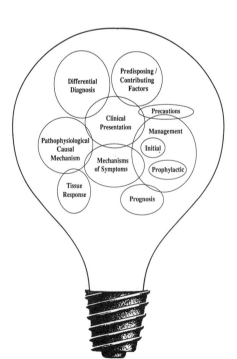

Fig. 6-2. Example of schema for identifying a clinical pattern of an acute locked cervical zygapophyseal joint.

Table 6-1. Subschema that Might Be Activated with Clinical Pattern of Acute Locked Cervical Zygapophyseal Joint

Clinical Presentation
    Sudden onset following unguarded movement
        of sustained posture
    Protective deformity of lateral flexion away
        from pain
    Active lateral flexion and rotation to painful
        side and extension limited by pain ±
        muscle spasm
    Passive physical and accommodative
        movements to close joint are mechanically
        blocked

Predisposing Factors
    Local hypermobility
    Adjacent hypomobility
    Poor muscle control
    Posture
    Lifestyle, work and sporting activities

Differential Diagnosis
    Muscular wry neck
    Acquired wry neck
    C1/C2 rotary fixation
    Spasmodic torticolis
    Hysterical torticolis
    Discogenic wry neck

Mechanisms of Symptoms
    Peripherally activated nociception ±
        sympathetic and affective components

Management
    Initial
        Passive movement
        Relaxation techniques
        Modalities
        Collar
    Prophylactic
        Stabilizing exercises
        Mobilizing exercises
        Activity modification

Pathophysiologic Mechanisms
    Synovial entrapment
    Meniscoid entrapment
    Muscle spasms
    Arthrotic articular surfaces
    Collagen disorder hypermobility

Tissue Response
    Inflammation
    Vasodilation
    Swelling
    Ischemia
    Fibrosis

Prognostic Factors
    Age
    Ease of onset
    Mechanism of onset (spont./trauma)
    Frequency of previous episodes
    Response to previous treatment
    Lifestyle
    Compliance

tific knowledge. This knowledge is linked in a network as presented through formal education. As more knowledge is added to the network, connections between concepts are formed, facilitating the development of clusters of related concepts. Clinical reasoning in this early stage is largely based on biomedical concepts, and students have difficulty in differentiating relevant from irrelevant patient findings, thus leading to excessive numbers of hypotheses. Schmidt and Boshuizen[42] refer to the development of clusters of related concepts as "knowledge encapsulation."

The second stage in the development of medical expertise involves the integration of biomedical knowledge into clinical knowledge. This occurs with students' increasing experience with patients. The knowledge structures drawn on in clinical reasoning at this stage contain little in the way of direct biomedical concepts. Rather, links are formed between patient findings and clinical concepts, enabling clinicians to form hypotheses and make diagnoses. Boshuizen and Schmidt[42] only describe examples of diagnostic concept clusters. Within physical therapy, diagnostic concept clusters, such as zygapophyseal joint arthralgia and variations of disc disorders, can be identified, but nondiagnostic clusters such as predisposing factors also exist, and these are discussed later, under the heading of "Hypothesis Categories." As students begin to recognize clinical patterns, their ability to differentiate relevant from irrelevant cues improves, and shortcuts in reasoning become evident for typical cases.

The third stage in developing expertise, is characterized by the development in the clinician's memory of stereotypical "illness scripts." These are analogous to the clinical patterns recognized by physical therapists, and include information about predisposing conditions (e.g., personal, social, and/or medical hereditary conditions that influence the patients' presentations), the pathophysiologic process taking place, and the presenting signs and symptoms typical of the condition. These illness scripts, or patterns, are activated as a whole in the clinician's memory, which increases the efficiency of the knowledge network as the amount of searching necessary to locate related information is decreased.[42]

According to Boshuizen and Schmidt,[42] the final stage in the development of expert knowledge content and structure involves the storage of real clinical encounters as "instance scripts" in memory. These memories of patient encounters are stored as discrete units in memory and are not merged with the stereotypical illness script or clinical pattern in memory. The more experience a clinician gathers, the better he or she is able to recognize the variations (stored as instance scripts) of basic clinical patterns seen in daily practice.

Research in physical therapy has yet to explore the knowledge structures that physical therapists utilize when reasoning through clinical cases. However, preliminary evidence suggests that a correlation exists between accumulated clinical experience and an improved ability to recognize clinical patterns in the field of physical therapy.[43] Certainly the illness script proposed in Boshuizen and Schmidt's stage theory of expertise[42] is consistent with the format in which some postgraduate orthopedic/manual therapy programs encourage students to assimilate clinical patterns.[44,45]

Boshuizen and Schmidt[42] suggest that to improve clinical reasoning, education must focus on the development of adequate knowledge structures. This requires further understanding of the knowledge structures that physical therapists use. The notion that biomedical knowledge is encapsulated in clinical knowledge is particularly relevant to education in physical therapy, which often has a similar structure of basic science subjects preceding clinical experience. This suggests that students of physical therapy are also likely to develop biomedical schema that must then be encapsulated into clinical patterns as the students gain clinical experience. Patel and Kaufman[26] cite a series of studies that are consistent with Boshuizen and Schmidt's theory that the use of biomedical concepts in clinical reasoning decreases with expertise. While this has not yet been demonstrated in physical therapists, it can be hypothesized that a similar phenomenon occurs as "textbook" information becomes altered or superseded by clinical experience.

Patel and Kaufman[26] see the key role of knowledge in biomedical science as facilitating explanation and coherent communication. This is typically not activated in the context of familiar conditions,[14,25] but in the context of complex, unfamiliar cases biomedical knowledge is utilized to understand and provide causal explanations for patient data.[25,46] As such, this knowledge assists in the organization of disjointed facts. Patel and Kaufman[26] purport that since well-organized, coherent information is easier to remember than disjointed facts, this use of biomedical knowledge should facilitate further clinical learning.

PROPOSED SYSTEM OF KNOWLEDGE ORGANIZATION: HYPOTHESIS CATEGORIES

Because the knowledge required in the practice of physical therapy is vast and diverse, the importance of a good organizational system is increased. Clinical experience in reasoning through a patient problem, as demonstrated by the clinical reasoning model, has the potential to expand, modify, and enhance the knowledge base of the physical therapist. However, this opportunity is lost if the new knowledge gained in the clinical encounter is stored in a disorganized fashion, for this knowledge will then not be easily accessible to the clinician in future experiences. The following discussion proposes an example of a way in which to organize information obtained from clinical encounters for immediate use, and for storing it accessibly in memory. In this system, clinical reasoning is characterized by the adoption of several hypothesis categories, including a category relating to the source of the symptoms or dysfunction and categories for contributing factors, precautions and contraindications to physical examination and treatment, management, prognosis, and mechanisms for the occurrence of symptoms. Each category represents clusters of related concepts. A case presentation follows, and will serve to illustrate these hypothesis categories.

Patient Presentation

A 28-year-old computer programmer presents with the complaint of a medial scapular ache on the right side at about the level of the spine of her scapula. She describes her ache as deep and intermittent. Before investigating the details of the patient's symptoms, the physical therapist notices that she has assumed a very slumped sitting posture, with her head thrust forward and shoulders rounded.

The patient experiences her ache after prolonged periods of working at her computer (e.g., 2 hours), and then notes difficulty (''stiffness'') in lifting her head up out of what she demonstrates to be a slightly flexed and right-rotated typing posture. Her ache resolves immediately when she is out of this posture during the morning, but occurs more quickly (e.g., within 10 minutes) toward the end of her working day, and by the time she leaves work there is a constant ache that takes several hours to resolve. While turning her neck does not hurt, she does note that it feels stiff to turn in either direction as the day progresses, and that at the end of the day her head feels heavy to hold up. She is not sure whether looking up is a problem, since she never really needs to, and thoracic and arm movements have no effect on her ache. The stiffness and heaviness continue through the evening but resolve after a night's sleep. Sleeping has never been a problem for the patient, and in the mornings she has no discomfort, but does complain of some general neck stiffness that lasts for 10 to 15 minutes on waking.

The patient reports that her ache began spontaneously about 3 weeks ago while she was typing at work. She is unaware of what might have caused it, but does recall gardening for several hours the previous day, something that she rarely does for more than half an hour at a time. The ache has gradually worsened in intensity over the 3 weeks since it began. The patient has never had a similar problem, but does report that she had a car accident about 6 months ago and had some generalized soreness and stiffness across the base of her neck following this for about 2 months. She received physical therapy at that time, consisting of mobilization and heat to the affected part of her neck, and instruction in home exercises. The treatment helped to relieve those symptoms but she has not continued with the exercise program that was given to her. Other than this medial scapular ache, the patient has no health problems or relevant past history.

Source of Symptoms or Dysfunction

The source of symptoms refers to the structure from which the symptoms are emanating. Information contributing to the formation of hypotheses about the source of a patient's symptoms or dysfunction is available from each of the major aspects of the patient's presentation. For example, from the patient information described above, a physical therapist might begin to generate hypotheses about the source of the patient's symptoms based on their site(s), since different structures are associated with different patterns of symptoms. In this patient, with a medial scapular ache, the therapist might consider the source of the ache to possibly include cervical spinal structures, thoracic spinal structures, and/or local soft tissues in the interscapular region.

The behavior of the symptoms (e.g., aggravating factors, irritability, easing factors, 24-hour pattern) can also help to implicate certain structures when the therapist considers which structures are most involved or compromised by a certain aggravating activity, or conversely, what stresses on what structures are reduced by a particular easing activity. In the case of the patient described above, the structures most implicated by typing in a sustained forward head posture and slumped sitting, difficulty in returning the head to neutral, symmetrical stiffness in turning the neck right and left, and heaviness of the head as the day progresses are the low cervical discs and neural structures. Since thoracic and arm movements have no effect on the ache, the thoracic joints and local muscles and soft tissues are less implicated, although specific physical tests of these structures are still required for confirmation of the source of the patient's condition. Structures more likely to be implicated by symptoms of spontaneous, gradual onset and the history of a car accident and cervical spine injury are cervical and/or neural. For this hypothesis category, as for all of the rest, each new item of information must be seen in the light of the information already obtained, and hypotheses in the category weighted accordingly, with those supported by most of the information heading the list of possibilities.

Contributing Factors

Contributing factors are any predisposing or associated factors involved in the development or maintenance of the patient's problem. These include environmental, emotional, physical, and/or biomechanical factors. In the case of the patient described above, contributing factors may include her poor posture and the nature of her job, which requires long periods in an activity that accentuates this posture. Her posture itself may be antalgic or be related to joint and neural hypomobility or poor muscle endurance. Hypotheses about contributing factors should be considered separately from the source of a patient's symptoms and evaluated specifically through physical testing and treatment to assess their involvement in the patient's symptoms. In this case, it is quite probable that the patient's symptoms are related to her gardening activities on the day before their onset, so that her previously nonaggravating work posture is now causing her difficulty. The correlation between the onset of her symptoms and the time at which the patient gave up doing her home exercises might also establish a relationship, implicating lack of exercise as a factor contributing to the symptoms.

Precautions and Contraindications to Physical Therapy

Hypotheses about precautions and contraindications to physical examination and treatment serve to determine the extent of physical examination that may safely be undertaken (i.e., how many physical tests are performed and whether provocation of symptoms is to be avoided or not). Additionally, these hypotheses help determine whether physical treatment is indicated, and if so, whether there are constraints to it (e.g., techniques done short of pain provocation versus techniques done with the intent of reproducing a patient's pain). Factors taken into consideration include the severity, irritability, and stability (i.e., predictability/variability) of the disorder. Also included are the progression of the disorder, rate of impairment, patient's general health, and other special screening questions, such as those relating to unexplained weight loss or any steroid use. In the context of the case example presented above, the presentation is not so severe that reproduction of the patient's symptoms would have to be avoided (i.e., the patient can continue working despite her ache); likewise, the irritability and stability of the symptoms do not indicate that any specific precautions in evaluation or treatment are necessary.

Management

The formation of management hypotheses is facilitated by clues gained in analysis of the patient's main complaint, site of symptoms, behavior of symptoms, precautionary questions, onset and progression of symptoms, mechanism of injury, past treatment, pain threshold, personality, physical examination, and ongoing management. These hypotheses assist in deciding whether or not physical therapy is indicated, and if so, what means should be tried. Decisions must be made about whether treatment should be directed primarily at the source of the symptoms or at the contributing factors. Preliminary management hypotheses that might be generated in light of the case example given above include manual techniques that address a cervical source for the symptoms (e.g., cervical disc), that address the postural contributing factor, or that include any appropriate stretching and/or strengthening exercises for the cervicothoracic complex. While physical testing will further implicate a potential source and contributing factor for the patient's condition, this information can only provide a general direction to the management of the patient. The specific passive movement techniques used in patient management will depend more on each patient's unique presentation, particularly the relationship of symptoms to resistance as revealed through passive movement testing. For further discussion of this issue, see Chapter 12.

Prognosis

Hypotheses about the prognosis for a patient enable the physical therapist to relay to the patient an estimate of the extent to which the patient's disorder appears amenable to physical therapy and of the time frame within which recovery can be expected. Many individual factors are considered and weighted as either "negative" (unfavorable), or "positive" (favorable) with respect to how the problem is likely to respond to physical therapy. Such factors include the mechanical (usually more positive) versus inflammatory (usually more negative) balance of the disorder, irritability of the disorder, degree of damage/injury (often reflected in the forces involved and immediate signs and symptoms of the disorder), the length of history and progression of the disorder, pre-existing disorders, the patient's expectations, personality, and lifestyle, and the patient's healing potential. The overall picture of a favorable or unfavorable prognosis is obtained by the combination of all of these factors. The case example given above demonstrates positive factors in that the patient is young and her condition does not appear to be predominantly inflammatory but rather mechanical. Her symptoms are not irritable, the history is recent, and the progression is gradual, all of which point to a more positive prognosis. Also positive is her history of a favorable response to physical therapy. Her history of a car accident and the nature of her job are relatively negative factors that must be weighed against the positive factors in the prognosis in this patient's case.

Mechanisms of Symptoms

The system of hypothesis categories presented in this chapter as an example of physical therapists' organization of knowledge must be viewed as an open-ended system, and those therapists adopting such a system must be alert and willing to expand the system to accommodate their growing knowledge bases. An excellent example of this is the hypothesis category "mechanisms of symptoms." In response to the work of Butler[47] (see Ch. 15), it is proposed that this hypothesis category be added to the five categories cited earlier. The aim of this hypothesis category is to encourage therapists to look beyond mere consideration of the structure at fault in a diagnostic sense, and to include a consideration of the mechanisms by which the patient's symptoms are being initiated and/or maintained neurologically. The development of this hypothesis category is a result of consideration of an enormous body of knowledge that exists in the literature on pain, not previously utilized in the building of most manual therapists' knowledge base of clinical patterns. Patient presentations that have traditionally been considered difficult to manage or perhaps unfairly labelled as not having an organic basis are being explained by some recent advances in the area of neural mechanisms.[48-50] The proposed hypothesis category of mechanisms of symptoms is composed of four subcategories, including peripherally evoked nociception, centrally evoked nociception, autonomic mechanisms, and affective mechanisms. A brief description of these is given below. For a more detailed account of the neural mechanisms referred to above, and for more clinical features stemming from such mechanisms, see Chapter 15.

Peripherally evoked nociception refers to nociception that is elicited in the peripheral nervous system, such as pain resulting from a noxious stimulus or following an acute zygapophyseal joint sprain. Where tissue damage has occurred, chemical and/or mechanical stimuli activate high-threshold sensory receptors. Pain-mediating afferents transmit impulses that enter the dorsal horn of the spinal cord and ascend via central nervous system pathways, terminating in the brain and resulting in pain perception and emotion. Such pain arising from tissue damage has been labelled "pathological pain."[51] The structures involved in peripherally evoked nociception may include joints, muscles, soft tissue, and/or nerves.

This clinical pattern of peripherally evoked nociception is easily recognized and may represent the majority of neuromusculoskeletal disorders seen by manual therapists. It is characterized by symptoms that present in clear neuroanatomic pattern(s) and behave "normally." There is typically a recognizable history accounting for the symptoms, and while an inflammatory component may produce constant irritation and hence constant symptoms, there is generally also a "mechanical" presentation in that symptoms are aggravated and eased by some variation of movement and rest. The pattern of peripherally evoked nociception is also characterized by the presence of clear physical signs existing in proportion to the presenting symptoms. The case example given above fits this category for mechanisms of symptoms.

Centrally evoked nociception refers to symptoms that are initiated or maintained by abnormal central nervous system processing. This can result from the increased excitability of dorsal horn interneurons and/or the effect of altered descending pain-control mechanisms. Symptoms provoked initially by a peripheral stimulus can be maintained by the excitation of spinal neurons long after the initial insult has ceased (healed). This excitation of spinal neurons may become so widespread that in addition to maintenance of the original symptoms, symptoms may be provoked by the stimulation of other, nonrelated areas. Other possibilities include the presentation of symptoms in a broad, somatically unconnected area or unrelated site (e.g., the unaffected limb) through stimulation of the site of an initial insult.[50]

The clinical pattern for centrally evoked nociception may be characterized by a bizarre presentation of symptoms as contrasted to the more easily recognized pattern of peripherally evoked nociception. In cases of centrally evoked nociception, symptoms may not fit the neuroanatomic patterns of typical tissue injury, and symptom behavior may not follow predictable mechanical patterns of aggravation and relief with movement and rest. In fact, symptoms may occur for no reason, such as with spontaneous stabs of pain. Pain may also be elicited by normally non-noxious stimuli. Similarly, the history of symptom onset may not provide a clear temporal or anatomic relationship between the precipitating event or injury and the presenting symptoms. Physical findings may not present the same proportional relationship to symptoms as exists in peripherally evoked nociception, providing further evidence of central influences in the production or maintenance of symptoms.

Autonomic mechanisms may also contribute to the genesis and maintenance of pain, through the peripheral interaction that is proposed to exist between sympathetic efferents and sensory afferents and altered central processing.[52] Peripheral tissue injury can elicit an abnormal sensory input. This has been explained through mechanisms by which local neural and non-neural inflammation induces peripheral sensitization.[51] This abnormal afferent input can contribute to altering normal central processing and in turn elicit an excessive ascending transmission of nociception and abnormal sympathetic responsiveness. Abnormal sympathetic activity is manifest in abnormal vasomotor, sudomotor, and trophic changes within peripheral tissues, which can themselves contribute to an increase in abnormal afferent activity. McMahon[52] proposed this vicious cycle, whereby abnormal afferent activity leads to altered signal processing in the dorsal horn, which can in turn elicit an abnormal sympathetic outflow that further contributes to abnormal afferent activity, as a general basis for the maintenance of sympathetic pain. The clinical features of abnormal sympathetic involvement include an altered circulation (temperature and color), swelling, sweating, and trophic changes. A change such as swelling may exist or persist out of proportion to a local tissue injury and, as implied by the vicious cycle described above, these changes may be accompanied by states in which pain is maintained.

The subcategory of an affective mechanism, or emotional involvement, encourages therapists to seek and attend to the emotional aspect of pain. The International Association for the Study of Pain has in part defined pain as "an unpleasant sensory and emotional experience associated with actual or potential tissue damage."[53] Neural pathways exist that relay the emotional element of pain. This can be seen in the results of frontal lobotomy, in which pain continues to be perceived by the patient, but no emotion is displayed in conjunction with the pain. A patient's present and past emotional history become relevant when one considers that emotionally traumatic events have been shown to influence supraspinal pain pathways, leading to exaggerated or abnormal responses to painful stimuli.[54] Thus, patients with no local signs related to their symptoms, those with bizarre symptoms, and those with an exaggerated focus on their symptoms may in fact be demonstrating a neurologic cause for these presentations rather than simply a behavioral disorder, which is the explanation frequently suggested.

The addition of the hypothesis category of mechanisms of symptoms to the system suggested here for organization of knowledge is an attempt to focus therapists' attention on an area that holds significant implications for reasoning in the areas of management and prognosis, thereby avoiding the tendency to focus only on the specific structure(s) at fault in a particular presentation. In considering the mechanisms of symptoms, however, care must be taken not to oversimplify the complex nor the still poorly understood area of pain. The complexities and inter-relationships of the neural mechanisms responsible for pain, and particularly abnormal pain states, mean that any division of these mechanisms will be artificial, and an overlap of mechanisms is likely within any clinical presentation. Thus, patients will present with disorders in which several mechanisms may be in evidence. Conversely, patients may also present with more straightforward disorders in which peripherally evoked nociception is the principal mechanism. There will always be some degree of an affective component to a patient's symptoms, but this will not be clinically relevant in many patients. Similarly, the autonomic nervous system will always be activated by nociceptive inputs, but in most patients this will not contribute significantly to the symptom presentation.

Categorization of the mechanisms of symptoms, as presented here, is useful only if it has clinical implications leading to improved patient management. Certain safety, management, and prognostic considerations will come with attention to the mechanisms of symptoms, but the discussion of these considerations is beyond the scope of this chapter.

During each clinical encounter, hypothesis categories such as those described above should be pursued concurrently as information is elicited about a patient's problem. The hypothesis categories can be used both as a means by which to organize this information and to facilitate access to the required relevant knowledge stored in the therapist's memory. Each new clue obtained while examining a patient should be considered in the light of relevant hypothesis categories, resulting in the building of a comprehensive clinical picture through the refinement of working hypotheses in each category.

CONCLUSION

Clinical reasoning in physical therapy, as in medicine, involves the processes of both hypothesis generation and testing and of pattern recognition. The extent to which either is used is largely related to a clinician's level of experience and in particular to the clinician's organization of knowledge. A model of the clinical reasoning process used by physical therapists is proposed to assist clinicians in conceptualizing this important skill. A structure for the organization of knowledge is put forward in the form of "hypothesis categories." While these categories will not necessarily be appropriate for all physical therapists in all settings, we strongly encourage physical therapists to consider the reasoning behind their inquiries, tests, and management interventions: this will help them to identify categories of hypotheses that reflect the clinical judgments typically encountered in the different areas of practice. Therapists can then critically analyze their own reasoning, with consideration given to the breadth of the hypotheses they consider, the means by which hypotheses will be tested, whether supporting and negating data are sought, and whether established clinical patterns are substantiated. This form of personal reflection and assessment should lead to more effective management for each patient, and a more rapid acquisition of expertise for the physical therapist.

REFERENCES

1. Jensen GM, Shepard KF, Hack LM: The novice versus the experienced clinician: insights into the work of the physical therapist. Phys Ther 70:314, 1990
2. Jensen GM, Shepard KF, Hack LM: Attribute dimensions that distinguish master and novice physical therapy clinicians in orthopedic settings. Phys Ther 72:711, 1993
3. May BJ, Dennis JK: Expert decision making in physical therapy: a survey of practitioners. Phys Ther 71:190, 1992
4. Payton OD: Clinical reasoning process in physical therapy. Phys Ther 65:924, 1985
5. Thomas-Edding D: Clinical problem solving in physical therapy and its implications for curriculum development. p. 100. In: Proceedings of the Tenth International Congress of the World Confederation for Physical Therapy; May 17–22, Sydney, Australia, 1987
6. Jones MA: Clinical reasoning in manual therapy. Phys Ther 72:875, 1992
7. Barrows HS, Feightner JW, Neufeld VR, Norman GR: Analysis of the clinical methods of medical students and physicians, Final Report, Ontario Department of Health, Hamilton, Ontario, Canada, 1978
8. Elstein AS, Shulman LS, Sprafka SS: Medical Problem Solving: an analysis of clinical reasoning. Harvard University Press, Cambridge, MA, 1978
9. Neufeld VR, Norman GR, Feightner JW, Barrows HS: Clinical problem-solving by medical students: A cross-sectional and longitudinal analysis. Med Educ 15:315, 1981
10. deGroot AD: Thought and Choice in Chess. Basic Books, New York, 1965
11. Barrows HS, Norman GR, Neufeld VR, Feightner JW: The clinical reasoning of

randomly selected physicians in general medical practice. Clin Invest Med 5:49, 1982

12. Barrows HS, Tamblyn RM: Problem-Based Learning: An Approach to Medical Education. Springer, New York, 1980
13. Groen GJ, Patel VL: Medical problem-solving: some questionable assumptions. J Med Ed 19:95, 1985
14. Patel VL, Groen GJ: Knowledge-based solution strategies in medical reasoning. Cogn Sci 10:91, 1986
15. Barrows HS, Feltovich PJ: The clinical reasoning process. Med Educ 12:86, 1987
16. Elstein AS, Shulman LS, Sprafka SA: Medical problem solving: a ten year retrospective. Eval Health Prof 13:5, 1990
17. Feltovich PJ, Barrows HS: Issues of generality in medical problem solving. p. 128. In Schmidt HG, DeVolder ML (eds): Tutorials in Problem-Based Learning. Van Gorcum, Assen/Maastricht, 1984
18. Arocha JF, Patel VL, Patel YC: Hypothesis generation and the coordination of theory and evidence in novice diagnostic reasoning. J Med Decision Making (In press)
19. Bordage G, Grant J, Marsden P: Quantitative assessment of diagnostic ability. Med Educ 24:413, 1990
20. Bordage G, Lemieux M: Semantic structures and diagnostic thinking of experts and novices. Acad Med, suppl. 66:S70, 1991
21. Grant J, Marsden P: The structure of memorized knowledge in students and clinicians: an explanation for medical expertise. Med Educ 21:92, 1987
22. Grant J, Marsden P: Primary knowledge, medical education and consultant expertise. Med Educ 22:173, 1988
23. Patel VL, Groen GJ, Frederiksen CH: Differences between medical students and doctors in memory for clinical cases. Med Educ 20:3, 1986
24. Patel VL, Groen GJ, Scott HS: Biomedical knowledge in explanations of clinical problems by medical students. Med Educ 22:398, 1988
25. Patel VL, Groen GJ, Arocha JF: Medical expertise as a function of task difficulty. Mem Cogn 18:394, 1990
26. Patel VL, Kaufman DR: Clinical reasoning and biomedical knowledge. In Higgs J, Jones MA (eds): Clinical Reasoning Skills. Butterworth-Heinemann, London (In press)
27. Hobus PPM, Schmidt HG, Boshuizen HPA, Patel VL: Contextual factors in the activation of first diagnostic hypotheses: Expert-novice differences. Med Educ 21: 471, 1987
28. Boshuizen HPA, Schmidt HG: On the role of biomedical knowledge in clinical reasoning by experts, intermediates and novices. Cogn Sci 16:153, 1992
29. Maitland GD: Vertebral Manipulation. 5th Ed. Butterworth, London, 1986
30. May BJ, Dennis JK: Teaching clinical decision making. In Higgs J, Jones MA (eds): Clinical Reasoning in the Health Professions. Butterworth-Heinemann, London (In press)
31. Anderson JR: Cognitive Psychology and its Implications, 3rd Ed. Freeman, New York, 1990
32. Rumelhart DE, Ortony E: The representation of knowledge in memory. In Anderson RC, Spiro RJ, Montague WE (eds): Schooling and the Acquisition of Knowledge. Lawrence Erlbaum, Hillsdale, NJ, 99, 1977
33. Chase WG, Simon HA: Perception in chess. Cogn Psychol 4:55, 1973
34. Chi MTH, Feltovich PJ, Glaser R: Categorization and representation of physics problems by experts and novices. Cogn Sci 5:121, 1981

35. Bordage G, Zacks R: The structure of medical knowledge in the memories of medical students and general practitioners: categories and prototypes. Med Educ 18:406, 1984
36. Ericsson A, Smith J (Eds): Toward a General Theory of Expertise: Prospects and Limits. Cambridge University Press, New York, 1991
37. Mattingly C: What is clinical reasoning? Am J Occup Ther 45:979, 1991
38. Maitland GD: The Maitland concept. In Twomey LT, Taylor JR (eds): Physical Therapy of the Low Back. Churchill Livingstone, New York, 1987
39. Boshuizen HPA, Schmidt HG, Coughlin LD: On the application of medical basic science in clinical reasoning: implications for structural knowledge differences between experts and novices. p. 517. In Patel VL, Groen GJ (eds): Proceedings of the Tenth Annual Conference of the Cognitive Science Society. August 17–19, 1988, Montreal, Quebec, Canada. Vol. 59. Lawrence Erlbaum Associates, Hillsdale, NJ, 1988
40. Boshuizen HPA, Schmidt HG: The development of clinical reasoning expertise: Implications for teaching. In Higgs J, Jones MA (eds): Clinical Reasoning Skills. Butterworth-Heinemann, London (In press)
41. Schmidt HG, Boshuizen HPA, Norman GR: Reflections on the nature of expertise in medicine. In Keravnou E (ed): Deep Models for Medical Knowledge Engineering. Elsevier Science Publishers, Amsterdam, 1992
42. Schmidt HG, Boshuizen HPA: On acquiring expertise in medicine. Educ Psychol Rev (In press)
43. Christensen N: Clinical Pattern Recognition in Physiotherapists—A Pilot Study Investigating the Effect of Different Levels of Clinical Experience. Unpublished Master of Applied Science thesis, University of South Australia, 1993
44. Harris BA, Dyrek DA: A model of orthopaedic dysfunction for clinical decision making in physical therapy practice. Phys Ther 69:548, 1989
45. Carr J, Jones MA, Higgs J: Experiential learning programs in physiotherapy clinical reasoning. In Higgs J, Jones MA (eds): Clinical Reasoning Skills. Butterworth-Heinemann, London (In press)
46. Joseph GM, Patel VL: Domain knowledge and hypothesis generation in diagnostic reasoning. Med Decision Making 10:31, 1990
47. Butler DS: Mobilisation of the Nervous System. Churchill Livingstone, Melbourne, 1991
48. Wells JCD, Woolf CJ (eds): Pain Mechanisms and Management. British Medical Bulletin, A Series of Expert Reviews. Vol. 47. Churchill Livingstone, Edinburgh, 1991
49. Wall PD: Neuropathic pain and injured nerve: central mechanisms. In Wells JCD, Woolf CJ (Eds): Pain Mechanisms and Management. British Medical Bulletin, A Series of Expert Reviews. Vol. 47. Churchill Livingstone, Edinburgh, 1991
50. Zusman M: Central nervous system contribution to mechanically produced motor and sensory responses. Aust J Physiother 38:245, 1992
51. Woolf CJ: Generation of acute pain: central mechanisms. In Wells JCD, Woolf CJ (eds): Pain Mechanisms and Management. British Medical Bulletin, A Series of Expert Reviews. Vol. 47. Churchill Livingstone, Edinburgh, 1991
52. McMahon SB: Mechanisms of sympathetic pain. In Wells JCD, Woolf CJ (Eds): Pain Mechanisms and Management. British Medical Bulletin, A Series of Expert Reviews. Vol. 47. Churchill Livingstone, Edinburgh, 1991
53. Merskey H (ed): Classifcation of Chronic Pain. Pain, suppl 3:S1, 1986
54. Fields H: Pain. McGraw Hill, New York, 1987

7 | Examination of the Cervical and Thoracic Spine

Mary E. Magarey

The cervical and thoracic sections of the vertebral column are closely related functionally and anatomically and, in many instances, should be examined as a single unit. Recent advances in understanding of the functions of the nervous system and its role in producing and maintaining nociception have led to a more global approach to the interpretation of clinical signs and symptoms, and consequently, also to their examination, than has been the case in the past. Emphasis is placed on understanding the underlying pathophysiology of symptoms of disorders of the cervicothoracic spine, with such consideration particularly relevant during physical examination and management. However, many mechanical problems seen by physical therapists have a principal component that is isolated to one section of the cervicothoracic spine, with possible predisposing factors in another section, rather than the principal problems involving the whole cervicothoracic complex. Consequently, this chapter considers examination of the cervical and thoracic areas separately, with reference where appropriate to the situations in which combined examination is indicated.

The examination of any patient presenting with symptoms of neuro-orthopaedic dysfunction consists of two main parts: a questioning/interview section, including inquiry about both the symptoms present, their history and that of any other symptoms that may be considered relevant to the presenting problem, and a physical examination section, in which structures implicated during the interview are examined. Both aspects of the evaluation are of equal importance in establishing a differential neuro-orthopaedic diagnosis and determining the appropriate course of treatment.

The system of subjective questioning and physical examination is so strongly based on the clinical reasoning process that the reader should become familiar with the hypothesis categories outlined in Chapter 6 before proceeding. These hypothesis categories are: mechanisms of symptoms, source of symptoms, contributing factors, precautions and contraindications, management, and prognosis. Further, the reader is assumed to be familiar with the concepts of peripherally evoked nociception, centrally evoked nociception, autonomic mechanisms, and affective mechanisms as defined and discussed in Chapters 6 and 15.

SUBJECTIVE EXAMINATION

The interview part of the evaluation, or subjective examination, aims to determine the patient's problems from the patient's perspective, interpreted in a way that provides the therapist with the means to perform an appropriate physical examination and, based on interpretation of the findings during that examination, to institute and continue management. The questioning done in the interview should be appropriate to the patient's specific situation. However, to enable the therapist to form hypotheses in the categories mentioned, some standard scanning questions are essential, particularly in the area of precautionary factors, and for the sake of efficiency, some basic routine in the interview process, adaptable to each situation, is advisable, although routines have the possible disadvantage of losing the potential for spontaneous, apparently unrelated but useful information. However, the skilled examiner can allow more freedom in the interview, providing an opportunity for such spontaneity.

In most situations, establishing immediately what the patient considers the main problem provides the opportunity for good communication between therapist and patient. From the outset, the patient recognizes that the therapist is interested in his/her personal concerns rather than those expressed by the referring doctor. This early information also provides a strong opportunity to form initial hypotheses related to the mechanism of the patient's symptoms, their source, and, potentially, to management and prognosis. Once the patient's main problem is established, the therapist should always attempt to use the patient's description of the symptoms, as this also enhances confidence in and rapport with the therapist.

Site, Character, Depth, and Severity of Symptoms

As indicated by Zusman,[1] localization of the source of a patient's symptoms on the basis of their site is dubious and may be inappropriate as a result of a centrally initiated stimulation of receptors. This is particularly so if the initial or residual pathologic processes are not clear. Consequently, the significance applied to the site of symptoms, and the precision with which that site should be identified, will depend on which category of mechanism of symptom production appears to be involved. The precise site of symptoms is likely to be of less significance in a centrally initiated nociceptive situation. However, this information should indicate a number of possible initial hypotheses in relation to the source of the symptoms, particularly those of peripheral initiation, that can then be further investigated once additional information is gained. Therefore, in most situations, a detailed analysis of the site of a patient's symptoms should be obtained, and this is best represented pictorially on a body chart, which also can be used to indicate the character, depth, constancy, and severity of the symptoms (Fig. 7-1). These additional factors all assist in devel-

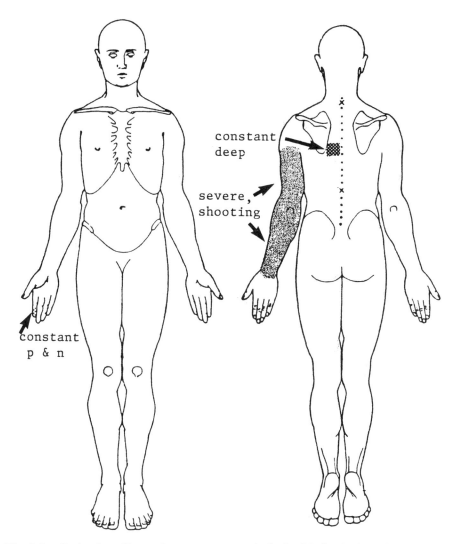

Fig. 7-1. Body chart illustrating symptoms typical of a C7 disc lesion with nerve root compression.

oping hypotheses related to the mechanism, source, and cause of the patient's symptoms and precautions or contraindications to examination and management of the patient, since disorders, particularly those of spontaneous onset, frequently demonstrate typical, predictable patterns. All symptoms present should be recorded on the body chart, even those that appear totally unrelated to the principal problem. The important possibility of multiple sites of symptoms related to altered function of the nervous system, and including sites unrelated somatically but potentially related via alteration in nervous system function, should be considered, so that this source is taken into account during the formation of hypotheses. Absence of symptoms in other areas should also be indicated on the body chart, and is important medicolegally. In the example given in Figure 7-1, constant deep pain adjacent to the medial border of the scapula opposite the seventh thoracic spinous process may implicate, among other structures, the C6-C7 intervertebral disc; severe, shooting pain on the posterior aspect of the arm and forearm with constant paresthesia of the tip of the index finger might implicate the C7 nerve root. The severity of the pain, coupled with its constancy, would indicate that the disorder is acute and that despite the mechanical variations in position and stress arising from the day's activities, some factor responsible for the symptoms is unrelenting, thus providing considerable information related to the hypothesis category of precautions and contraindications. The physical therapist viewing the body chart would immediately consider an acute C6-C7 disc protrusion causing pressure on, or irritation of, the C7 nerve root as the most likely hypothesis related to the source and cause of this patient's symptoms, and would direct the remainder of the subjective examination to confirming or disproving this hypothesis. The chapters on innervation and pain patterns of the cervical and thoracic spine (Chs. 4 and 5) should be read in conjunction with this section.

The character of symptoms, particularly pain, may help to identify their source, because specific structures and systems often appear to produce typical kinds of pain. For example, the pain from an acute nerve root irritation tends to be severe, burning, shooting, and unrelenting, whereas chronic nerve root pain is frequently described as "annoying, nagging, of nuisance value." The same kinds of words tend to be used by different patients to describe pain that appears to come from a similar source.

A similar situation arises with depth. While the patient's estimation of the depth of symptoms need bear no relation to the depth of their source, the descriptions given again tend to be consistent among patients. Discogenic pain is described as deep, whereas local zygapophyseal joint pain tends to be more superficial (e.g., "I can put my finger right on it.").

The severity of the symptoms can be a guide to the state of the disorder, but since many factors are responsible for an individual's perception of pain, severity is most useful as an indicator of the degree of restriction of normal activities imposed by the symptoms. The perceived severity and that assessed by the physical therapist during the interview may not correlate, but this information alone is a guide to the way in which the patient may need to be managed, and may provide a clue to the presence of affective mechanisms in the patient's symptoms. Knowledge of the severity of the symptoms, coupled with information about their behavior, helps to determine in what detail the patient can safely be examined at the first visit.

The Behavior of Symptoms

The way in which symptoms behave during the day, and their response to activity, provide the physical therapist with information related to all hypothesis categories.

Mechanical Stimuli

Symptoms that respond to mechanical stimuli in a predictable manner are usually considered to have a mechanical course. For example, pain that is provoked each time the patient turns, and which is relieved by returning to a neutral position, can be assumed to be a result of mechanical stress related to turning. Zusman[1] warned of the danger of overemphasizing the attribution of structural sources to symptoms that are mechanically evoked, owing to the intricate and complex interconnections and the potential for altered responses in the spinal and supraspinal neuron pools. Consequently, while in many situations the assumption of a mechanical source for mechanically provoked symptoms may be valid, the therapist should always be aware of the potential for this assumption to be invalid. Symptoms that show no predictable response to mechanical stimuli are unlikely to be mechanical in origin, and their presence should alert the therapist to the possibility of a more sinister disorder or one of central initiation, autonomic, or affective nature. Thus, for example, cervical pain that is constant and unaltered by rest or activity may be inflammatory in origin, in which case physical therapy, and particularly manual therapy, may be an inappropriate form of management.

Night Pain

Symptoms of mechanical origin may worsen initially on retiring for the night, but are usually relieved by rest, and will therefore be less severe on waking in the morning. The exceptions are those mechanical disorders that are aggravated by postures adopted or movements taking place during sleep. If sleeping posture or movement is a problem, the patient may waken with pain, but this soon eases with a change of position. Symptoms of inflammatory origin are unrelieved, and frequently worsened, by rest, so that the patient has difficulty sleeping and often needs to get out of bed and move around to gain any relief. If the patient is able to sleep, rising in the morning is difficult because of stiffness, usually with associated discomfort, and both of these problems may take several hours to ease.

Twenty-four-hour Pattern

Establishing the pattern followed by symptoms during a 24-hour period provides information about the degree of restriction the disorder is imposing on the patient; the response to mechanical stimuli, the importance of which is discussed above; indications about the presence of different components to the problem, and particularly any inflammatory component; and any factors contributing to production or continuation of the symptoms. It also provides an indication of the predictability of symptoms, thereby assisting in the formation of hypotheses about mechanisms for the symptoms and an effective approach to examination and management of the patient. The severity and irritability of the disorder can also be established, providing additional information related to precautions and contraindications, management, and prognosis. The kinds of activities or postures that aggravate and ease the symptoms provide information related to both the source and cause of the symptoms, and can give useful information about possible management strategies. The example given earlier of the zygapophyseal joint as the source of pain, with differing aggravating and easing factors, indicates different causes of pain within the same source.

Precautions/Contraindications to Treatment by Physical Modalities

Regardless of the hypotheses developing during the interview relating to the mechanism, source, and cause of the patient's symptoms, scanning questions relating to precautions and contraindications to examination or treatment by physical modalities should be asked routinely with every patient. The specific relevant information is outlined below, and adequate recording of the responses to the individual questions is important medicolegally, in addition to its significance to patient safety.

The Structural Stability of the Source of Symptoms or of Adjacent Structures

Any indication of structural instability of the spine, such as may be present after a rear-end motor vehicle collision, clearly indicates a need for caution in examination and management, since stress on an unstable segment may lead to the compromise of adjacent neural or vascular structures. Hypermobility of the craniovertebral junction has been described in a paper by Aspinall[2] that should be read in conjunction with this chapter. Aspinall described the following subjective complaints and clinical signs, which may indicate the presence of craniovertebral hypermobility or instability:

1. Occipital numbness or parasthesia, which may indicate trespass on the second cervical nerve root.

2.   Symptoms of vertebrobasilar insufficiency (VB1), such as vertigo, nausea, tinnitus, and visual disturbances.

3.   Signs of spinal cord compromise, including delayed myelopathy ranging from paraparesis to Brown–Sequard syndrome; dysesthesia in the hands with clumsiness and weakness of the lower limbs, or spastic weakness of the lower limbs with slight general wasting and hyperreflexia; ankle clonus and extensor plantar reflexes; difficulty with walking and possible effects on sphincter control.

4.   History of recent upper cervical or cranial trauma or unguarded movement.

5.   Marked inability to resist upper cervical flexion or extension.

6.   Increased range of contralateral rotation following a traumatic injury involving flexion and rotation, in which the alar ligaments may be stretched. Right rotation is limited by the left alar ligament and vice versa.

Since cardiac and respiratory centers lie at the level of the atlas, craniovertebral instability is potentially life-threatening. Consequently, an important feature of the scanning questions related to precautions and contraindications concerns the symptoms or historical features outlined above. Instability may also occur at the C4-C5 or C5-C6 levels in association with hypomobility of the cervicothoracic junction and a forward head posture, particularly if trauma such as whiplash is superimposed. Inquiry about radiographic investigations is also important, since evidence of structural instability, indicating the need for caution, may be seen. Plain radiographs, however, may not demonstrate craniovertebral hypermobility, with computed tomography (CT) the more reliable assessment.

The Integrity of Vital Structures in the Area, Particularly the Vertebrobasilar and Carotid Arterial Systems and the Spinal Cord

The vertebrobasilar system is covered in Chapter 8, which should be read in conjunction with this chapter. The carotid system is not compromised to the same extent in examination and treatment of the cervical spine as is the vertebrobasilar system, but symptoms indicating its involvement should still be considered a potential for caution in examination and management, particularly in relation to anterior cervical examination. Loss of integrity of the spinal cord is likely to be manifested initially by the presence of bilateral paresthesia or anesthesia of the hands and/or feet, with the altered sensation presenting in a glove or stocking distribution. Hypertonicity may lead to unsteadiness or clumsiness of gait or of other physical tasks.

The General Health of the Subject

General health questions provide information about the status of the cardiopulmonary system and the presence or absence of systemic disease or illness, such as diabetes mellitus or cancer. Past medical history may be relevant, particularly in the cervical area, where juvenile rheumatoid arthritis or rheumatic fever may lead to weakening of the ligaments of the upper cervical spine. A history of cancer may alert the therapist to the possibility of secondary deposits in bone. Previous radiotherapy, such as for the treatment of carcinoma of the breast, may result in localized sternal and costal osteoporosis. Systemic diseases such as ankylosing spondylitis may also lead to ligamentous weakening in the upper cervical spine.

The Pharmacologic Status of the Patient

The pharmacologic status of the patient should be considered, particularly in relation to the following medications:

1. Oral steroids. One side effect of prolonged use of corticosteroids is a decrease in bone density. Even the use of corticosteroids many years in the past can lead to a long-term loss of bone density, the significance of which depends on the patient's pretreatment bone density.

2. Anticoagulant medication. A patient undergoing anticoagulant therapy has a reduction in clotting ability. Consequently, any firm techniques may cause bruising or haemarthrosis.

3. Aspirin. A patient who has taken even small doses of aspirin in the 2 weeks prior to examination will demonstrate some anticoagulant effect. Consequently, care should be taken with any firm technique.

4. Analgesics. These drugs may mask potentially harmful effects of physical examination and management by reducing the perception of pain. Conversely, if a patient has a considerable amount of pain, appropriate use of these drugs may enhance treatment, allowing more rapid progression than would otherwise be possible.

5. Nonsteroidal anti-inflammatory drugs (NSAIDs). The anti-inflammatory effect of NSAIDs may mask harmful effects of physical evaluation and management in a manner similar to that with analgesics. However, knowledge of the response to NSAIDs provides an indication of the degree of inflammation associated with a patient's disorder, and therefore some indication of appropriate management and prognosis. As with analgesics, some disorders can tolerate and benefit from physical treatment if it is undertaken with a cover of NSAIDs, whereas such treatment would not be possible in their absence.

The Status of the Patient in Relation to Medical Evaluation

The therapist should know before undertaking a physical examination or beginning treatment whether the patient has seen a medical practitioner about the presenting problem and, in particular, whether any medical evaluations have been undertaken and the results of any such evaluations. Radiographic evaluation may provide indications of structural problems in addition to instability requiring caution in examination and management. With the advent of sophisticated radiographic methods of evaluation, inquiry only about plain radiography is inadequate. The patient should be asked about investigation with CT, magnetic resonance imaging (MRI), and bone scans, and the films and radiologic reports viewed if possible. Blood tests, nerve function tests, Doppler studies, and myelograms and their results can give an indication that medical personnel consider the patient's problem to be potentially one of greater significance than an uncomplicated musculoskeletal disorder, and favorable results of these tests may strengthen the confidence with which the physical therapist can proceed with the examination.

The information from the subjective examination provides an evolving clinical picture in which supporting and negating evidence leads to continuing modification of the initial and subsequent hypotheses.

HISTORY

While a hypothesis-testing approach to the subjective examination eliminates the concept of a standardized format for questioning regardless of the responses, the timing of history taking can be crucial to the understanding of a problem and to efficient management of time. If a disorder is of recent or sudden onset and the symptoms are severe, taking the history immediately after establishing the patient's main problem is beneficial, whereas a knowledge of the behavior and location of symptoms makes history taking from a patient with a chronic condition more succinct. The examiner, having gained some insight into the problem, will be better able to recognize the significant information in the history than if the history is taken with little knowledge of the nature of the disorder. Similarly, in most instances, taking the history of the patient's current problem before that of previous episodes is also advisable, since irrelevant information from the past history can then be sifted out. The detail with which the intervening period is investigated depends on the type of problem and the relationship between the initial episode and the current symptoms.

In addition to the history of symptoms related to the patient's current problem, inquiry into previous symptoms and traumatic episodes may be relevant, particularly if there are any indications of a central, autonomic or affective component. A further reason for inquiry about previous problems is the potential for the presenting symptoms to be part of a multiple crush phenomenon (see Ch. 11), in which the history, characteristics, behavior, and response to treatment of previous problems may be significant, providing useful clues to this potential cause of the presenting problem. This may be particularly relevant with respect to symptoms in the thoracic area, since the thoracic spine has strong anatomic connections with the sympathetic trunk[3] and is an area in which relatively high tension is produced in the neuraxis[4] (see Ch. 15).

The history should be taken in considerable detail, determining both the mechanism of injury, if traumatic, and the presence of any possible predisposing factors. The relationship between local and referred or radicular symptoms, or two different areas or types of symptoms, and the severity and nature of the patient's pathology, may be determined in part by the history of each symptom relative to the others. The skill and importance of history taking have been discussed comprehensively by Maitland.[5]

PLANNING THE PHYSICAL EXAMINATION

Once the subjective examination is complete, the physical therapist will have reached a series of working hypotheses related to the various hypothesis categories. On the basis of those hypotheses, the structures that require examination should be determined. In addition, the need for specific testing related to precautionary factors, such as vertebrobasilar insufficiency (VBI), is identified and a decision made about the extent of examination that can be performed without exacerbation of the patient's disorder.

Patients may be classified into two broad categories, those in whom a limited examination is appropriate at the first consultation and those in whom a full examination is possible.

Limited Examination

Examination procedures are taken only to the point at which symptoms are provoked or begin to increase if they are present at rest. The number of examination procedures may also have to be limited.

The decision to limit the examination is made on the basis of any subjective features that indicate the need for caution. These features include:

An irritable or severe disorder.
Worsening symptoms.
A history of a recent, traumatic onset of symptoms.
Subjective evidence of potential involvement of vital structures, such as the vertebrobasilar system, spinal cord, or nerve roots.
A history of systemic disorders or general health considerations that may lead to alteration in the integrity of the structures to be examined, such as underlying rheumatoid arthritis.
A history of corticosteroid use, or current use of aspirin or anticoagulant medication.
Indications that the symptoms do not behave in a predictable pattern, and that the response to examination procedures is therefore likely to be unpredictable.
Indications of potential structural instability.

In situations in which the decision to limit an examination is based on factors related to symptoms rather than underlying medical or structural concerns, the examination procedures should be limited to the point of onset of symptoms or initial exacerbation of symptoms during rest. In addition, return to the resting level of symptoms should be ensured before proceeding to the next examination procedure. If symptoms do not resolve, further examination should be omitted. If a movement is found that relieves symptoms, it may be further examined with the addition of other movement components in different combinations to determine whether a particular combination may be useful as a treatment technique (see Ch. 9). All examination procedures should be limited according to the same principles. For example, if a neurologic examination is considered necessary but contraction of muscles increased the patient's pain, that aspect of the neurologic examination should be omitted. Similarly, if there are indications of potential VBI but a full range of active rotation or extension is not possible, the tests for VBI should be deferred until the range of movement is increased and the severity of symptoms reduced. Passive examination should also be modified, perhaps by being performed only with the patient supine and with additional support to ensure a pain-free resting position. The depth and extent of such examination should follow the same principles as apply to active examination procedures.

When examination is limited because of potential structural injury or general health considerations, such as possible upper cervical ligamentous weakening related to general mild rheumatoid arthritis, exacerbation of symptoms may not be as significant. If the potential exists for loss of ligamentous or bony integrity, a movement should not be taken to full range and overpressure applied, even if that movement provokes no symptoms. Consequently, in this situation examination may be limited not by the onset of symptoms but by the onset of ligamentous tightening or resistance to movement, or the lack of such resistance when it should be present. If pain were also a significant factor, the onset of either pain or tissue resistance would determine the extent of each examination procedure. All aspects of the examination need to be limited in the same way.

Similarly, examination limited on the basis of symptoms related to the spinal cord or vascular system should not go further than the initial onset of these symptoms, whatever they are. In this situation, full examination, with overpressure applied to active and passive movements in certain directions, may be safe and appropriate if symptoms are not reproduced, whereas movements in other directions must be limited either by the onset of symptoms or by soft-tissue resistance. Such is the case with a patient who experiences severe dizziness only when looking upward. Examination of cervical extension and of any movement with a component of extension should be done with extreme care not to provoke dizziness, while other movements may be examined fully, provided no dizziness is provoked.

While examination limited in these ways does not provide the physical therapist with knowledge about the behavior of pain, joint resistance, or muscle spasm beyond the point at which the examination procedure was abandoned, information can still be gained about the relative involvement of the joint, muscular, neural, or vascular systems without aggravation of the symptoms. Therefore, initiation of treatment is possible in a safe, symptom-free environment at the first consultation, and this is a major priority. The additional information can be gained as the symptoms ease and examination can be taken further. When examination is limited by factors other than symptoms, treatment must continue to be restricted to those procedures that can be performed safely within the limitations of the relevant features.

Full Examination

Examination procedures may be taken to their full extent with overpressure applied to the limit of movement, neurologic and vascular testing performed fully, muscle tests undertaken to the maximum capacity necessary, and passive examination taken to the fullest extent necessary to confirm the hypotheses evolving through the subjective examination. If routine examination procedures are inadequate to provide the necessary information, examination may be taken further, such as by the addition of compression to movement, movements performed at speed, movements sustained at the limit, and combinations of movements. Such an evaluation is possible if the subjective examination has indicated that no exacerbation of symptoms is likely because the condition is non-irritable, not severe, its nature and progression are stable and predictable, and there are not other precautionary factors present. A full examination allows the physical therapist to obtain a complete clinical picture on which to base treatment and management decisions, and provides the optimal situation for physical methods of treatment. With availability of all of the information about the mechanism, source, and cause of the symptoms and the factors predisposing or contributing to them, the choice of treatment and priority of each factor in management of the patient can be made with considerable confidence.

During examination, the relative significance of symptoms provoked at the limit of a range of motion and their relationship to soft-tissue resistance can be determined by comparison with the physical therapist's knowledge of comparable normal movement and comparison with the contralateral movement. For a movement of the spine to be considered normal, a full physiologic and intervertebral range of motion must be present, with the application of overpressure provoking the same amount of discomfort and producing the same pattern of ligamentous tightening as the corresponding contralateral movement or as much as would be expected for the patient's age and somatotype.

Despite the freedom to fully examine all components, some priorities must be set, since a single consultation frequently does not provide enough time for such a detailed assessment. Consequently, the physical therapist must decide on those features that should be examined as having a high priority and those that can be left until the following consultation. The examination should be completed within two or three consultations. Those features most likely to be responsible for producing symptoms and therefore related to the hypothesis categories of mechanism, source, and cause are likely to receive highest priority, while the examination of those possibly related to contributing or predisposing factors may be delayed. Those features related to treatment safety should always be examined at the first consultation.

While two clear categories of patients have been described with regard to physical examination, the decision about the extent of examination is based on the reasoning process undertaken through the subjective examination, and may involve a combination of test procedures in which some may be fully used while others are restricted or omitted. Therefore, a continuum exists from the time of presentation, in which at one end extreme care is required to avoid exacerbating symptoms while at the other end additional examination procedures are needed to reproduce symptoms and provide appropriate information related to the hypothesis categories.

PHYSICAL EXAMINATION

The physical examination should not involve the indiscriminate application of a standardized set of procedures, but should be a continuation of the clinical reasoning process undertaken during the subjective examination. While there are core examination procedures undertaken with most patients, the physical examination should, within the limitations of the extent of appropriate examination, be personalized, thus providing an assessment unique to the individual patient. The physical therapist should continue the process of hypothesis testing in all categories, with the examination findings either confirming or negating the hypotheses and providing useful clues to appropriate management.

Jones and Jones[6] have provided an excellent presentation on the principles of the physical examination, which should be read in conjunction with this chapter. They present the particular examination procedures relevant to the cervical and thoracic spine and clinical patterns related to the areas. However, those structures and systems extrinsic to the local area but which could be classified as contributing to a disorder in the cervicothoracic region must also be considered and examined in sufficient depth to determine their involvement.

If physical examination is to fulfill its aim of determining an appropriate management approach, the physical therapist must be aware of the clinical patterns that may be seen in patients who present with symptoms in the cervical or thoracic area, or sites to which these spinal regions can refer, either somatically or autonomically. As discussed earlier, the ability to identify the source of symptoms is not by itself sufficient, since different causes of symptoms within the same source may present with different physical signs and respond to different approaches to management. Consequently, maintenance of an open mind in addition to recognition of clinical patterns will allow the development of new patterns and variations of those already recognized. Such reflective thinking and analysis allows continued growth and enables the therapist to build a knowledge base of clinical patterns from which to draw with each new patient evaluated. Acknowledgment of the need to consider involvement of systems rather than particular individual structures also provides opportunities for varying the emphasis on or depth of examination of individual structures. If a central mechanism is indicated, detailed examination of local structures may be inappropriate, with more emphasis placed on evaluation of the nervous system and those vertebral structures closely associated with it. Considerable detail of examination is necessary if subtle variations in clinical patterns and new patterns are to be recognized.[6]

The Structures to Be Examined

In the cervical and thoracic areas, all potential sources implicated during the subjective examination should be tested during the physical examination. These include all structures underlying the area of symptoms; all structures that can refer to the area of symptoms; and all structures that could potentially be implicated in causing the symptoms.

All potential contributing factors implicated during the subjective examination should also be tested. These include

1. All structures that can mechanically affect other structures contributing to symptom production (e.g., weakness of upper cervical flexors, leading to a forward head posture and development of symptoms in the cervicothoracic junction),
2. All structures that can affect symptom production either chemically or nutritionally from sites remote from the symptomatic area (e.g., vascular compromise or chemical effects in the nervous system, such as the double crush phenomenon).[6]

Consequently, while the focus of this chapter is on the cervical and thoracic spine, the entire body may potentially have to be assessed to determine the possible contribution to cervical or thoracic symptoms of altered pelvic and lower limb biomechanics, through their potential to produce abnormal cervical posture and abnormal neural biomechanics and chemical responses.

To reach a confident differential physical diagnosis, evaluation of these structures that are less likely to be involved in a patient's condition is as important as evaluation of the most likely sources. Knowledge of lack of involvement is as important in the decision-making process as knowledge of involvement. However, the examination should still be directed as appropriate for the individual patient rather than following a textbook approach.

Physical Signs of Potential Involvement

Many physical signs, which must be interpreted in relation to the patient's age and somatotype, may be present to alert the physical therapist to the involvement of a particular structure in the production of symptoms. These include

1. Abnormal appearance (e.g., bony asymmetry, abnormal muscle contours, and trophic changes).
2. Abnormal movement (functional, active, passive, and resistive).
3. Abnormal characteristics on palpation (e.g., temperature, swelling, thickening, and tightness).

The potential involvement of a structure is strengthened if

1. Alteration of the abnormality potentially associated with that structure (e.g., asymmetry or pattern of movement) affects the patient's symptoms.
2. Direct or indirect stress on a structure reproduces the patient's symptoms.
3. Direct or indirect stress on a structure that is capable of referring symptoms, either somatically or autonomically, to the symptomatic area demonstrates abnormality of that structure (e.g., hypomobility and local pain on stress of the Occ-C1 joint in a patient with unilateral headaches).
4. Direct or indirect stress on a structure that is capable of contributing to the predisposition to symptom development demonstrates abnormality of that structure (e.g., tightness of upper trapezius in a patient complaining of cervical pain).

Reproduction of symptoms by direct or indirect stress on structures that could be implicated in a patient's condition is not essential, and is in many cases unlikely to be possible. Demonstration of an abnormality in the implicated structure is sufficient, and the relevance of that abnormality to the disorder will be determined during management, when the effect on the disorder of alteration of the abnormality can be seen. Understanding the relationship between posture, movement, and symptoms and their association with pathophysiology and pathomechanics assists in determining the relative importance of physical abnormalities. Consequently, continual assessment of these relationships during examination is essential, and their interpretation in relation to the hypotheses that have been formulated about the patient's condition is a significant clinical skill.

Components of the Physical Examination

The components of the physical examination of the cervical or thoracic spine include observation of the patient, both during the subjective examination and, more formally, during the physical examination, and analysis of posture; the functional activity that provokes the patient's symptoms; physiologic movements, both active and passive; passive accessory movements; soft tissues; the nervous system; muscle performance; the vascular system; the upper extremities; and the viscera.

Assessment of the lumbar spine, pelvis and lower extremities may be necessary as part of an evaluation of factors contributing to the production of symptoms in the neck or thoracic region.

Each component of the physical examination offers opportunities to test the hypotheses developed during the subjective examination, and the information gained will lead to the modification of existing hypotheses or the development of new ones.

Observation and Posture

The patient's cervical and thoracic posture and willingness to move should be observed while the patient is undressing and during the subjective examination. The patient should be sufficiently undressed that the spine, shoulder girdles, upper limbs, and trunk are readily visible, and preferably also the lower extremities while an evaluation of posture is undertaken. For an initial assessment of posture, the patient should be viewed in the standing position, so that an indication of the total body posture can be gained, including the potential involvement of abnormal lower body posture as a factor predisposing to the development of cervical or thoracic symptoms.

Posture should be viewed from in front, behind, and laterally. The position of the head on the neck and neck on the thorax, the degree of scapular protraction, and kyphosis of the thoracic spine may all be observed in the frontal plane, making sure that the patient's hair does not obscure the contour of the neck. The degree of lumbar lordosis, particularly that relative to the thoracic kyphosis, and the general contour of the abdomen and buttocks, pelvic posture, and degree of hyperextension of the knees can also be assessed. In the sagittal plane posteriorly, the symmetry of the head, position of the spinous processes and shoulder girdles, symmetry and degree of development or tightness of posterior muscle groups, and amount of rotation of the arms can be seen. Anteriorly, symmetry of the head and neck position, bony symmetry of the chest, symmetry of development, tone and tightness of anterior muscle groups, height of the nipples, and position of the umbilicus may be assessed.

Having viewed the entire body in the standing position, further assessment of the effect of sitting on the cervical and thoracic posture should be performed prior to an analysis of active physiologic movements.

Active Examination

Analysis of the Functional Provoking Activity and Differentiation of Movements

The ability of a patient to reproduce symptoms with a particular movement, activity, or posture should be analyzed. Functional activities consist of combinations of different movements that can be examined initially in isolation and then in different combinations in an attempt to determine the principal provocative component. For example, a tennis player has midthoracic pain at late cocking and early acceleration of a serve. At this point in the swing, the player's thoracic spine is likely to be in a position of extension, rotation, and lateral flexion toward the serving arm. Limitation of any, or a combination, of these components may be the cause of the pain. With the patient adopting the position of discomfort, the therapist increases each component of the provoking activity individually, assessing any alteration of symptoms. Thoracic rotation in the neutral position may be without pain, but when performed with the spine already in an extension/lateral flexion posture, it may provoke pain. Further analysis related to the potential involvement of the nervous system in the production of symptoms during the serve may be tested by placing the arm in the serving position of late cocking, with shoulder abduction, extension, and lateral rotation, and by then altering the position either of the wrist and hand or the elbow, to determine whether these maneuvers alter the thoracic symptoms.

Similar principles of differentiation may be applied to any movement that provokes symptoms but in which more than one structure or system may be implicated. Differentiation may take several forms, as follows:

1. Taking the combined movement to the point of production of symptoms and then maintaining one component while altering the other in a way that increases the stress on one and decreases it correspondingly in the other. For example, if combined cervical and thoracic rotation provokes pain, the movement can be held at a point in the range within which pain is produced. The shoulder girdle is then rotated slightly further, increasing the stress on thoracic rotation but decreasing stress on cervical rotation. The response to this procedure may be confirmed by derotating the shoulder girdle, leading to a decrease in stress on thoracic rotation and a corresponding increase in stress on cervical rotation.

2. Examining one of the implicated movements while the other is maintained in a neutral position and comparing the symptom response with that in a similar examination of the other implicated movement. For example, if combined cervical and thoracic rotation is painful, as described above, the symptom response to thoracic rotation can be compared with that to cervical rotation. This procedure and the one described above are frequently used together, with one procedure confirming the response found in the other.

3. Movement of a noninvolved structure may be added to a painful position or movement to determine the involvement of other systems, particularly the nervous system, in the production of symptoms. The example given above of addition of wrist and finger extension to the arm position during the act of serving, in order to determine involvement of the nervous system, falls into this category.

4. If a joint is implicated, differentiation of an intra-articular or periarticular source may be undertaken by examination of a movement with and without the application of compression across the joint surfaces. If pain on movement is exacerbated by the addition of minor joint compression, intra-articular struc-

tures are implicated. The specific structures involved are not yet known, but possible explanations have been proposed.[7]

Analysis of a provoking factor and differentiation of movement in this way can assist in determination of the source of symptoms and in directing the remainder of the examination appropriately. If the symptoms can be reproduced, the movements most significant to the patient's problem are determined, and they can be further examined in more detail, rather than attention being given to other less significant aspects of the evaluation. The information gained can also be useful in selecting management strategies, and the provoking factor becomes a valuable reassessment test. However, if the condition is severe or irritable, examination of the provoking factor may be omitted or assessed by taking each component only to the onset of symptoms.

Active Physiologic Movements

The standard movements to be examined in the cervical or thoracic region are flexion, extension, lateral flexion, and rotation. If the examination is to be limited, particularly if limited by the onset of pain, the procedure must be explained to the patient, since cooperation is necessary to avoid exacerbation of symptoms. Determination of the gross range of physiologic movement and the production or lack of production of symptoms is inadequate to both a limited and a full examination. Details of symptoms at rest, the quality of active movement, and the relationship between changes in symptoms and the quality and range of movement provide useful information. If a movement is limited by pain (or other symptoms), the therapist should note the range and quality of the movement, return the spine to a neutral position, and clarify site and character of the symptoms produced. If a movement covers the normal full range and is pain free, or is restricted but pain free, overpressure should be applied. Overpressure may stress the entire cervical or thoracic spine or may stress different portions separately, depending on which is relevant to the particular patient. The relationship between symptoms and soft-tissue resistance is assessed during the application of passive overpressure. To simplify this text, all test movements are described, assuming that they can be taken to the end of the normal range and overpressure applied.

Cervical Spine. When examining routine active cervical movements, the patient should be sitting with the thighs fully supported, arms resting comfortably on the thighs, and shoulders relaxed. The benefits of this standard positioning for examining are consistency for later re-evaluation and stability and comfort for the patient. All movements should be observed from in front to note any deviation that occurs with a movement (e.g., any lateral flexion or rotation associated with flexion or extension), as well as from the side, to note the gross range of movement and intersegmental movement, particularly that of the upper (head on neck) and lower (neck on thorax) cervical regions. Movement of the whole cervical spine should be examined first, with the examination later being isolated to the upper or lower portions if indicated. Overpressure also may isolate the upper or lower portion, depending on the relevance to a particular patient (Fig. 7-2).

Thoracic Spine. Movements of the thoracic spine should be observed both from behind, to note any deviation that occurs with a movement and to observe intersegmental movement, and from the side to observe the gross and interseg-mental ranges of movement.

Upper Thoracic Spine (T1 to T4). The upper thoracic area is examined in the same way as the low cervical spine, with overpressure localizing the move-ment to the thoracic area. If the patient's problem is one that is difficult to reproduce, and overpressure on low cervical movements alone demonstrates no abnormality, these movements may need to be combined with those of the thoracic spine to put sufficient stress on the joint at fault to reproduce symptoms.

Mid-thoracic Spine (T4 to T8). The mid-thoracic area is examined with the patient sitting and thighs fully supported. Flexion and extension are examined with the patient's hands clasped behind the cervicothoracic junction and elbows held together.

Flexion involves approximation of the shoulders to the groin, creating a bowing effect that is further emphasized by the direction of overpressure (Fig. 7-3). Lumbar extension should be kept to a minimum during the examination of thoracic extension, which is then easier to localize. Overpressure should localize the movement to individual intervertebral levels (Fig. 7-4).

Lateral flexion is examined with the hands again linked behind the cervico-thoracic junction, but this time with the elbows in the frontal plane. Again, lumbar movement should be minimized so that thoracic lateral flexion is empha-sized. Overpressure on the angle of each rib further localizes the movement (Fig. 7-5).

Rotation of the mid-thoracic spine is maximal with the spine in flexion. Rotation with the spine in neutral occurs more in the low thoracic area. There-fore, mid-thoracic rotation is examined by asking the patient to rotate while in flexion (e.g., asking the patient to "bend under my arm" while the therapist holds the patient's shoulders). This movement is best performed with the pa-tient's arms folded across the chest. Overpressure is applied through the shoul-ders (Fig. 7-6).

Low Thoracic Spine (T8 to 12). The low thoracic spine is examined with the patient standing, feet together and arms by the sides. The standard active movements scanned are flexion, extension, and lateral flexion, and these are examined in the same way as for the lumbar spine, the direction of overpressure emphasizing movement in the low thoracic area. Rotation is examined in the

Fig. 7-2. Cervical extension; **(A)** general cervical extension, **(B)** upper cervical extension, **(C)** lower cervical extension.

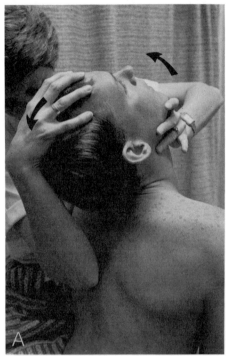

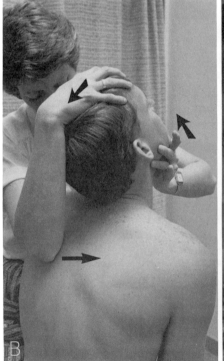

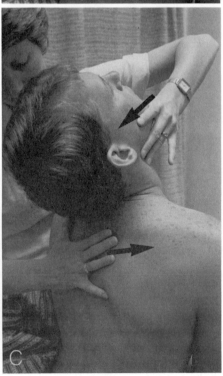

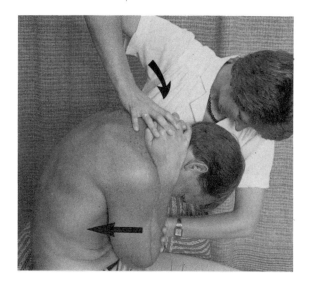

Fig. 7-3. Thoracic flexion illustrating the direction of overpressure.

sitting position, with the thighs fully supported and arms folded across the chest. Overpressure is applied through the shoulders. More detail and pictorial representation of these movements may be found elsewhere.[5,8]

Additional Movement Tests when Appropriate

If a clinical reasoning approach is used during the physical examination, the need for further examination becomes obvious. Provided the examination is not limited by precautionary factors, additional movement tests may be appropriate if:

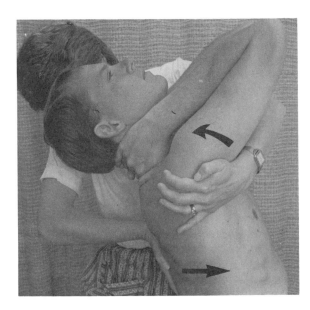

Fig. 7-4. Thoracic extension with localized overpressure.

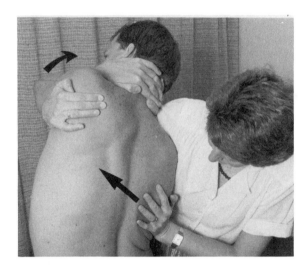

Fig. 7-5. Thoracic lateral flexion with localized overpressure.

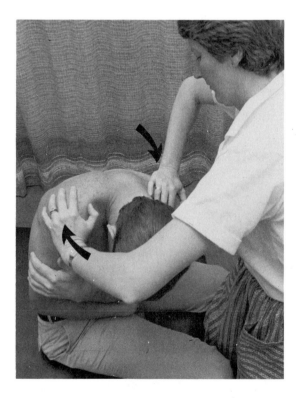

Fig. 7-6. Midthoracic rotation with overpressure.

Local Symptoms have not been reproduced with standard test movements, in an attempt to find a source of these symptoms.

Symptoms remote to a hypothesised local source have not been reproduced, in an attempt to confirm the local site as the source of the remote symptoms (e.g., headache or supraspinous pain with a potential local cervical source).

Abnormal movement, either gross or intersegmental, has been detected but its relevance to the presenting disorder is unclear.

The standard scanning movement tests have not revealed sufficient information about any of the hypothesis categories.

These additional movement tests may take any form, depending on the subjective indications in a particular case, but some test procedures are indicated and used frequently.

Combined Movements. Most natural movements occur in combinations of pure anatomic movement, and any combination of movements can be responsible for the production of symptoms. In the cervical and thoracic spine, those combinations that either stretch or compress one side of the spine frequently become symptomatic, particularly when a condition is of spontaneous onset rather than traumatic. Movement combinations that compress the articular surfaces and narrow the intervertebral foramina are useful in reproducing referred symptoms; this is particularly true for the combinations of extension with ipsilateral lateral flexion and with rotation. The rotation and lateral flexion should be localized to the area implicated in causing the symptoms (Fig. 7-7). Examination of combined movements in the cervical spine is covered in detail in Chapter 9.

The addition of neural tensioning procedures. The addition of neural tensioning procedures to movements that demonstrate abnormalities can provide

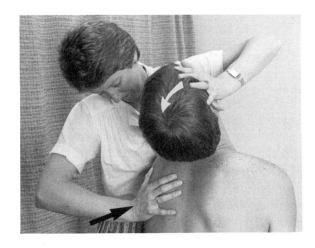

Fig. 7-7. A combination of low cervical extension, rotation, and lateral flexion to the same side.

an indication of the involvement in the abnormal movement of adverse neural tension (see Ch. 11). For example supraspinous pain that is provoked during cervical flexion may be associated with a somatic referral from a local zygapophyseal joint, among other possibilities. Equally possible is an association with limited movement of the neural structures. Such involvement could be determined by the addition of minimal ankle dorsiflexion or knee extension to the position of painful cervical flexion. This movement of the ankles or knees alters the tension in and movement of the nervous system without altering local structures. Consequently, if a change in symptoms is observed, the nervous system is implicated.

Sustained Positions. Sustaining a movement at its limit may be diagnostically useful, particularly if the subjective indications are that symptoms are provoked either in this way or following return from a sustained position, in which situation a latent response to the examination procedure may be anticipated.

Headaches are frequently reproduced by upper cervical extension, or by the combination of such extension with ipsilateral lateral flexion and rotation (Fig. 7-8) if the position is sustained. Similarly, arm or medial scapular pain may be reproduced with sustained ipsilateral rotation, extension, or the combination of low cervical extension with ipsilateral rotation and lateral flexion.

The movement examined should be held at its limit, with overpressure applied in the form of small oscillations, for the length of time appropriate for the individual patient and circumstances, or for a period sufficient to allow an alteration of viscous tissues in a way that might provoke symptoms. Once the

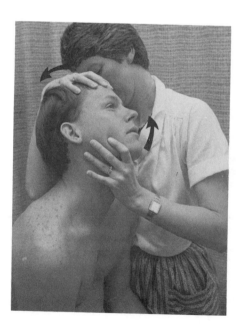

Fig. 7-8. A combination of upper cervical extension, rotation, and lateral flexion to the same side.

position is released, a similar period should elapse before the next test procedure is performed, in order to allow for the possibility of a latent response to the movement.

Speed of Movements. Frequently, a movement is performed during examination more slowly than during the activity that aggravates symptoms, in which case symptoms are not necessarily provoked. If the movement is repeated at greater speed the symptoms will often appear.

Repeated Movements. A patient's symptoms may be provoked only with repetition of a movement. By examining the movement a number of times, the examiner can obtain an accurate count of the number of repetitions needed to provoke the symptoms, a fact that may be valuable in reassessment.

Examination Following Provocation. Occasionally, an examination will fail to reproduce a patient's symptoms because the clinical assessment cannot stress the affected structures sufficiently. When this occurs, the patient should be asked to report again for examination, this time following a provocation of symptoms. While the symptoms are present, examination should reveal some abnormality of movement or position. Thus, for example, examination of a computer operator with upper thoracic pain that is provoked only at the end of a working day may be negative if undertaken on a non-working day. The patient should be advised to return for reassessment after work, when the symptoms should be easy to reproduce.

Compression/Distraction. In the cervical spine, and particularly the upper cervical area, symptoms are often reproduced by compression and, somewhat less frequently, eased by distraction. Consequently, compression and distraction should be considered as additional, high priority examination procedures for the cervical spine.

Compression may be applied to the cervical spine in such a way that it affects each intervertebral segment equally on both sides, or affects one side more than the other. In order for it to affect the neck symmetrically, pressure is applied with the spine in the neutral position, whereas for a more unilateral effect the neck is flexed laterally to the level being tested and compression is added. The compression is then transmitted through the articular pillar on the concave side of the neck. Compression to the thoracic spine is usually added in such a way that its effect is symmetrical, although it is not as useful in producing symptoms in this area as in the cervical area. Distraction may also be applied symmetrically or with a unilateral bias.

Movements with Compression/Distraction. If compression or distraction alone is unhelpful, and the subjective examination indicates that either may be a component of the patient's problem, movements performed with the addition of compression or distraction forces may be helpful. Headaches of upper cervical origin are frequently reproduced by cervical rotation or lateral flexion under compression, while medial scapular pain is often provoked by adding compression to a combined position of low cervical extension and lateral flexion.

Examination of the Nervous System

Involvement of the nervous system in a patient's symptoms may be manifested by an impairment of conduction demonstrated by an alteration in sensation, muscle power, and reflexes, and by signs of adverse tension or abnormal movement manifested by abnormal responses to neural tension tests, such as the upper limb tension tests and the slump.

Examination for Impairment of Neural Conduction

Descriptions of the tests for impairment of conduction are presented in detail elsewhere.[4,5,8] Tests for upper and lower motor neuron and peripheral nerve function should be included. A neurologic assessment should be included when the patient presents with symptoms of a neural character, when symptoms are present in the limbs, and for any disorder with a history of trauma or in which the patient's condition is worsening. Butler[4] advocated the addition of an assessment of two-point discrimination, vibration sense, and proprioception to the evaluation of sensation. The cervical and thoracic spinal segments and their dermatomes, representative muscles, joint action, and reflexes may be found in most textbooks of anatomy and are neatly presented by Butler.[4] Tests of nerve conduction must be done with finesse to detect minimal differences that may indicate the early stages of a loss of integrity of nervous tissue.

Tests for Adverse Neural Tension

Because of the potential involvement of central nervous system structures in a significant number of nociceptive disorders, and the apparent relationship between adverse neural tension and nociceptive symptoms, an assessment of movement of, and the ability to transmit tension through, the nervous system should be a routine part of the examination of all patients who present with symptoms in or related to the cervicothoracic region. Such an assessment should involve testing of the neuraxis and lower limbs with the slump test and its derivatives, and of the upper limbs by the upper limb tension tests. Potential involvement of the autonomic nervous system may be assessed by modifications of the traditional tension tests in which emphasis is put on the sympathetic trunk. Those tests appropriate to the individual are determined by clues from the subjective and previous physical examinations.

Tension testing is discussed in detail in Butler[4] and in Chapter 11. Butler suggested that a system of easily repeatable base tests with known normative responses should be used as routine starting points, with further examination dependent on the specific presentation of the patient. The most sensitive of these base tests with a principal effect on the neuraxis and lower limbs is the slump test.

The Slump Test. The base slump test involves a maximal spinal flexion combined with maximum available hip flexion, knee extension, and ankle and foot dorsiflexion. The confirming procedure of release of cervical flexion is commonly used, with other sensitizing and confirmatory movements used as indicated.

The Upper Limb Tension Tests. Testing of adverse neural tension (ANT) in the upper limbs is undertaken by means of the upper limb tension tests (ULTTs). Four base ULTTs have been developed, and these are described in Chapter 11.

Sensitizing procedures for all ULTTs include contralateral cervical lateral flexion, while other movements can be added to each test as appropriate for the individual patient's problem, and should reflect the anatomic pathway of the nerve(s) implicated in the patient's symptoms.

Testing for Adverse Neural Tension in the Sympathetic Trunk

The potential relationship between ANT in the sympathetic trunk and sympathetically maintained pain syndromes is discussed in detail in Chapter 15. Space does not allow discussion of this important and exciting new area of tension testing here. Trunk lateral flexion as added to the base slump test, and cervical extension rather than cervical flexion, are both movements that potentially enhance ANT in the sympathetic trunk. Butler and Slater (Ch. 15) also suggest that because of the close association between the thoracic spine and the sympathetic trunk, potential sympathetic involvement should lead to additional assessment of the thoracic spine, including the movement of skeletal structures in positions of ANT (e.g., the application of posteroanterior pressure over the costotransverse joints with the arm in a ULTT position).

In addition to the assessment of ANT, Butler[4] advocated the palpation of nerves where they are accessible. A normal nerve should feel hard and round and should be movable transversely. This movement may be reduced if the nerve is under tension or adherent to adjacent interface tissues. Swelling or thickening may be detected, indicating abnormality of the nerve. The symptomatic response to palpation could also assist in localizing the site of ANT, with specific types of responses apparently related to specific types of involvement of the nerve.

Muscle Performance

The cervical and thoracic muscles may be a source of symptoms in conjunction with or independent of underlying vertebral disorders. However, structures within each vertebral segment are capable of referring pain to the adjacent muscles, establishing areas of local tenderness and even tissue changes with no intrinsic muscle disorder. Static contraction of the paraspinal muscles is impossible without some stress on the adjacent noncontractile structures. Therefore, differentiation of contractile tissue as a source of symptoms is difficult, and can often be done only in retrospect, when the effect on one structure of treating another can be assessed.

Clues to the involvement of muscle as a factor contributing to symptoms can be found in the subjective examination. For example, a cervicothoracic ache that develops only toward the end of a day in a patient working at a computer may indicate a "postural" component in which poor muscular endurance leads to fatigue, in turn causing increasingly poor posture and excessive stress on underlying structures. The hypothesis of muscle involvement is further tested during the physical examination.

Chronic disorders of the cervicothoracic region commonly produce typical patterns of muscle imbalance. These can be seen initially during an assessment of posture. The characteristic forward head posture with elevated and protracted scapulae is typically associated with tightness in the upper cervical extensor, sternocleidomastoid, scalene, upper trapezius, levator scapulae, pectoral and shoulder medial rotator muscles and weakness of the deep cervical flexors, long cervical extensors, lower scapular stabilizers, and shoulder lateral rotators.

The hypothesis of muscle imbalance should be tested with a specific assessment of muscle length, strength, and endurance. Muscle imbalance, its effects, and the tests used to establish it are discussed in Chapters 10, 13, and 16, as well as in other texts.[6,9]

Precautionary Procedures

The integrity of vital structures must be established prior to beginning the management of disorders of the cervical or thoracic area. The systems and structures that need to be tested include the nervous system, already discussed, and the vascular system, including testing for VBI and the involvement of peripheral vascular tissue either locally or in the thoracic outlet. Testing for instability of the upper cervical spine is a further consideration. These tests need be performed only if there are clues in the subjective examination or early part of the physical examination that indicate a need for their inclusion.

The Vascular System

Testing for Vertebrobasilar Insufficiency. A realization is growing within the international community of the need for testing for VBI prior to cervical manipulation.[10] The Australian Physiotherapy Association has produced a protocol for premanipulative testing of the cervical spine. This document[11], outlines the various steps that should be undertaken before considering the use of cervical manipulation. The document also includes appropriate examination procedures for the provocation of symptoms of VBI in patients presenting with these symptoms, and tests to determine whether stress on the vertebrobasilar artery provokes previously unreported symptoms in patients presenting with no complaints of symptoms of VBI. The steps involved and the reasoning behind the protocol are covered in Chapter 8.

The Thoracic Outlet Syndrome. The thoracic outlet syndrome may affect neural structures, particularly the C8 or T1 nerve roots, or vascular structures such as the subclavian artery. Symptoms related to the C8 or T1 nerve roots may be provoked by sustained shoulder girdle elevation or one of the ULTTs (see Ch. 15), while subclavian involvement may be tested by palpating the radial pulse in a number of positions.[12]

If the subclavian artery is affected, the radial pulse will be reduced or obliterated with the tests discussed, and symptoms may be provoked. Manual compression of the subclavian artery against the first rib in such a way that the radial pulse is obliterated may also provoke symptoms. Anteroposterior pressures and/or posteroanterior pressures over the first rib are likely to reveal restriction and be locally painful, and may reproduce symptoms of vascular or neurogenic origin.

Peripheral Pulses. If evidence of poor circulation is present, the autonomic nervous system or vascular system itself may be implicated. As part of the assessment, the patient's peripheral pulses should be examined. The pulses in the affected area should be checked and compared with those in the other arm to determine the integrity of blood flow through the arm. This assessment should be performed both in the resting position and in aggravating positions in which flow may be compromised.

Tests for Craniovertebral Hypermobility

Aspinall[2] described a set of tests for craniovertebral hypermobility. Detailed descriptions of the test methods and the underlying applied anatomy and biomechanics can be found in her paper and will not be repeated here. The tests described include the Sharp-purser test, alar ligament test, transverse ligament test, alar ligament and dens/atlas osseous stability test, and tectorial membrane test.

No validity studies have been performed on these ligamentous tests, and their use is not yet widespread. They are potent tests that have led to the provocation of nausea, fainting, and a general sense of apprehension when performed on asymptomatic individuals during class demonstrations. However, subjective or historical indications of upper cervical hypermobility or instability should alert the therapist to the need for assessment, and if the tests for these effects are used appropriately, fatal or significant vascular or neurologic compromise from inappropriate management should be avoided.

Examination of Associated Structures

Peripheral Joints

Symptoms that spread from the neck or thoracic spine into the upper limb or head and face may have a source that is entirely within the spine, or may have some component from one or more of the peripheral structures, including the joints over which the symptoms pass. Examination of all joints within the area of symptoms will determine the degree to which each contributes to the overall problem. Detailed examination of the peripheral joints is unnecessary, since signs related to these joints are likely to be minimal. The protocol for brief examination of the peripheral joints has been described.[5]

The degree of involvement of a peripheral joint and the spine in a patient's symptoms should be assessed by examining the passive movements of both structures. If abnormalities are found in both structures, treatment of one (usually the spine first) and assessment of alteration in the other will determine the relative contribution of each to the symptoms.

For a comparative evaluation to be most effective, an appropriate interpretation of passive movement testing is essential. The relationship between soft-tissue resistance to passive movement and symptoms during the movement is fundamental in such an interpretation. For example, if during the testing of a peripheral joint a high degree of tissue resistance is encountered before the onset of symptoms, whereas, during testing of the cervical spine, pain is provoked early in the range of motion with little or no tissue resistance detected, the neck is the more likely source of the patient's symptoms. A passive movement is more likely to be stressing the source of symptoms if pain is the dominant feature throughout the movement, with or without abnormal resistance (see Ch. 12), although the evidence presented by Zusman[1] would suggest that care should be taken in such interpretations, particularly with patients with a chronic condition, who may have a component of centrally initiated nociception.

The Viscera

Indications of potential involvement of the thoracic or abdominal viscera will be found in the subjective examination, with clues related to visceral function. Detailed examination of the viscera is beyond the scope of the physical therapist, but the differentiation of intrinsic visceral pain from pain related to overlying contractile tissue or pain referred from the thoracic spine is possible. If palpation of the abdominal wall reproduces the patient's pain, it should be repeated with the abdominal muscles contracted, thereby removing the pressure from the viscera. If the pain is unchanged, it is unlikely to be of visceral origin, but probably arises from the abdominal wall or thoracic spine. If the pain originates in the abdominal wall, resisted contraction should be painful, with local tenderness accompanied by palpable alterations in tissue texture. If the pain is referred from the spine, changes in the soft tissues and joint movement in the appropriate segment will be evident.

Passive Examination

Passive examination has the advantage of permitting a correlation between the range of motion of a structure, the patient's symptoms, and the feel of tissue resistance and texture. As mentioned earlier, interpretation of the relationship between tissue resistance to movement and symptoms is fundamental. The abnormalities that can be detected with passive movement include:

Alterations in the range of movement, with either hyper- or hypomobility.
An abnormal quality of resistance to passive movement, such as the early and rapidly developing resistance associated with a gross restriction of movement; a lack of normal resistance—the "empty" endfeel of instability; the subtle difference in behavior of resistance in joints often associated with minor symptoms; and the "almost unyielding" quality of muscle spasm.
Provocation of symptoms (local or remote). If symptoms are reproduced, the direct involvement of the structure being moved can be assumed, with the reservations outlined above. That these symptoms are abnormal can be determined by comparing them with the effects produced by the movement of other, related structures. A provocation of local symptoms that differ from the presenting problem may still be relevant. If intersegmental movement at a level capable of referring to the symptomatic area is locally painful, a spinal source or component may be implicated.

The relationship between soft-tissue resistance to movement and symptom response is of greatest significance in seeking the source of a presenting problem. A structure may demonstrate abnormal movement that has no relevance to the problem. Similarly, a structure may be painful when moved or pressed, but show no intrinsic abnormality. Abnormality of movement associated with an abnormal symptom response in structures capable of producing the presenting symptoms is a significant finding. When these related abnormalities are also associated with changes in the texture of related soft tissue, indications of their relevance are even stronger.

Passive Physiologic Intervertebral Movements

The physiologic movements of which the vertebral column is capable (i.e., flexion, extension, lateral flexion, and rotation and their combinations) can be examined at each intervertebral level. The examination of such passive physiologic intervertebral movements (PPIVMs) may be used to:

1. Confirm a restriction of movement seen on gross active testing. The amount of restriction, the level(s) involved, and the direction of the restriction can be confirmed and therefore localized.
2. Detect restriction of physiologic movement not obvious on gross testing.
3. Detect increases (either hypermobility or instability) or decreases in physiologic movement and associated joint play. For example, in the cervical spine, the addition of a lateral glide may demonstrate a loss of movement not obvious on lateral flexion, but which may be significant in producing symptoms.

The range of movement of one vertebrae level, quality of movement through the range, and endfeel must be determined and compared with those of adjacent vertebrae and the expected norm for the patient. As with all examinations of passive movement, the ability to interpret the relationship between soft-tissue resistance to movement and symptoms during movement is important. Movements in the coronal plane must also be compared with those of the opposite side. The basic movements of flexion, extension, lateral flexion, and rotation are routinely assessed and, when appropriate, combinations of these movements are also examined.

A description of individual techniques for examining PPIVMs is beyond the scope of this chapter, but detailed descriptions can be found elsewhere.[5,8]

Palpation Examination

Palpation examination is extremely informative and therefore an essential aspect of the evaluation of symptoms. An inflammatory disorder may cause a local increase in skin temperature and perspiration, both of which may be detected by palpation. The non-bony tissues should be palpated to detect thickening, swelling, muscle spasm, tightness, fibrous bands, or nodules. The position of the vertebrae and the presence of any bony anomalies should also be assessed, since an alteration in position may result in significant biomechanical changes that may in time generate sufficient stress to provoke symptoms. Alterations in vertebral position are often observed in the thoracic area.

Soft Tissues. The following areas are of particular significance in the palpation examination, since changes in tissue texture are frequently found in them.

These changes often alter with treatment, and would therefore appear to be related to the presenting symptoms.

Upper cervical (Occiput to C3), including the capsule of the atlanto-occipital joint; the occipital soft tissues from medial to lateral; the suboccipital tissues overlying the atlas and between the atlas and occiput; the tissues immediately adjacent to the spinous process of the axis; the interlaminar space of C1-C2 and C2-C3 zygapophyseal joints; the tissues overlying and immediately anterior to the transverse processes of the atlas and axis.

Mid-cervical (C3 to C5), including the tissues immediately adjacent to the spinous process; the area extending laterally between the spinous processes; the interlaminar spaces and capsules of the mid-cervical zygapophyseal joints; the area laterally overlying and anterior to the transverse processes.

Low cervical (C5 to T1), comprising the C7 to T1 area, where changes associated with a dowager's hump may be found.

Thoracic spine, including the area immediately adjacent to the spinous processes; the area extending laterally between spinous processes; the area further laterally, over the transverse processes and costotransverse joints; the angle of the ribs; intercostally, depending on the area of symptoms.

Vertebral Position and Bony Anomalies. The following abnormalities are frequently found. Positional abnormalities are relevant to the patient's symptoms if they change with treatment.

Upper cervical: slight rotation or displacement of the atlas relative to the occiput, as shown by asymmetry of depth and prominence of the atlantal transverse processes; absence or asymmetry of the bifid processes of the axial spinous process; exostoses at the C2-C3 zygapophyseal joints.

Mid-cervical: prominence of the C3 spinous process, frequently associated with chronic headaches; prominence of the C4 spinous process, usually associated with mid-cervical pain; exostoses at the mid-cervical zygapophyseal joints.

Low cervical: the spinous process of C6 is frequently very close to that of C7 and therefore a long way from that of C5, giving the impression of prominence of the C5 spinous process.

Thoracic: one spinous process is deviated laterally, either as a result of vertebral rotation or bony asymmetry; two spinous processes are very close together, creating a large interspinous space at the level below; one or more spinous processes are deep-set, with those on either side appearing prominent. The symptoms in such cases usually arise predominantly from the deep-set level.

Passive Accessory Intervertebral Movements

The earliest detectable changes in movement that occur with aging are changes in the quality of the accessory movements.[13-15] Therefore, accessory movements are the most sensitive indicators of abnormality of movement in a joint.

Accessory movements are routinely examined throughout the spine by postero-anterior oscillatory pressures (PAs) on the spinous process of each vertebra; PAs over the laminae on each side of the spinous process and over the transverse processes where they are palpable; and transverse oscillatory pressures against the lateral aspect of the spinous process.

In addition, in the cervical area, the following movements are routinely examined: transverse pressures against the transverse process and the laminae; and anteroposterior oscillatory pressures (APs) unilaterally over the area of the anterior and posterior tubercles.

In the thoracic area, unilateral PAs and APs on the ribs and APs on the sternum, sternocostal joints, or costochondral junctions may be indicated in particular patients.

Central movement at any level should be compared with the movement at the level above and below, and with the expected norm for the patient's age and somatotype; unilateral movements should also be compared with the corresponding movement on the opposite side.

The variations in the basic movements of the spine are endless, each providing information that may be useful in confirming the source of symptoms or a contribution to symptom production, and in directing treatment. Indications for the use of variations in basic movements come from a number of sources, including the movements that aggravate the patient's symptoms, particular movements found to be significant during the active examination, abnormalities found with PPIVMs, and interpretation of the basic passive accessory intervertebral movements (PAIVMs). If a particular spinal level is suspected as a source or contributing factor in a patient's symptoms, and routine movements do not reveal any abnormality, the examination should be taken further, with variations in the direction of movement and/or an assessment of PAIVMs in positions other than neutral. Any abnormalities that are detected should be relevant to the presenting symptoms. For example, a C2-C3 zygapophyseal source may be suspected for unilateral headaches, whereas unilateral PAs, APs, and transverse pressures do not demonstrate abnormalities proportional to the degree of symptoms. Unilateral PAs over the most lateral available aspect of the zygapophyseal joint, with a bias in a cephalad direction and performed with the head in ipsilateral rotation, may demonstrate a significant difference in the quality of movement and symptom production relevant to headache when compared with the response to the same movement on the opposite side. With an irritable or severe disorder in which a limited examination is indicated, the examination of PAIVMs may be modified in order to avoid provocation of symptoms. Indications for appropriate positions will be gained from positions that ease symptoms. Common examples of modifications include a posterior examination performed with the patient supine, a posterior examination with the patient prone but with the neck in slight flexion, and unilateral PAs performed in slight ipsilateral rotation.

Palpation and PAIVMs can help differentiate between an intervertebral source of symptoms, a contributing factor, and irrelevant findings. Soft-tissue thickening adjacent to a zygapophyseal joint, with a feel similar to that of old leather and combined with painless restriction as evidenced by unilateral PAs, indicates a chronic abnormality that is not the direct source of symptoms. If the soft tissue at an adjacent level is soft and feels swollen, and unilateral PAs demonstrate hypermobility with pain through the range of motion of this level, this joint is likely to be the source of the pain. However, the adjacent stiff, hypomobile joint could be hypothesized to be a contributing factor. Abnormalities found in levels more remote from the symptomatic area, or in areas that cannot be somatically connected with it, may still be relevant, either as contributing factors or as indicators of underlying neural involvement, particularly if the original abnormality is in the midthoracic region. However, their relevance can be determined only in retrospect, following appropriate treatment and a reassessment of all presenting signs and symptoms.

ASSESSMENT

The process of clinical reasoning is not complete with completion of the physical examination, but is a continual process throughout the course of management. Continuing assessment during and following the physical examination and subsequent treatment sessions allows development and modification of the hypotheses formed during the initial evaluation. Because complete examination is not always possible during the initial evaluation, aspects omitted should be addressed during the following one or two sessions.

In addition to the ongoing reasoning process, continuous assessment minimizes the chances of exacerbation of symptoms following examination, with its concomitant harmful effects. Assessment during the examination also helps the patient to develop confidence in the physical therapist, a factor that greatly enhances the chances of successful treatment.

The approach described here of ongoing clinical reasoning combined with an understanding of clinical patterns, good examination skills, and a mind that is sufficiently open to recognize subtle variations in familiar patterns and any new patterns that emerge, and to challenge and question assumed knowledge in order to enhance the understanding of underlying pathophysiology, allows physical therapists the opportunity for constant professional growth. If this approach is also combined with a degree of reflective thinking and good treatment skills, it provides the patient with optimal management.

REFERENCES

1. Zusman M: Central nervous system contribution to mechanically produced motor and sensory responses. Aust J Physiother 38:245, 1992
2. Aspinall W: Clinical testing for the craniovertebral hypermobility syndrome. JOSPT 12:47, 1990
3. Williams PL, Warwick R, Dyson M, Bannister LH (eds): Gray's Anatomy. 37th Ed. Churchill Livingstone, Edinburgh, 1989
4. Butler DS: Mobilisation of the Nervous System. Churchill Livingstone, Melbourne, 1991
5. Maitland GD: Vertebral Manipulation. 6th Ed. Butterworths, London, 1986
6. Jones MA, Jones HM: Principles of the physical examination. In Boyling JD and Palastanga N (eds): Grieve's Modern Manual Therapy. Churchill Livingstone, Edinburgh (In press).
7. Austin L, Maitland GD, Magarey ME: Manual therapy: what, when and why? In Australian Physiotherapy Association (Victorian Branch) (eds.): Sports Physiotherapy: Applied Science and Practice. Churchill Livingstone, Melbourne, (In press).
8. Grieve GP: Common Vertebral Joint Problems. 2nd Ed. Churchill Livingstone, Edinburgh, 1988
9. Kendall FP, McCreary EK: Muscle Testing and Function. 3rd Ed. Williams & Wilkins, Baltimore, 1983
10. Grant R, Trott PH: Pre-manipulative testing of the cervical spine—The APA protocol three years on. In Proceedings, Seventh Biennial Conference of the Manipulative Physiotherapists Association of Australia, Blue Mountains, November 1991
11. Australian Physiotherapy Association: protocol for pre-manipulative testing of the cervical spine. Aust J Physiother 34:97, 1988
12. Phillips H, Grieve GP: The thoracic outlet syndrome. In: Grieve GP (ed): Modern Manual Therapy of the Vertebral Column. Churchill Livingstone, Edinburgh, 1986
13. Trott PH: Mobility study of the trapezio-metacarpal joint. In Proceedings of the Second Biennial Conference of the Manipulative Therapists Association of Australia, Adelaide, August 1980
14. Milde MR: Accessory movements of the glenohumeral joint—a pilot study of accessory movements in asymptomatic shoulders and the changes related to ageing and hand dominance. Unpublished Graduate Diploma thesis, School of Physiotherapy, South Australian Institute of Technology, 1981
15. Thurnwald PA: The effect of age and gender on normal temporomandibular movement. Physiotherapy Theory and Practice 7:209, 1991

8 | Vertebral Artery Concerns: Premanipulative Testing of the Cervical Spine

Ruth Grant

SETTING THE SCENE

The use of manipulative techniques in the management of spinal disorders is not the province by right of any one profession. What is the province of the clinician, however, is the responsibility that attends the use of these techniques, namely, the responsibility to recognize what is expected of the prudent, careful practitioner in providing care and in avoiding untoward outcomes of treatment.

But what might be expected of the prudent careful practitioner and what might be determined to be an unexpected outcome of treatment? The answer to both aspects of the question lies in the conducting of screening tests prior to undertaking manipulative treatment.

Grant[1,2] reviewed cases of vertebrobasilar complications of a serious nature following cervical manipulation that were reported in the English language literature from 1947 to 1986. That review of cases allowed a distinction to be made between unexpected consequences in patients otherwise seemingly normal and healthy, in whom previous manipulation had been performed without apparent incident, and those patients in whom manipulative techniques should never have been used, either because signs and symptoms of vertebrobasilar insufficiency (VBI) were present following previous manipulation or before the implicated treatment session.

In this series, premanipulative testing for dizziness was reported in one case only.[3] This case involved a physical therapist. Although published case reports of serious complications following cervical manipulation involving physical therapists remain rare,[3-5] the issue is not how few or how many cases may be laid at the door of any particular profession, but rather what can be learned from all relevant reports; and further, what is each professional group that uses manipulative thrust techniques in treatment doing about the issue of quality control?

Testing for dizziness has been a part of patient screening by manipulative physical therapists for many years, and was first described by Maitland in 1968.[6] However, the work by Grant[1,2] highlighted the need for the Australian Physiotherapy Association (APA) to formalize a protocol for premanipulative testing of the cervical spine[7] and to recommend its use for all patients prior to cervical manipulation. In January 1988, the Biennial Conference of Manipulative Physiotherapy Teachers of Australia drew up the Protocol; the APA approved the Protocol in March 1988, and the APA Protocol was published in September 1988.[7] In doing this, the APA became the first professional group of any who use manipulative techniques in patient treatment in Australia (and as far as is known, worldwide) to have such a formalized protocol. Since that time, other countries' physical therapy associations or special interest groups have formalized similar protocols. At the time of this writing, these countries include Canada, the Netherlands, South Africa, and the United Kingdom.

WHAT CAN BE LEARNED FROM INCIDENTS AND ACCIDENTS INVOLVING THE VERTEBRAL ARTERY?

Tens of thousands of manipulative techniques are performed across the world in a single day. Serious consequences following cervical manipulation are reportedly rare. Hosek[8] estimated that such consequences occur once in 1 million cervical manipulations, and Dvorak and Orelli[9] estimated that they occur once in 400,000 (based on the results of a questionnaire sent to doctors of the Swiss Association of Manual Medicine). While the exact incidence of vascular accidents following cervical manipulation is unknown, what can be deduced is that many serious complications go unreported and that many transient deficits and/or instances of exacerbations of patients' symptoms following manipulation do occur.[5,10,11]

What can be deduced from these published case reports?[1,2,9,11] Complications were experienced predominantly by young adults, who often underwent multiple manipulative procedures at the incident session and not infrequently had warning symptoms or signs of potential VBI prior to the incident session. The most frequent description was of a rotation manipulation. Early onset of neurologic symptoms following manipulation (within minutes) was common, in many instances progressing to permanent deficit or death. In the 58 cases of VBI reviewed by Grant,[1,2] 23 of the 26 cases in which radiographs of the cervical spine were taken after the incident were reported as normal or showing only minor degenerative changes.

PREDISPOSING FACTORS AND MECHANISM OF INJURY

Stretching and momentary occlusion of the vertebral artery occurs in normal daily activities, and is asymptomatic. Indeed, the extracranial portion of the vertebral artery (parts 1, 2, and 3 in Fig. 8-1.) appear to be designed for movement and in some parts designed to compensate for lack of support. This extracranial section has a well-developed external elastic lamina and media.[12–14] Interestingly, after the artery penetrates the dura (in its fourth part) and joins with its contralateral fellow to form the basilar artery, the adventitia becomes much reduced, the external elastic lamina disappears, and the elastic fibrils in the media become very rare.

The vertebral arteries contribute about 11 percent of the total cerebral

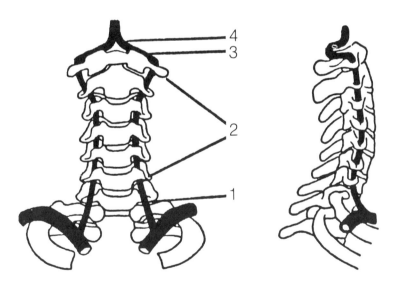

Fig. 8-1.   Anterior and lateral views of the vertebral artery. The course of the vertebral artery may be described in four parts. *(1)* The first part extends from the subclavian artery to the C6 foramen transversarium. *(2)* The second part runs vertically through the foramina transversaria of the upper six cervical vertebrae. *(3)* The third part passes through the foramen transversarium of the C1 vertebra and turns horizontally across it. *(4)* The fourth part enters the foramen magnum to join the opposite artery to form the basilar artery. (From Bogduk,[53] with permission.)

blood flow, the remaining 89 percent being supplied by the carotid system.[15] Asymmetry in the size of the two vertebral arteries is exceedingly common.[16,17] Indeed, complete interruption of blood flow in one vertebral artery, such as follows its ligation,[18] may be asymptomatic as long as there is adequate flow through the other vertebral artery and a normal configuration of the circle of Willis. Thus we can say that while blood flow may be affected by a variety of circumstances both intrinsic (e.g., atherosclerosis) and extrinsic (e.g., osteophyte impingement), the mere presence of a stenotic or occlusive lesion does not necessarily imply the presence of symptoms. Symptoms will occur when the blood supply to an area is critically reduced. This will depend ultimately upon a balance between compromising and compensatory factors.

The major vascular complications following cervical manipulation occurred predominantly in young adults (mean age, 37 years).[1,2,11] This finding suggests that neither cervical spondylotic and osteoarthrotic changes nor atheroma of the vertebrobasilar system would be pathognomonic in the majority of these cases. Bony changes, when present, are most likely to compromise the vertebral artery in its second part (Fig. 8-1). Compromise of the vertebral artery in the vertical portion through the foramina tranversaria of the upper six cervical vertebrae was infrequently reported in the case studies reviewed. Trauma to the vertebral artery following cervical manipulation occurred predominantly in its third part, the atlantoaxial component (Fig. 8-2), and was in most cases related to a manipulative thrust technique with a strong rotary component. This part of the artery is subject to stretching as a result of the large range of rotation that occurs at the C1-2 level. As early as 1884 Gerlach[19] recognized from his

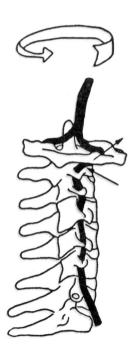

Fig. 8-2. A sketch of the right vertebral artery, demonstrating how the atlantoaxial segment *(arrow)* is stretched forward by left rotation of the atlas. (From Bogduk,[53] with permission.)

cadaver studies that rotation of the neck resulted in stretching of the contralateral vertebral artery at this level, and many other authors have since confirmed this.[20–23]

It can be deduced that the extent of the trauma to the vertebral artery following a strong rotary manipulation would be greater in the more mobile neck of the young adult than in the older person, in whom spondylotic, osteoarthritic or normal degenerative changes would limit the extent to which the neck could be rotated, thereby according some protection to the atlantoaxial segment of the artery in the older age group.

The nature of the arterial insult may be such that spasm of the artery ensues. This may be transient or it may persist, resulting in brain stem ischemia. If transient it may render the affected artery irritable, such that a manipulation done some time later may result in a major sequela. The trauma of the manipulation may actually damage the artery wall, resulting in subintimal tearing, hematoma, perivascular haemorrhage, thrombosis, or embolus formation. The extent of the damage may well determine the extent of the resulting brain stem ischemia. An understanding of the mechanism of injury highlights the degree of concern raised by those case histories in which practitioners (chiropractors in the main) continued to manipulate, in part to relieve the additional symptoms that were created. Indeed, Terrett's recounting of some of these case reports makes chilling reading.[24]

Cervical extension has been less consistently reported as narrowing the vertebral artery, than rotary manipulation, with such compromise as was reported occurring at the atlanto-occipital and atlantoaxial levels.[25,25a,25b] On the other hand, extension combined with cervical rotation produced occlusion of the vertebral artery whereas extension alone did not.[21,22] The addition of traction to this combined procedure increased the number of occlusions in the vertebral artery from 5 to 32, or by another 27 occlusions in 18 subjects.[22] All of these occlusions occurred at or above the level of C2. The most common site of occlusion was at the atlantoaxial level in the vertebral artery contralateral to the direction of rotation (in 26 out of 32 cases).

DIZZINESS AND VERTEBROBASILAR INSUFFICIENCY

Vertebrobasilar insufficiency (VBI) may be described as episodes of relative ischemia in the area of distribution of the vertebrobasilar system that result from a temporary alteration in flow in the vertebrobasilar system and its branches, and which gives rise to symptoms. As might be expected, a wide spectrum of symptoms and signs may be attributed to critical alterations in the vertebrobasilar circulation.

Dizziness is the most common and usually the predominant symptom of VBI. It may be the only presenting symptom in VBI, and while its presentation in isolation is less common, various investigators agree that this does occur.[26–29] Coman[30] has designated the major symptoms associated with VBI as the "five Ds": dizziness, diplopia, drop attacks, dysarthria, and dysphagia. While this makes for easy recall, the list is by no means complete. A major review by Williams and Wilson[26] of what they termed basilar insufficiency is instructive. These authors reviewed symptoms in 20 cases of major basilar insufficiency and 65 patients with minor syndromes of basilar insufficiency. The minor syndromes were defined as the "occurrence of transient symptoms disturbing otherwise normal health." Williams and Wilson considered the latter group not to be uncommon, particularly in later life, and their 65 cases were found in a thousand consecutive cases in their neurologic practice. It may well be that their minor syndrome is what Oostendorp et al. described as "functional vertebrobasilar insufficiency."[31] In any event, there appears to be a continuum here, rather than two quite separate subgroups.

Dizziness (vertigo) occurred in two-thirds of the minor cases described by Williams and Wilson,[26] and was by far the most common presenting symptom. The most convincing association was of vertigo with visual perceptual disturbances (including spots before the eyes, blurred vision, hallucinations, illusions, and field defects), diplopia, ataxia, and drop attacks. Half the patients reported visual disturbances and one-fifth reported visceral and vasomotor disturbances such as nausea, faintness, and lightheadedness. In addition, the authors found perioral dysaesthesia (tingling around the lips) to be much more common in the minor cases than the demonstrable changes in the territory of the trigeminal nerve that were considered to be more typical of major syndromes of basilar insufficiency. Perioral changes in sensation have also been reported by other authors.[27,29] Nystagmus, hemianesthesia, and hemiplegia are other symptoms and signs that have been described. Williams and Wilson[26] found that the vertigo they observed was unlikely to be associated with deafness or tinnitus in cases of basilar insufficiency.

Dizziness may arise as a result of distortion or diminution of the normal afferent input to the vestibular nuclei from receptors in the neck (termed *cervical* or *reflex vertigo*). These receptors are thought to be in the capsules of the upper three cervical joints, particularly the atlanto-occipital and atlantoaxial joints and in the neck musculature.[32-38] Signs of restriction of movement in the upper cervical joints, with or without pain, will be found on examination using passive accessory and passive intervertebral movement tests. However, such findings do not aid in differential diagnosis, because many patients with VBI and benign positional vertigo also exhibit such findings on examination.

While it may be stated that the essential difference between dizziness of vascular origin and cervical vertigo is that the latter is not accompanied by other features of brain stem ischemia or cardiovascular disease,[29,39] it still may be difficult to differentiate the two when dizziness is an initial, unaccompanied symptom. Some authors, like Troost,[27] considered that a latent response to a sustained position or head posture differentiates peripheral causes of vertigo (like benign positional vertigo or cervical vertigo) from dizziness due to central causes. However, Hulse,[40-42] who has written extensively in the European literature, is not in agreement, describing no latency time for cervical vertigo. Others consider that dizziness occurring latently may also be a feature of brain stem ischaemia.[38,43] All agree however, that fatigability is a characteristic of peripheral causes of vertigo.

"Dizziness sometimes cannot be simply classified as peripheral, central, or systemic," wrote Troost. "The symptom complex may well represent a combination of abnormalities, including incomplete adaption. This is particularly true when vertebrobasilar disease is a contributing factor."[27]

CLINICAL PROTOCOL FOR VERTEBRAL ARTERY TESTING AND FOR PREMANIPULATIVE TESTING

This section draws heavily upon previous work by the author,[1,2] and upon the Australian Physiotherapy Association Protocol for Premanipulative Testing of the Cervical Spine.[7]

Clinical Evaluation

In any patient for whom treatment of the cervical spine is to be undertaken, the presence or development of dizziness or other symptoms of VBI is carefully assessed. The four aspects of this assessment are subjective examination; physical examination; onset of symptoms during treatment; and onset of symptoms following treatment.

Subjective Examination

In every patient presenting with upper-quarter dysfunction, questions are specifically asked to ascertain the presence of dizziness or other symptoms suggestive of VBI. (These symptoms were outlined earlier in the chapter.) Should the patient respond in the affirmative, a detailed profile of each symptom must be obtained. Questioning should reveal

The type, degree, frequency, and duration of the dizziness; the occurrence or aggravation of dizziness by head movements and by sustained positions of the head and neck, particularly rotation, extension, or a combination of these movements; and any other movement, posture, or position volunteered by the patient.

The nature and type of any other symptom that may or may not be associated with dizziness but which may suggest VBI.

The history of dizziness vis à vis the history of the neck, headache, or other symptoms.

The status of the dizziness: is it improving, worsening, or staying the same?

The status of associated symptoms.

Previous treatment (if any) and its effect in relieving, exacerbating, or producing dizziness and/or associated symptoms.

Physical Examination

Many tests for the detection of VBI or tests to be undertaken prior to cervical manipulation have been described.[1,6,11,31,39,44,45] In some of these reports the tests were many and/or were sustained for 40 seconds or more. There has been a need to find a balance between what is done in clinical practice, the many tests reported, and the knowledge that the test procedures themselves hold certain risks, including a potentially additive effect on the vertebral artery. On this basis the tests described in the following sections are recommended.

Tests Undertaken in Patients With No History of Dizziness or Other Symptoms of VBI, But in Whom Cervical Manipulation is the Treatment of Choice

These tests are undertaken with the patient in the sitting and/or supine position (as deemed appropriate for each patient). With the supine position it is often possible to gain a greater range of movement, particularly if pain is a prominent presenting symptom. These tests comprise sustained extension (Fig. 8-3); sustained rotation to the left and right (Fig. 8-4); sustained rotation with extension to left and right (Fig. 8-5); a simulated manipulation position, in which the patient's head and neck are held in the position of the manipulative technique that the physical therapist proposes to use in treatment. An example is illustrated (Fig. 8-6).

The patient is questioned about dizziness both during each test and after each test position has been released. The physical therapist also observes the patient's eyes for the presence of nystagmus. Each position is maintained with over-pressure for a minimum of 10 seconds (or less if symptoms are evoked),

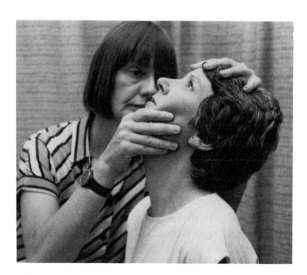

Fig. 8-3. Sustained cervical extension in sitting.

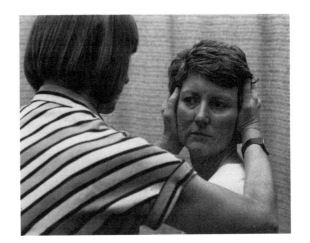

Fig. 8-4. Sustained cervical rotation in sitting. While both rotations are performed, only left rotation is illustrated.

and upon release, a period of at least 10 seconds should elapse to allow for any latent response to the sustained position.

If any of these tests produce dizziness or any other symptom suggestive of VBI, then cervical manipulation is not undertaken. If the tests are negative and no contraindications to manipulation have been elicited on specific overall assessment, then informed consent is obtained from the patient and the manipulative technique is carried out.

Tests Undertaken in Patients in Whom Dizziness is a Presenting Symptom

These tests are undertaken in sitting. The physical therapist may decide to proceed to test the patient in the supine position if all tests that follow are negative. These tests comprise sustained extension (Fig. 8-3); sustained rotation

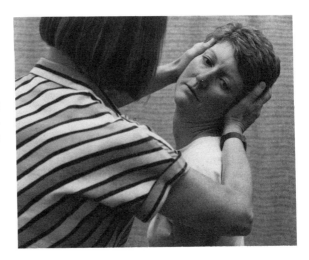

Fig. 8-5. Sustained cervical rotation with extension in sitting. Only left rotation with extension is illustrated.

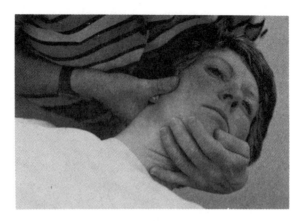

Fig. 8-6. Simulated manipulation position (simulation of transverse thrust technique to "gap" the left C2-3 zygapophyseal joint).

to left and right (Fig. 8-4); sustained rotation with extension to left and right (Fig. 8-5); testing the position or movement that provokes dizziness as described by the patient (if different from the above); and rapid movement of the head through the available range of the relevant movement, such as rotation. This test is done only when the patient relates dizziness in response to rapid movements of the head, rather than to head postures or positions.

When dizziness is provoked upon rotation, or rotation with extension, either during the sustained tests or the rapid movement test, these tests are further explored in the standing position. This is done to differentiate dizziness arising from the vestibular apparatus of the inner ear from that elicited by neck movement (whether the latter is due to cervical vertigo or symptomatic compromise of the vertebral artery). The tests in the standing position are head held still, sustained trunk rotation to the left and right (Fig. 8-7); head held still, repetitive trunk rotation to the left and right. When positive, these standing tests suggest that the patient's dizziness is not caused by labyrinth disturbance.

It is acknowledged that the stabilization of the head in these standing tests may be difficult, particularly with the latter test. If this is a concern, then the tests should be repeated with the patient seated in a rotating chair (a secretary's chair may be used). With the help of an assistant to rotate the chair, this position ensures good head stabilization.

In all tests for this group of patients in which dizziness is a presenting symptom, sustained positions are adopted for a minimum of 10 seconds or less if symptoms are provoked, and a pause follows each test to allow for any latent responses to occur before proceeding with the next test.

In summary, if during the physical examination any test is positive, producing or reproducing dizziness and/or associated symptoms that may be due to VBI, then cervical manipulation is contraindicated as a treatment option.

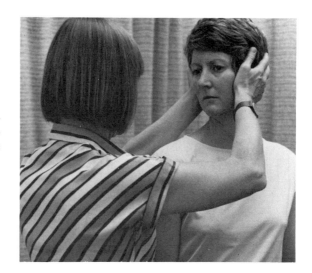

Fig. 8-7. Head held still, sustained trunk rotation in standing. Only trunk rotation to the left is illustrated.

Symptoms Provoked During Or After Treatment Procedures

Positive findings provoked while the patient adopts a treatment position, during any treatment procedure, or after any treatment procedure are considered contraindications to cervical manipulation. However, when these findings disappear and all tests become negative, manipulation may be reconsidered as a treatment of choice.

Choice Of Technique and Method Of Application

For those patients who present with dizziness and/or other symptoms that may be due to VBI but in whom the tests outlined previously are negative, there are some points of caution, as follows:

Any treatment technique that provokes the dizziness should be avoided or the technique performed with care and without reproducing dizziness, and its effect assessed over a 24-hour period before any decision about progression of that technique is made. Passive mobilization techniques can be most beneficial in the management of all forms of vertigo if there is a relevant cervical component to the symptomatology. Often a diagnosis of cervical vertigo will be made in retrospect in this way, and illustrates a prudent and responsible approach.

Passive mobilizing techniques (or other appropriate treatments) should be used in the initial treatment, and their effect over a 24-hour period should be known before the use of cervical manipulation is even considered

When manipulation is chosen as the method of treatment, a single, gentle, localized manipulation should be undertaken providing that all relevant tests previously described remain negative.

For any patient in whom cervical manipulation is the treatment of choice, these guidelines should be followed:

Informed consent should be gained from the patient. The patient must give verbal consent before the manipulative procedure is undertaken. It is therefore important that the patient understands what the procedure entails, that manipulation does hold certain risks, albeit very rare, and that all precautionary tests have been done and little risk is deemed to be operative in the patient's case. The APA Protocol (1987) advises the use of standardized wording for obtaining informed consent.

A generalized rotary manipulation of the cervical spine is potentially dangerous and must not be used. Rotation was the directional component common to almost all of the cases reviewed by Grant and Terrett in which a major incident followed cervical manipulation.[2,24]

The use of strong axial traction during a manipulative procedure must be avoided. The reports of Brown and Tatlow,[22] Parkin et al.,[3] Bourdillon,[46] and Gutmann (1983)[47] should be considered in this light.

At the first treatment session a single (not multiple) manipulation is performed. It is well to consider whether multiple cervical manipulations at a single treatment session are ever necessary in view of the potential cumulative effect on the vertebral artery.[2,11,23]

Vertebral Artery Testing At Subsequent Visits

The APA Protocol specifies that dizziness testing in the simulated manipulation position should be performed at all subsequent visits by the patient (not just at the initial consultation) in which cervical manipulation is used. In 13 of the 58 cases of vertebrobasilar complications following cervical manipulation reviewed by Grant in 1987,[1] previous cervical manipulation had been carried out without apparent incident. However, it must also be remembered that while the premanipulative tests described earlier seek to simulate some of the stresses imposed on the cervical structures when a manipulation is performed, the rapid thrust component cannot be simulated. This should always be borne in mind, and forceful manipulative techniques avoided. The section that follows, describes research undertaken with respect to the APA Protocol which suggests that the full vertebral artery testing procedure should be performed at all subsequent visits in which cervical manipulation is to be undertaken. Physical therapists are encouraged to do this.

Recording

It is vital that the premanipulative tests undertaken and the response to these on the part of the patient be recorded. It is also necessary to record that informed consent has been obtained.

THE APA PROTOCOL FOR PREMANIPULATIVE TESTING OF THE CERVICAL SPINE UNDER SCRUTINY

Survey of APA Members Regarding The Protocol

In 1991, two and a half years after the APA formalized the Protocol for Premanipulative Testing of the Cervical Spine and recommended its use with all patients before cervical manipulation, Grant and Trott[48] undertook a survey of APA members. They formulated a detailed questionnaire and tested item consistency in a pretrial on a small sample of 20 physical therapists from a variety of fields of practice.

The questionnaire established the fields in which the members practiced; their gender; their knowledge of the APA Protocol; their attitudinal responses to statements commonly made about the Protocol; whether they used manipulative techniques in treatment; their compliance with the subjective and physical examination components of the Protocol; whether informed consent was obtained prior to cervical manipulation; whether screening tests undertaken and informed consent gained were recorded; and whether the format suggested in the Protocol was used.

Systematic stratified random sampling of 10 percent of the APA membership nationwide yielded 727 names. Questionnaires were sent to these physical therapists and 455 (63 percent) responded. The fields of practice in which those who responded worked are outlined in Table 8-1. It may be seen that a wide

Table 8-1. Fields of Practice of Respondents to Survey of APA Members Regarding the Protocol for Premanipulative Testing of the Cervical Spine

Fields of Practice	Number of Respondents (%)
Cardiopulmonary	183 (40)
Gerontology	153 (34)
Manipulative physiotherapy	198 (44)
Neurology	179 (39)
Occupational Health	107 (24)
Orthopedics	331 (73)
Pediatrics	106 (23)
Psychiatry	11 (2)
Sports physiotherapy	246 (54)
Women's Health	123 (27)
Other Fields	62 (14)

variety of fields of practice was represented. (It should be noted that many respondents worked in more than one field of practice).

Seventy-nine percent of the respondents were female and 21 percent were male. Eighty-nine percent (406) of the respondents knew there was an APA Protocol. Nineteen percent (84) of the respondents used manipulative techniques occasionally, often, or very often in the treatment of upper-quarter disorders. Of these physical therapists, 98 percent (82) knew there was an APA Protocol and 92 percent (77) had read it.

The responses of those individuals who knew there was an APA Protocol to statements commonly made about it are presented in Figures 8-8 through 8-11 (with the five-point scale "strongly disagree" to "strongly agree" collapsed to three categories). This comprised 406 physical therapists in the whole group and 82 in the manipulation (sub)group, or those respondents who used manipulative techniques in treatment. (Missing responses to these statements were few).

It may be seen from Figure 8-8 that two thirds of the respondents in both groups agreed with the statement, *"The APA Protocol for premanipulative testing of the cervical spine places appropriate medicolegal restrictions upon the physiotherapy practitioner."*

Of those physical therapists who used manipulation in the treatment of upper-quarter disorders, 41 percent considered that *"The APA Protocol for premanipulative testing of the cervical spine is too time consuming to be under-*

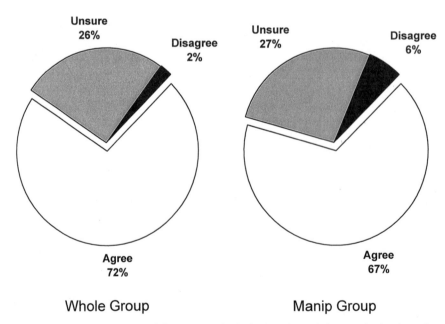

Whole Group   Manip Group

Fig. 8-8.   "The APA Protocol for premanipulative testing of the cervical spine places appropriate medicolegal restrictions upon the physiotherapy practitioner."

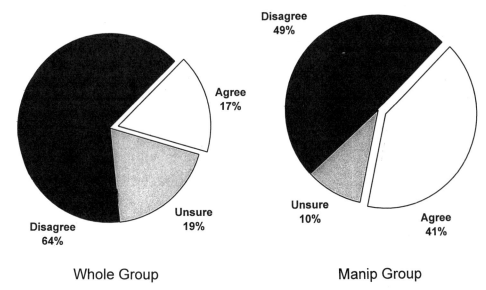

Whole Group   Manip Group

Fig. 8-9. "The APA Protocol for premanipulative testing of the cervical spine is too time consuming to be undertaken with every patient prior to cervical manipulation."

taken with every patient prior to cervical manipulation" (Fig. 8-9). Just under half of these physical therapists (49 percent) disagreed with the statement. By contrast, 65 percent of the group as a whole disagreed, and only 17 percent agreed.

"The requirement of informed consent on the part of the patient prior to undergoing cervical manipulation will mean that fewer patients will agree to manipulation as a form of treatment and as a consequence a valuable method of treatment will be used less frequently." Twice as many respondents in the whole group disagreed with this statement as compared with those who agreed with it, with 31 percent unsure (Fig. 8–10). However, in the group that used manipulative techniques in treatment, a slightly greater percentage was of the opinion that the requirement for informed consent on the part of the patient would lead to a valuable method of treatment (manipulation) being used less frequently (44 percent), as compared to the percentage who disagreed with this (40 percent).

It may be seen from Figure 8-11 that at least two-thirds of each group agreed with the statement, *"The APA Protocol for premanipulative testing of the cervical spine is an important initiative and should be retained."* However, a greater percentage of those physical therapists using manipulative techniques in practice were unsure with respect to this statement than was the case for the group as a whole.

Thus, in summary, two-thirds of the group of respondents who used manipulative techniques in treatment agreed both that the APA Protocol placed appropriate medicolegal restrictions on the practitioner and that it was an important

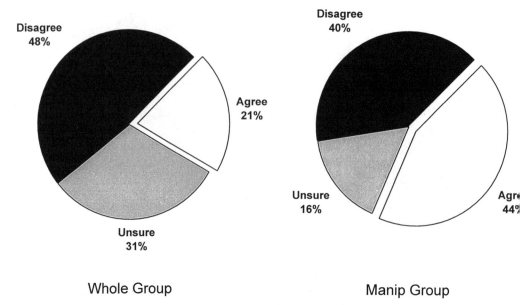

Whole Group   Manip Group

Fig. 8-10. ''The requirement of informed consent on the part of the patient prior to undergoing cervical manipulation will mean that fewer patients will agree to manipulation and as a consequence a valuable method of treatment will be used less frequently.''

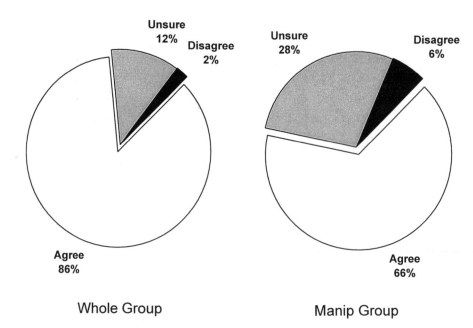

Whole Group   Manip Group

Fig. 8-11. ''The APA Protocol for premanipulative testing of the cervical spine is an important initiative and should be retained.''

initiative and should be retained. However, many of these respondents were of the opinion that the Protocol was too time consuming and that its requirement for informed consent would mean that manipulation as a form of treatment would be used less often.

Of the 84 physiotherapists who used manipulative techniques in the treatment of upper-quarter disorders, 100 percent complied with the subjective examination component of the Protocol. Eighty-one respondents (96 percent) performed some or all of the recommended screening tests prior to the first treatment using cervical manipulation, with 88 percent (71) utilizing two or more of the tests and 64 percent (52) using all of the tests. Before subsequent treatments using cervical manipulation, 89 percent of the respondents (75) performed screening tests, with 91 percent of these using the simulated manipulation position (SMP). The SMP is the test recommended in the Protocol for use prior to subsequent treatments employing cervical manipulation. The frequency of recording of the tests done at the first visit was 90 percent while at subsequent visits it was 60 percent.

Informed consent was reported as being obtained from patients by 93 percent (78) of the 84 physiotherapists before they undertook cervical manipulation. Of these only 58 percent gained informed consent in every case, and only 50 percent recorded that such consent had been obtained. Where informed consent gained was recorded, 33 percent of the respondents used the wording suggested in the APA Protocol, while 67 percent either did not use this wording or didn't know whether the wording they used was the same as that in the Protocol.

In summary, it may be deduced that knowledge of the existence of the APA Protocol was widespread. With regard to those physiotherapists who used manipulative techniques in the treatment of upper-quarter disorders, a high percentage complied with the Protocol in terms of the screening procedures they used. However, the obtaining of informed consent, and particularly the use of the wording suggested for this in the APA Protocol, were areas in which there was less compliance. This reflects the distribution of the attitudinal responses to the statement on informed consent (Fig. 8-10). Modification of this section of the Protocol, at least to allow practitioners to gain informed consent using phraseology of their own choice, is currently being considered.

Other Research Undertaken Using The APA Protocol

Forty-one percent of respondents who used manipulative techniques in the treatment of upper-quarter disorders felt that the APA Protocol was too time consuming to be undertaken with every patient prior to manipulation, although a very high percentage complied with most components of the Protocol. It is therefore useful to consider the two unpublished studies in which the testing procedures outlined in the protocol have been investigated in patients with symptomatic disorders of the cervical spine.[49,50] Both studies showed that it was important to retest, since the dizziness testing response (DTR) changed from negative to positive in some patients at the second assessment. Further, Hutchison found that the testing procedures reproduced the patients' dizziness and/or other symptoms of VBI, especially when these were related to cervical movement, and also that they produced dizziness in 20 percent of patients in the absence of dizziness as a presenting symptom.

While there was no significant difference between the sensitivity of the tests in producing a positive DTR, the combined rotation/extension test was found to be the most sensitive of the bilateral tests and more sensitive than the SMP. (The SMP is the test recommended in the Protocol for use during subsequent visits prior to cervical manipulation, and, as might be expected, was the test most commonly reported to be undertaken in follow-up by respondents to the survey). Oostendorp[31,51] used a more detailed and more time consuming screening procedure that incorporated the elements of the APA Protocol but also included sustained flexion, lateral flexion, and lateral flexion combined with extension/rotation and flexion/rotation in examining 90 patients with headache, dizziness, and neck pain. The mean percentage of positive responses was highest for sustained extension/rotation and sustained extension/rotation/lateral flexion to either side. There was very little difference between these combined movement tests in the incidence of positive responses, suggesting perhaps that both tests need not be undertaken. The sensitivity of the bilateral extension/rotation test finds support in the later work of Hutchison.[49] Unlike Hutchison, Oostendorp found a high percentage of positive responses to bilateral rotation as well. It must, however, be said that the mean onset of symptoms in Oostendorp's study was 55 seconds—a long time to sustain each test.

Further research is required to ascertain which of the initial screening tests needs to be carried out, and which need to be carried out at each subsequent visit.

CONCLUSION

The clinical protocol for premanipulative testing of the cervical spine as outlined in this chapter more than adequately meets the concerns arising from the reported cases of vertebrobasilar incidents that have been reviewed. All physical therapists and indeed all other clinicians who use manipulative techniques in the management of upper-quarter disorders should perform premanipulative testing of the cervical spine with every patient prior to cervical manipulation.

The Protocol formalized by the APA is put forward as a model. However, more research needs to be undertaken to establish the discriminative validity of the Protocol.

While the clinical protocol outlined in this chapter should ensure that we responsibly use the effective manipulative techniques at our disposal, it is important for us to remember that:

An element of unpredictability remains and incidents do occur, even when all premanipulative tests are negative and even when the patient has responded favorably to manipulative treatment in the past.[2,52]

The test procedures themselves hold certain risks.

There is a need to carefully and accurately record all dizziness tests and premanipulative testing procedures and the responses to them on the part of the patient.

Even when the patient is made aware of the risks attached to the manipulative procedure, (i.e., when informed consent is obtained), the physical therapist (or indeed any professional performing manipulative procedures) may still remain legally liable if reasonable care, defined as the care expected of the average competent and prudent practitioner, is not employed.

REFERENCES

1. Grant ER: Clinical testing before cervical manipulation—can we recognise the patient at risk? p. 192. Proceedings of the Tenth International Congress of the World Confederation for Physical Therapy, Sydney, May 17–22, 1987
2. Grant R: Dizziness testing and manipulation of the cervical spine. In Grant R (ed): Physical Therapy of the Cervical and Thoracic Spine. Churchill Livingstone, New York, 1988
3. Parkin PJ, Wallis WE, Wilson JL: Vertebral artery occlusion following manipulation of the neck. NZMedJ 88:441, 1978
4. Fritz VU, Maloon A, Tuch P: Neck manipulation causing stroke. South Af Med J 66:844, 1984
5. Michaeli A: Dizziness testing of the cervical spine: can complications of manipulations be prevented? Physiother Theory Pract 7:243, 1991
6. Maitland GD: Vertebral Manipulation. 2nd Ed. Butterworths, London, 1968
7. Protocol for pre-manipulative testing of the cervical spine. Aust J Physiother 34: 97, 1988
8. Hosek RS, Schram SB, Silverman H: Cervical manipulation. JAMA 245:922, 1981
9. Dvorak J, Orelli F: How dangerous is manipulation of the cervical spine? Manual Med 2:1, 1985
10. Grieve GP: Incidents and accidents of manipulation. In Grieve GP (ed): Modern Manual Therapy of the Vertebral Column. Churchill Livingstone, Edinburgh, 1986
11. Terrett AGJ: Vascular accidents from cervical spine manipulation: Report on 107 cases. J Aust Chirop Assoc 17:15, 1987
12. Wilkinson IMS: The vertebral artery. Extracranial and intracranial structure. Arch Neurol 27:392, 1972
13. Winkler G: Remarques sur la structure de l'artere vertebrale. Quad Anat Prac 28: 105, 1972
14. George B, Laurian C: The Vertebral Artery. Pathology and Surgery. Springer-Verlag, Vienna, 1987
15. Hardesty WH, Whitacre WB, Toole JF, et al: Studies on vertebral artery blood flow in man. Surg Gyn Obstet 116:662, 1963
16. Franke JP, Dimarina V, Pannier M, et al: Les artéres vertébrales. Segments atlanto-axoidiens V3 et intra-cranien V4 collatérales. Anat Clin 2:229, 1980

17. Cavdar S, Arisan E: Variations in the extracranial origin of the human vertebral artery. Acta Anat 135:236, 1989
18. Shintani A, Zervas NT: Consequence of ligation of the vertebral artery. J Neurosurg 36:447, 1972
19. Gerlach L: Ueber die bewegungen in den atlasgelenken und deren beziehungen zu der blutstromung in den vertebralarterien. Beitr Morphol 1: 104, 1884, cited by George B, Laurian C, 1987
20. Dekleyn A, Nieuwenhuyse P: Schwindelanfaelle und Nystagmus bei einer Destimmten Stellung des Kopfes. Acta Otolaryng 11:155, 1927
21. Toole JF, Tucker SH: Influence of head position upon cerebral circulation. Studies on blood flow in cadavers. Arch Neurol 2:616, 1960
22. Brown BSJ, Tatlow WFT: Radiographic studies of the vertebral arteries in cadavers. Radiology 81:80, 1963
23. Krueger BR, Okazaki H: Vertebrobasilar distribution infarction following chiropractic vertical manipulation. Mayo Clinic Proc 55:322, 1980
24. Terrett AGJ: Vascular accidents from cervical spine manipulation: The mechanisms. ACA J Chirop 22:59, 1988
25. Lewis RC, Coburn DF: The vertebral artery. Missouri Med 53:1059, 1956
25a. Mehalic T, Farhat SM: Vertebral artery injury from chiropractic manipulation of the neck. Surg Neurol 2:125, 1974
25b. Okawara S, Nibbelink D: Vertebral artery occlusion following hyperextension and rotation of the neck. Stroke 5:640, 1974
26. Williams D, Wilson TG: The diagnosis of the major and minor syndromes of basilar insufficiency. Brain 85:741, 1962
27. Troost BT: Dizziness and vertigo in vertebrobasilar disease. II: Central causes and vertebrobasilar disease. Stroke 11:413, 1980
28. Ausman JI, Shrontz CE, Pearce JE, et al: Vertebrobasilar insufficiency. A review. Arch Neurol 42:803, 1985
29. Bogduk N: Cervical causes of headache and dizziness. In Grieve GP (ed): Modern Manual Therapy of the Vertebral Column. Churchill Livingstone, Edinburgh, 1986
30. Coman WB: Dizziness related to ENT conditions. In Grieve GP (ed): Modern Manual Therapy of the Vertebral Column. Churchill Livingstone, Edinburgh, 1986
31. Oostendorp RAB, Bernards JA, Clarijs JP, Elvers JWH: Functional vertebrobasilar insufficiency. Ned T Fysiother 99:181 1989
32. McCouch GP, Derring ID, Ling TH: Location of receptors for tonic neck reflexes. J Neurophysiol 14:191, 1951
33. Cohen LA: Role of eye and neck proprioceptive mechanisms in body orientation and motor coordination. J Neurophysiol 24:1, 1961
34. Norrse M, Stevens A: Cervical nystagmus and functional disorders of the cervical column. Acta Otorhinolaryngol Belg 30:457, 1976
35. De jong PTVM, De Jong JMBV, Cohen B, Jongkees LBW: Ataxia and nystagmus induced by injection of local anesthetics in the neck. Ann Neurol 1:240, 1977
36. Wyke B: Neurology of the cervical spinal joints. Physiotherapy 65:72, 1979
37. Abrahams VC: Sensory and motor specialization in some muscles of the neck. Trends Neurosci: 24, 1981
38. Reker V: Cervical nystagmus caused by proprioceptors of the neck. Laryngol Rhinol Otol (Stuttg) 62:312, 1983
39. Aspinall W: Clinical testing for cervical mechanical disorders which produce ischemic vertigo. J Orthop Sports Phys Ther 11:176, 1989
40. Hülse M: Die differentialdiagnostische auswertung des zervikalnystagmus HNO 30: 192, 1982

41. Hülse M: Die Cervikalen Gleichgewichtsstörungen. Springer-Verlag, Berlin, 1983
42. Hülse M: Zervikale gleichgewichtsstörungen. In von Wolff HD (ed): Die Sonderstellung des Kofpgelenkbereich. Springer-Verlag, Berlin, 1988
43. Scherer H: Neck induced vertigo. Arch Otorhinolaryngol, suppl. 2:107, 1985
44. Maigne R: Orthopaedic Medicine: A New Approach to Vertebral Manipulation. Charles C Thomas, Springfield, IL 1972
45. Maitland GD: Vertebral Manipulation. 5th Ed. Butterworths, London, 1986
46. Bourdillon JF, Day EA: Spinal Manipulation. 4th Ed. Heinemann, London, 1987
47. Gutmann G: Injuries to the vertebral artery caused by manual therapy. Manuelle Mediz 21:2, 1983
48. Grant ER, Trott PH: Premanipulative testing of the cervical spine—The APA Protocol and its aftermath. p. 378. Proceedings of 11th International Congress of the World Confederation for Physical Therapy, London, July 28–August 2, 1991
49. Hutchison MS: An investigation of pre-manipulative dizziness testing. p. 104. Proceedings of Sixth Biennial Conference of Manipulative Therapists Association of Australia, Adelaide, July 25–29, 1989
50. Powell VJ: An investigation of testing procedures for vertebrobasilar insufficiency (abstract). Aust J Physiother 36:31, 1990
51. Oostendorp RAB: Vertebrobasilar insufficiency. p. 42. Proceedings of the International Federation of Orthopaedic Manipulative Therapists Congress, Cambridge, September 4–9, 1988
52. Bolton PS, Stick PE, Lord RSA: Failure of clinical tests to predict cerebral ischemia before neck manipulation. J Manip Physiol Ther 12:304, 1990
53. Bogduk N: Dizziness and the vertebral artery. The Cervical Spine and Headache Symposium. p. 61. Manipulative Therapists Association of Australia, Brisbane, April 11–12, 1981

9 | Combined Movements of the Cervical Spine in Examination and Treatment

Brian C. Edwards

The shape of the articular surfaces and the symptoms associated with joint dysfunction vary quite distinctly at different levels in the cervical spine. Because of this the examination of the cervical spine needs to be divided into the following three compartments: high cervical—occiput to C2; middle cervical—C3 to C5; low cervical—C6 to T1.

HIGH CERVICAL SPINE (OCCIPUT TO C2)

This is an area of the vertebral column that does not easily lend itself to physical examination, while at the same time being subject to a wide variety of mechanical disorders. Hence, a considerable proportion of this chapter will be devoted to the examination of the high cervical spine.

Headaches of cervical origin commonly arise from these levels.[1-3] These types of headaches are presented in detail in Chapter 13.

The anatomy of the high cervical spine is unique and to some degree more complicated than that of the rest of the vertebral column. The shapes of the bones and their articulations are quite distinctly different between the occiput and atlas, atlas and axis, and axis and C3. Such marked changes in anatomic configuration in such close proximity occur nowhere else in the vertebral column.

It is interesting to note that the articulations of the occipitoatlantal and atlantoaxial joints are situated approximately 1 cm anteriorly to the articulations of the second and third cervical vertebrae. Although the articular surfaces of the occipitoatlantal and atlantoaxial joints vary somewhat, those between the occiput and atlas are as a general rule, concavoconvex, and those between the atlas and axis are slightly biconvex (excluding the articulation between the odontoid peg and the anterior arch of the atlas).

The main movements that occur between the occiput and atlas are flexion and extension. Although there is some dispute about whether any rotation occurs between the occiput and atlas, a small amount of rotation may be felt between the mastoid process and the transverse process of C1 on passive testing. Lateral flexion of the occiput on the atlas causes the condyles of the occiput to move in a direction opposite to that in which the head is laterally flexed.

Braakman and Penning[4] suggest that lateral flexion is combined with rotation to the opposite side. When examining the occipitoatlantal complex with combined movements, flexion or extension in combination with rotation, rather than lateral flexion, is more effective in increasing or decreasing stretch or compressive effects.

It has been suggested that the occiput and axis should be considered as a segment, rather than the atlas and axis,[5] because of the ligamentous attachments from the axis to the occiput, consisting of the superior longitudinal band of the cruciform ligament, the apical ligament, and the alar ligaments. While this is a useful concept, the examination of the high cervical spine is not complete without the testing of movements between the atlas and axis both singly and in combination.

Examination by Combined Movements

The combining of movements when examining the cervical and lumbar spine has been presented previously.[6-10] The principle underlying the use of combined movements in the high cervical spine—the effecting of stretch or compression of specific joints and surrounding structures—is the same as for the rest of the vertebral column. It is rare for headache symptoms to be reproduced by standard physiologic movements of the high cervical spine alone; often it is only by combining these movements that sufficient tension can be placed on high cervical structures to produce the patient's symptoms.

The Occipitoatlantal Complex

Testing in Flexion and Right Rotation. On flexion, the condyles of the occiput move backward in relation to the articular surface of the atlas. When this

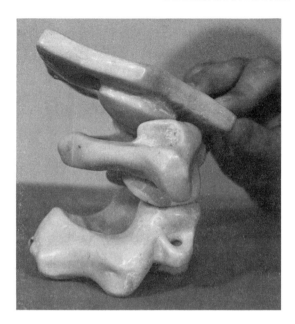

Fig. 9-1. Flexion and right rotation: occipitoatlantal complex. (From Edwards,[9] with permission.)

is combined with rotation to the right, an increased stretch is placed on the posterior aspect of the capsule of the right occipitoatlantal joint (Fig. 9-1).

Method of Testing. The therapist supinates the patient's left forearm and extends the left wrist. The web between the left index finger and left thumb is placed over the symphysis menti. The right hand is placed over the crown of the head with the finger tips extending down to grasp the skull below the external occipital protuberance. The head is flexed on the cervical spine. Right rotation is added in such a manner as to increase the stretch on the right posterior atlanto-occipital membrane (Fig. 9-2).

Testing in Extension and Right Rotation. On extension, the condyles of the occiput move forward in relation to the articular surface of the atlas. When combined with rotation to the right, an increase in the stretch on the anterior capsule of the left occipitoatlantal joint is obtained (Fig. 9-3).

Method of Testing. The left hand is placed over the crown of the head and the right hand under the chin. The head is then extended on the neck, and right rotation of the head is added so as to increase the stretch of the anterior part of the capsule of the left occipitoatlantal joint (Fig. 9-4).

The Atlas-Axis Complex

Testing in Right Rotation and Flexion. On right rotation of the atlas on the axis, the left inferior articular surface of the atlas moves forward on the left superior articular surface of the axis, with the opposite movement occurring

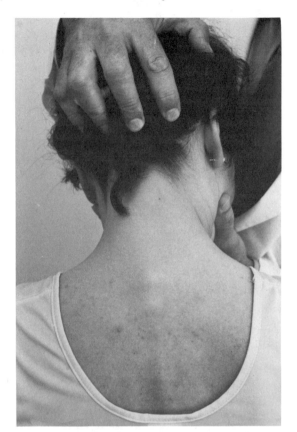

Fig. 9-2. Testing flexion and right rotation: occipitoatlantal complex.

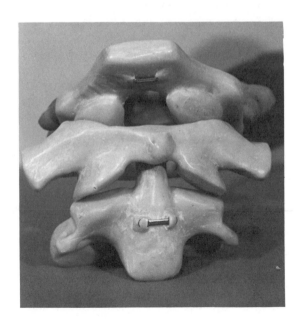

Fig. 9-3. Extension and right rotation: occipitoatlantal complex. (From Edwards,[9] with permission.)

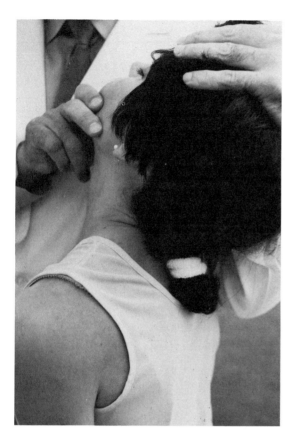

Fig. 9-4. Testing extension and right rotation: occipitoatlantal complex.

on the right side. If flexion is then added, an increased stretch of the posterior aspect of the left and right atlantoaxial joints is obtained (Fig. 9-5).

Method of Testing. The therapist's left hand is placed over the posterior aspect of C2 so that the left middle finger is over the anterior aspect of the left transverse process of C2. The left index finger is placed on the left side of the spine of C2 and the left thumb is placed over the posterior aspect of the superior articulation of C2. The right hand and arm take hold of the patient's head so that the right little finger comes around the arch of C1. The head is then rotated to the right until C2 just starts to rotate. Flexion of the occiput and C1 is then added, thereby increasing the stretch on the posterior aspects of both atlantoaxial joints (Fig. 9-6).

Testing in Right Rotation and Extension. On rotation to the right of the atlas on the axis, the left inferior articular surface of the atlas moves forward on the left superior articular surface of the axis, and the opposite occurs on

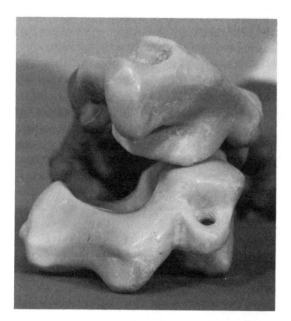

Fig. 9-5.   Right rotation and flexion: atlas-axis complex. (From Edwards,[9] with permission.)

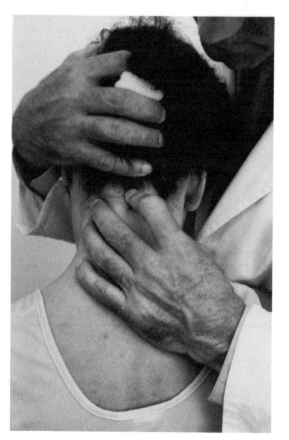

Fig. 9-6.   Testing right rotation and flexion: atlas-axis complex.

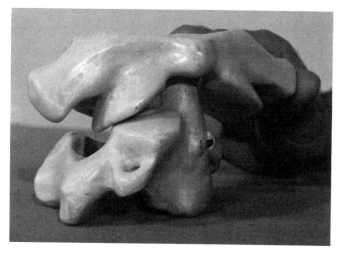

Fig. 9-7. Right rotation and extension: atlas-axis complex. (From Edwards,[9] with permission.)

the right side. If extension is added, there is an increase in the stretch on the anterior part of the capsule of the right and left atlantoaxial joints (Fig. 9-7).

Method of Testing. The same hand positions are adopted as in Figure 9-6, however, extension is added, so that there is an increased stretch of the anterior capsule of both atlantoaxial joints (Fig. 9-8).

Confirmation of Findings by Palpation

The passive testing procedures described above will elicit signs that are more related to restriction than to reproduction of pain. Thus, following the examination of physiologic movements, the next step is to either confirm the findings by palpation or, where the appropriate symptoms have not been reproduced by combined movements, identify them by palpation. Very often, specific signs and symptoms will be more easily isolated by palpation.

When performing palpation, close attention must be given to placing the joint to be examined in the appropriate combined position. This position must be strongly maintained while the palpation procedure is performed.

The Occipitoatlantal Complex

Flexion and Right Rotation. Stressing the posterior aspect of the right atlanto-occipital joint by manual palpation is achieved in the manner illustrated in Figure 9-9. With the patient in the prone position, the patient's head is flexed

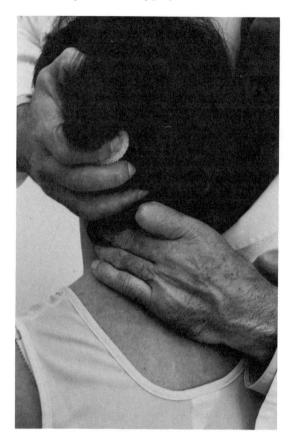

Fig. 9-8.   Testing right rotation and extension: atlas–axis complex.

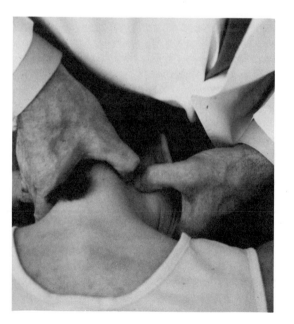

Fig. 9-9.   Posterior palpation on the right of C1 in flexion and right rotation.

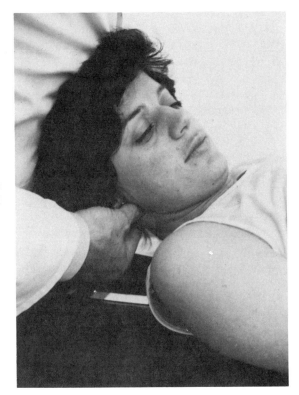

Fig. 9-10. Anterior palpation on the right of C1 in flexion and right rotation.

and rotated to the right. The therapist's thumb tips, placed over the right posterior arch of C1, apply oscillatory pressures so as to increase the stretch on the right occipitoatlantal articulation (Fig. 9-9). Palpation over the anterior aspect of the right transverse process of C1 with the patient's head in flexion and right rotation will decrease the stretch on the right occipitoatlantal joint (Fig. 9-10).

Extension and Right Rotation. The stretch on the anterior aspect of the left occipitoatlantal joint will decrease when oscillatory pressures are applied over the left posterior arch of C1 with the patient's head in extension and right rotation, as illustrated in Figure 9–11.

Palpation over the anterior aspect of the left transverse process of C1 with the patient's head in extension and right rotation will increase the stretch on the anterior aspect of the left occipitoatlantal joint (Fig. 9-12).

The Atlas-Axis Complex

Left Rotation and Flexion. With the C1-2 in left rotation and flexion, palpation over the anterior aspect of the right transverse process of C1 will decrease rotation between the atlas and axis and therefore decrease the stretch on the posterior aspect of the left and right atlantoaxial articulations (Fig. 9-13).

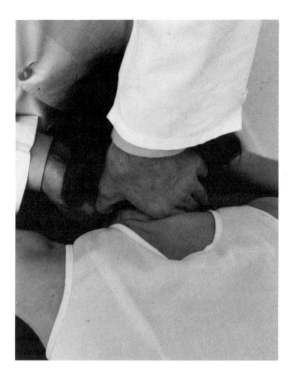

Fig. 9-11.   Posterior palpation on the left of C1 in extension and right rotation.

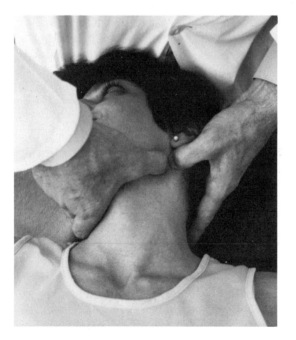

Fig. 9-12.   Anterior palpation on the left of C1 in extension and right rotation.

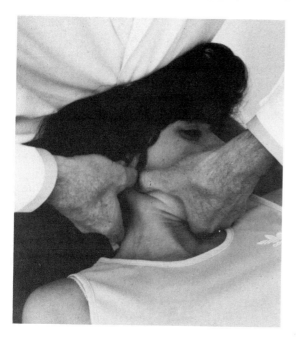

Fig. 9-13. Anterior palpation on the right of C1 in left rotation and flexion.

With the patient in the same position as illustrated in Figure 9-13, palpation over the anterior aspect of the right transverse process of C2 will increase the stretch on the posterior aspects of the left and right atlantoaxial articulations (Fig. 9-14).

When oscillatory pressures are applied over the right posterior aspect of C1, the stretch on the posterior aspect of the atlantoaxial articulations is increased. The palpation position is illustrated in Figure 9-15.

Palpation over the right posterior aspect of C2, by decreasing right rotation, also decreases the stretch on the posterior aspect of the atlantoaxial articulations (Fig. 9-16).

Right Rotation and Extension. In right rotation and extension, palpation over the anterior aspect of the right transverse process of C1 will increase the rotation of C1 on C2, thereby increasing the stretch on the anterior aspect of the right and left atlantoaxial joints, as illustrated in Figure 9-17.

Palpation over the anterior aspect of the right transverse process of C2 decreases right rotation and decreases the stretch on the anterior aspect of both atlantoaxial joints (Fig. 9-18). Palpation over the posterior aspect of the right transverse process of C1 with the head in right rotation and extension will decrease the rotation of C1 on C2, thereby decreasing the stretch on the anterior aspect of both the right and left atlantoaxial joints (Fig. 9-19).

Palpatory pressure over the posterior aspect of the right transverse process of C2 increases right rotation and increases the stretch on the anterior aspect of the atlantoaxial articulations (Fig. 9-20).

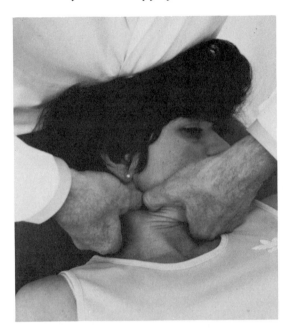

Fig. 9-14. Anterior palpation on the right transverse process of C2 in left rotation and flexion.

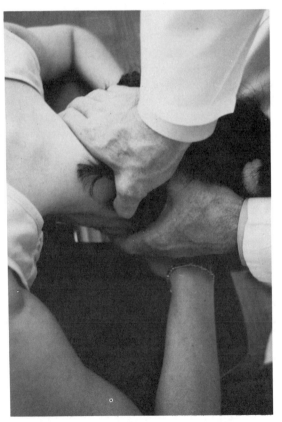

Fig. 9-15. Posterior palpation on the right of C1 in left rotation and flexion.

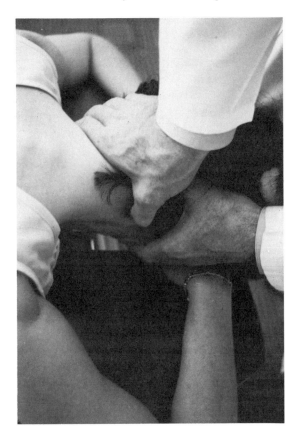

Fig. 9-16. Posterior palpation on the right of C2 in right rotation and flexion.

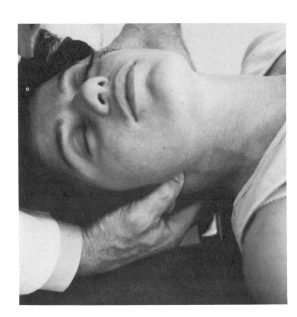

Fig. 9-17. Anterior palpation on the right of C1 in right rotation and extension.

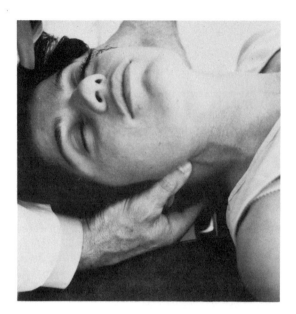

Fig. 9-18. Anterior palpation on the right transverse process of C2 in right rotation and extension.

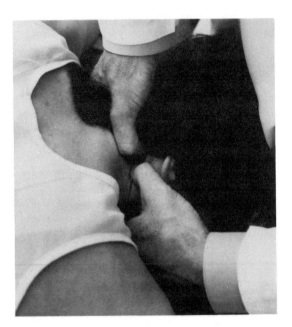

Fig. 9-19. Posterior palpation on the right of C1 in right rotation and extension.

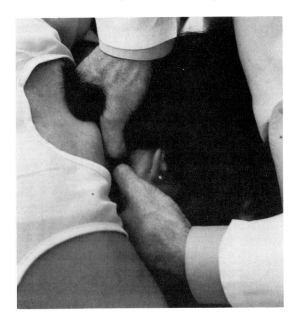

Fig. 9-20. Posterior palpation on the right of C2 in right rotation and extension.

Treatment

The examination procedures described are those primarily for headaches of cervical origin. One of the essentials of the physical examination for cervical headaches is the reproduction of part or all of the headache symptoms with physiologic movement, palpation, or a combination of both.

In the case of unilateral headache symptoms, the palpation procedure should be performed on the side of the symptoms. If tenderness is the main sign elicited, the response of the symptomatic side must be compared with that of the unaffected side using the same oscillatory pressure. If the headache symptoms are reproduced, the technique chosen for treatment is the reciprocal or opposite movement to the painful direction found on examination; alternatively, the head and neck can be placed in the neutral position with movement in the painful direction. Examples of this approach for the occipitoatlantal and atlas-axis complex follow.

The Occipitoatlantal Complex

Flexion and right rotation of the occiput on the atlas reproduces the patient's right-sided headache symptoms. Posterior pressure over the right transverse process of the atlas with the head in flexion and right rotation in relation to the atlas also reproduces the symptoms.

Anterior pressure over the right transverse process of the atlas with the head in flexion and right rotation is the first choice of technique, with progression to posterior pressure as the symptoms improve. An alternative treatment approach is to use posterior pressure over the right transverse process of the atlas with the head in neutral, and to progress the position of the head to right rotation and flexion as the symptoms improve.

The Atlas-Axis Complex

Right rotation and flexion reproduces the headache on the right. Anterior pressure over the transverse process of C1 on the right, with the head in the same position as above, also produces the headache. The first choice of technique may be anterior pressure over the right transverse process of C1 with the head in the neutral position, progressing to the position of right rotation and flexion as the symptoms improve. Another choice may be anterior pressure over the right of C2 with the head in right rotation and flexion, progressing to anterior pressure over C1 in this position.

It can be seen that there are a number of different choices for localizing the source of headache by movement and palpation of the cervical spine; however, care must be taken to relate the choice of technique to the position in relation to physiologic movements as well as to the reproduction of symptoms by palpation.

The treatment progression described relates to improvement of symptoms. However, if symptoms do not improve, the same progression is made. If finally there is no improvement with this progression, then the position that reproduces the symptoms most strongly is combined with the treatment techniques that also increase the symptoms. If still no improvement is forthcoming, then passive movement procedures will not help the patient's symptoms.

MIDDLE CERVICAL SPINE (C3 TO C5)

In the middle cervical spine (C3 to C5), the movements of rotation and lateral flexion occur together. It seems most likely that the movements of lateral flexion and rotation occur in the same direction, with lateral flexion to the right being combined with rotation to the right.[1] This is at least partly due to the shape of the joint surfaces, but is also affected by the soft-tissue structures between the bony articulations and the structures between the neural foramina and vertebral canal. Different movements of the cervical spine, such as flexion with lateral flexion in one direction and rotation in the same direction, can cause stretching or compressing effects of the intervertebral joints on either side. When flexion is performed in the sagittal plane, the articular surfaces of the zygapophyseal joint slide on one another, with the inferior articular facet of the superior vertebra sliding cephalad on the superior articular facet of the inferior vertebra, while at the same time the interbody space is narrowed anteriorly and widened posteriorly. Rotation to the left and left lateral flexion cause the right zygapophyseal joint to open. While these movements of lateral flexion and rotation result in a similar upward motion of the superior on the inferior facet, they are not identical movements to those that occur with flexion.

Consider the movements of the cervical spine in relation to the facet joints. With the movement of lateral flexion and rotation to the right, such as of the fourth cervical vertebra (C4) on the fifth (C5), the right inferior facet of C4 slides down the right superior facet of C5. A similar movement on the right side occurs in extension. Therefore, there is some similarity in terms of direction of movement of the right facet joint in movements of extension, right lateral flexion, and right rotation. The facet joint on the opposite side moves upward during each movement (except with extension).

Examination by Combined Movements

Because of the combination of movements that occurs in the cervical spine, the examination of a patient's movements must be expanded to incorporate these principles. There are times when it is inadequate to examine the basic movements of flexion, extension, lateral flexion, and rotation, and other movements combining these basic movements must be examined. Aspects of this concept have been described previously.[7] The symptoms and signs produced by examining movements involving rotatory or lateral flexion, performed while the spine is maintained in the neutral position in relation to other movements, can be quite different from the signs and symptoms produced when the same movements are performed with the spine in flexion or extension. Testing movements while the spine is maintained in flexion or extension may accentuate or reduce symptoms or may even change local spinal pain to referred pain.[7,10]

The range of movement possible in the neutral position will be different from that obtained when movements are done in combined positions. For example, the range of rotation or lateral flexion may be greater when these movements are performed in the neutral position than when they are performed in the fully flexed position. In addition to differences in range of movement, there is also much greater stretching or compression of structures on either side.

Examining the cervical spine by combining movements will assist in the treatment program[7,10]

By establishing the type of movement pattern that is present.

By assisting in the selection of a treatment technique, the direction of the technique, and the position of the joint on which the technique is to be performed.

By predicting the response of the patient's symptoms to a treatment technique.

Movement Patterns

There are two types of patterns. These are (1) regular, and (2) irregular.

Regular Patterns

These are patterns in which similar movements at the intervertebral joint produce the same symptoms whenever they are performed, although the symptoms may differ in quality or severity. Regular patterns can further be subdivided into compressing or stretching patterns. If the patient's symptoms are produced on the side to which the movement is directed, then the pattern is a compressing pattern. That is, compressing movements produce the symptoms. If the symptoms are produced on the side opposite to that to which the movement is directed, then the pattern can be considered a stretching pattern. Examples of regular compressing patterns are:

1. Right cervical rotation produces right suprascapular pain, which is made worse when the same movement is performed in extension and eased when it is performed in flexion.
2. Cervical extension produces right suprascapular pain, which is made worse when right rotation is added to the extension and further increased when right lateral flexion is added.

Examples of regular stretching patterns are:

1. Right lateral flexion of the cervical spine produces left suprascapular pain, which is accentuated when the same movement is performed in flexion and eased when it is performed in extension.
2. Flexion of the cervical spine produces left suprascapular pain which is made worse when right lateral flexion is added and further increased when right rotation is added.

This simple explanation cannot be universally applied because the biomechanics of spinal movement are complex and have yet to be fully described. Influences such as the changing instantaneous axes of rotation of the vertebrae complicate the situation. The explanation conveyed in this chapter refers to simple physiologic patterns of movement and to those patterns that occur in association with accessory movements; for example, pain and restriction of movement on extension of the lower cervical spine being matched by similar restriction with posterior/anterior pressure over the spinous process of C5.

Irregular Patterns

All patterns of movement that are not regular as defined above fall into the category of irregular patterns. With irregular patterns there is not the same consistency of symptoms as described, and stretching and compressing movements do not follow any recognizable pattern. There does not appear to be a regular relationship between the examination findings obtained when combining movements with either the compressing or stretching components of the movements. Rather, there is an apparent random reproduction of symptoms despite the combining of movements that have similar stretching and compressing effects on the structure on either side of the spine. An example of an irregular pattern of movement is as follows: right rotation of the cervical spine produces right suprascapular pain (a compressing test movement), which is made worse when right rotation is performed in flexion (a stretching movement), and eased when the movement is performed in extension (a compressing movement).

There are many examples of irregular patterns, which frequently indicate that there is more than one component to a particular disorder; for example, the zygapophyseal joint, interbody joint, and canal and foraminal structures may all contribute to symptoms. Generally, traumatic injuries, such as whiplash and other traumatic causes of pain, do not exhibit regular patterns of movement. Nontraumatic zygapophyseal and interbody joint disorders on the other hand, tend to be manifest with regular patterns of movement.

Confirmation of Findings by Palpation

As with the high cervical spine, signs found on physiologic movements can be confirmed by palpation. If, for example, right-sided mid-cervical pain occurs with right rotation and this pain is accentuated when right rotation is performed in extension, these findings may be confirmed by comparing responses to anterior and posterior palpation. Using this example and assuming an articular problem between C4 and C5, anterior pressure on the right, directed caudally over the anterior tubercle of C4, will increase the symptoms, whereas anterior pressure on the right directed caudally over C5 will decrease the symptoms. A comparison of these findings with those found by posterior palpation is useful. Posterior palpation directed caudally over the right inferior articulation of C4 will increase the symptoms, while posterior pressure directed caudally over the right superior articulation of C5 will decrease the symptoms.

Treatment

The use of combined movements assists in selecting the technique of treatment by indicating to the therapist how the symptoms vary when similar movements are performed in different positions.

Regular Patterns

When a patient presents with symptoms related to a regular pattern of movement, the treatment technique chosen is usually the one that is found on examination to involve the most painful direction of movement, but it is performed in the least painful way. For example, in a patient with right suprascapular pain, right lateral flexion of the cervical spine will reproduce the pain, and the pain will be further increased when the movement of right lateral flexion is performed in extension, and will be eased when it is performed in flexion. Similarly, when right lateral flexion is sustained (a movement that produced the right suprascapular pain) and flexion is added, the pain eases, and when extension is added the pain increases. When each of these movements is done in extension, the pain is increased, but when the movements are performed in flexion the pain is eased. Thus the general technique of right lateral flexion is initially performed in flexion and then progressed to extension as the symptoms improve.

Similar principles can apply when using accessory movements. Considering the same example used previously, unilateral posteroanterior pressure on the right C4-C5 zygapophyseal joint may produce maximum symptoms when the cervical spine is placed in the position of right lateral flexion and right rotation. Unilateral pressure on the right of C4, pushing the inferior articulation of C4 caudad, may be performed with the head and neck in the neutral position, and this can be progressed to performing the same procedure with the head and neck in right lateral flexion and right rotation as the symptoms improve. The physical therapist would commence by performing the technique in the neutral position, then progress to the most painful combined position.

Irregular Patterns

The direction of movement chosen for treatment in cases in which there are irregular patterns of movement may also be the most painful movement performed in the least painful way. For example, if right lateral flexion produces right suprascapular pain that eases when done in extension and worsens when performed in flexion, then the chosen direction of treatment would be right lateral flexion in extension. However, when there is an irregular pattern of combined movements, the response to treatment is less predictable. In other words, performing right lateral flexion in extension (the least painful position) may improve the most painful examination movement (lateral flexion in flexion), or the treatment technique may actually increase the pain experienced (i.e., there may be a random response to the technique).

When the disorder is characterized by severe pain or is very irritable, the least painful direction of movement should be used as a technique in the least painful combined position.

Techniques of Treatment

It is not possible in an introductory chapter such as this to describe the many positions that may be selected in treatment. A manual of technique would be required for that purpose.[10] However, five treatment techniques are described. Most cervical physiologic movements are examined in the upright position. As a consequence, the first four techniques described are performed in that position and are described for C4-C5.

Right Rotation in the Neutral Position (Fig. 9-21). The therapist stands on the right side of the patient. The pad of the left middle finger is placed over the left superior articulation of C5. The pad of the left index finger is placed on the left side of the spinous process of C4, with the left thumb on the right superior articulation of C5. The right arm holds the head so that the right middle finger is placed on the left inferior articulation of C4. In this position mobilization of C4 is performed by moving the right arm while stabilizing C5 with the left hand.

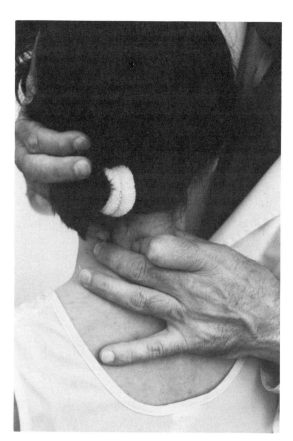

Fig. 9-21. Right rotation in the neutral position.

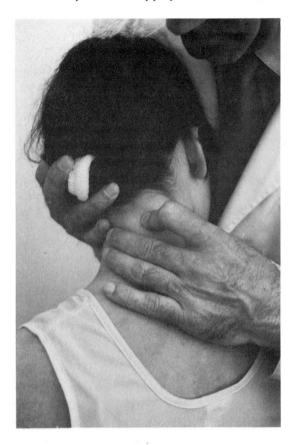

Fig. 9-22.   Right rotation in the flexion position.

Right Rotation in the Flexion Position (Fig. 9-22). The same hand positions are adopted as described for right rotation in neutral, but the cervical spine is in flexion.

Right Lateral Flexion in the Neutral Position (Fig. 9-23). The therapist's left hand is placed in the same position as described previously. The therapist's right little finger is placed over the left inferior articulation of C4, with the fingers of the right hand spread over the left side of the cervical spine. Right lateral flexion is done with the right hand laterally flexing at C4, while C5 is fixed by the left hand.

Right Lateral Flexion in the Flexion Position (Fig. 9-24). The same hand positions are adopted as described for right lateral flexion in neutral, but the cervical spine is in flexion.

Right Unilateral Posteroanterior Pressure in Right Rotation and Flexion (Fig. 9-25). The patient lies prone with the neck flexed and rotated to the right. The therapist's thumbs are placed on the right C4-5 zygapophyseal joint, with the

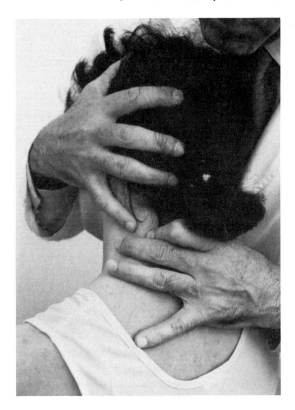

Fig. 9-23. Right lateral flexion in the neutral position.

fingers placed lightly over either side of the cervical spine. The direction of the mobilization is cephalad.

Predicting the Response to a Technique

The use of combined movements and movement patterns can assist in predicting the result of treatment. With regular patterns of movement, the least painful movement on examination improves before the most painful. For example, if right lateral flexion in a neutral position produces the patient's right suprascapular pain, and this pain is made worse when the movement is done in extension, then right lateral flexion in neutral will improve before right lateral flexion in extension.

It may also be expected that a treatment technique of right lateral flexion done in flexion, found on examination to be a painless position, will be unlikely to make the symptoms worse.

The response in the case of irregular patterns of movement is not as predictable, and the improvement in the symptoms may occur in an apparently random fashion. Most examinations of the cervical spine are done with the patient in the upright position; however, the treatment techniques for problems involving

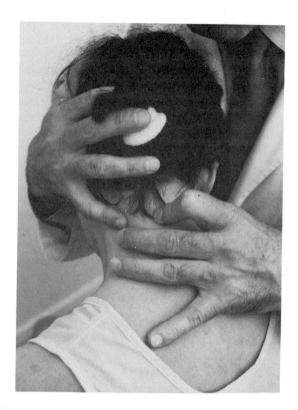

Fig. 9-24. Right lateral flexion in the flexion position.

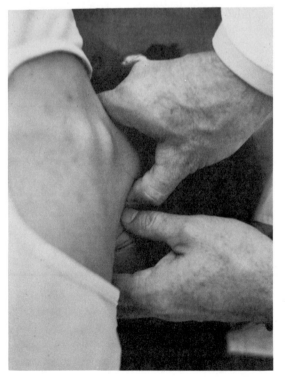

Fig. 9-25. Right unilateral posteroanterior pressure in right rotation and flexion.

this area are frequently performed with the patient prone or supine. Because of the altered weight distribution and position of canal structures when adopting the supine, prone, or side-lying positions, there may be some alteration in the pain response when the movements are compared with those in the upright position. Consequently, for a technique chosen because it produced particular symptoms in the upright position, it is important that the treatment position adopted must be adjusted in such a way as to produce the same signs and symptoms.

LOWER CERVICAL SPINE (C6 TO T1)

Because of the change in shape from lordosis in the mid-cervical spine to kyphosis in the thoracic spine, the change in shape of the vertebral bodies, and the attachment of the first rib to the first thoracic vertebra, the lower cervical spine should be examined as a separate unit.

Examination by Combined Movements

The same principles of combining movements apply to the lower cervical spine as for the mid-cervical spine (C2 to C5); however, the first rib limits the amount of movement available. The techniques of examination, while the same as for the mid-cervical unit, must include palpation of the first rib. This should be performed with the lower cervical spine in combined movement positions. Figures 9-26 and 9-27 illustrate palpation techniques for the lower cervical spine.

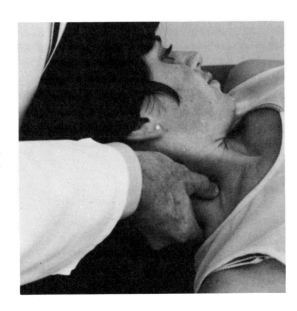

Fig. 9-26. Anterior palpation of the right lower cervical spine in flexion and left rotation.

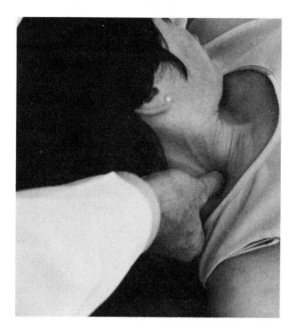

Fig. 9-27. Anterior palpation of the right first rib with the neck in flexion and left rotation.

Anterior Palpation of the Right Lower Cervical Spine with the Head and Neck in Flexion and Left Rotation

With the patient supine, the therapist's left hand placed under the occiput flexes and rotates the patient's head and neck to the left (Fig. 9-26). The therapist's right thumb pad is placed over the right inferior articulation of C6 anteriorly. If pressure is directed caudally at this level, it will tend to decrease the effect of the right rotation between C6 and C7.

Anterior Palpation of the Right First Rib with the Head and Neck in Flexion and Left Rotation

The position of the patient and of the therapist's left hand is as described for Figure 9-26. With this technique however, the therapist's right thumb pad is placed over the first rib anteriorly and mobilization is performed (Fig. 9-27). The lower cervical spine, including the first rib, is an area that causes a large percentage of symptoms distributed to the upper thoracic and upper limb areas. Anterior palpation in combined positions of the neck, as well as palpation of the first rib, is an important diagnostic procedure for pain distributed to the upper limb. In performing these testing procedures, care must be taken that the shoulder and arm remain in the neutral position.

Treatment

The palpation procedures are performed in the neutral position for the offending joint, and as the symptoms improve, the position is progressively changed to the most painful position.

In summary, the importance of relating symptoms and signs to physiologic movements in combined positions has been emphasized. Not only will combined movements highlight clinical findings, but they will also reveal patterns of movement that will assist in selecting treatment techniques and in predicting the response to treatment.

ACKNOWLEDGMENTS

I would like to thank Mr. D. Watkins, photographer, School of Physiotherapy, Curtin University of Technology, for his assistance with the photographs.

REFERENCES

1. Stoddard A: Manual of Osteopathic Practice. Hutchinson, London, 1969
2. Stoddard A: Manual of Osteopathic Technique, Hutchinson, London, 1962
3. Jackson R: Headaches associated with disorders of the cervical spine. Headache 6:175, 1967
4. Braakman R, Penning L: Injuries of the Cervical Spine. Excerpta Medica, Amsterdam, 1971
5. Worth DR, Selvik G: Movements of the craniovertebral joints. p. 53. In Grieve GP (ed): Modern Manual Therapy of the Vertebral Column. Churchill Livingstone, Edinburgh, 1986
6. Edwards BC: Combined movements of the lumbar spine. Examination and clinical significance. Aust J Physiother 24:147, 1979
7. Edwards BC: Combined movements in the cervical spine (C2–7). Their value in examination and technique choice. Aust J Physiother 26:165, 1980
8. Edwards BC: Combined movements in the lumbar spine: their use in examination and treatment, p. 561. In Grieve GP (ed): Modern Manual Therapy of the Vertebral Column. Churchill Livingstone, Edinburgh, 1986
9. Edwards BC: Examination of the high cervical spine (Occiput–C2) using combined movements, p. 512. In Grieve GP (ed): Modern Manual Therapy of the Vertebral Column. Churchill Livingstone, Edinburgh, 1986
10. Edwards BC: Manual of Combined Movements. Churchill Livingstone, Edinburgh, 1992

10 | Muscles and Motor Control in Cervicogenic Disorders: Assessment and Management

Vladimir Janda

It is no longer necessary to stress the importance of muscles in the pathogenesis of various pain syndromes of the musculoskeletal system. This is because of the now well recognized fact, applied in clinical practice, that effective protection of the joints depends largely on the appropriate functioning of the muscle system. It has also been recognized that the dysfunctions of muscles and joints are so closely related that the two should be considered as a single, inseparable functional unit, and should be assessed, analyzed, and treated together. Although the causal relationship of muscles and joints in the pathogenesis of individual syndromes may still be a matter of discussion, practical clinical experience shows that the predominant influence of all (or almost all) techniques used in modern manual therapy is on muscles. Improvement of joint function depends to a large extent on the improvement in function of those muscles that have an anatomic or functional relationship to that joint. This is true even for those manipulative techniques employing high-velocity thrust (with impulse), which were initially thought to influence the restriction of joint movement only. It is even more true for the soft mobilization techniques, muscle energy procedures, and post-isometric relaxation or myofascial release techniques, to mention only those most frequently used. In this respect, the entire philosophy of how a particular therapeutic procedure works has to be re-evaluated.

In conditions with acute pain, the increase in muscle tone plays the decisive role in pain production. In this respect, it has been suggested[1,2] that the increased muscle tone (muscle spasm) is probably the link in the pathogenetic chain that is necessary to perceive a joint dysfunction as a painful condition. Without the development of muscle spasm, the joint dysfunction usually remains painless. For this reason, muscle spasm should be given special attention in both the assessment and treatment of painful disorders of the cervical and thoracic spine. According to this view, use of the term "painful joint" within the range of musculoskeletal disorders may be simplistic and misleading, and it should perhaps be used as a clinical descriptor only, when analyzing the function of many body structures.

Muscles play an extremely important role in the pathogenesis and management of various syndromes. It is therefore surprising that the analysis of muscle function has not been developed as precisely as the examination of joints. Many therapists underestimate the importance of precise muscle analysis, and are therefore likely to misinterpret clinical findings. For example, painful areas on the occiput are often considered to reflect periosteal pain or a painful posterior arch of the atlas,[2a] despite the fact that they may well be occurring at the insertions of muscles in spasm.

While the treatment of acute painful dysfunctions are less challenging, the treatment of chronic disorders, and particularly the prevention of recurrences of acute pain, are major challenges. It should be mentioned that from the socioeconomic aspect, chronic disorders of the spine are extremely costly. Although they represent only about 6 to 10 percent of all painful conditions of the musculoskeletal system, they consume about 80 percent of the costs.[3] The high incidence of neck pain in the community demands that special attention be given to determining its origin, so that appropriate preventive and therapeutic measures may be taken.

THE ROLE OF MUSCLES AS A PATHOGENETIC FACTOR IN PAIN PRODUCTION

When considering the role of muscles in a specific syndrome, at least two factors have to be taken into consideration: the presence of an acutely painful condition and the background against which this painful condition developed.

In acute pain, the role of a muscle as a pathogenetic factor can be explained in the following ways:

- Irritation from pain produces increased muscle tone, which leads to the placing of the involved spinal segment in a painless position.[4] In this case, the irritation and altered proprioceptive input from the joint are probably essential in producing muscle spasm, while a decrease in spasm leads to the relief of pain.

- An initial increase in muscle tone decreases mobility in the involved spinal segment (joint blockage) and causes pain. This is illustrated by the tension headache, which is triggered by increased muscle tone, such as in stress-induced situations (through increased activity of the limbic system) or as a defensive reaction associated with overactivation of virtually all of the neck muscles.
- Trigger points develop in predictable locations, with local and referred pain occurring in typical patterns.[5] The trigger points also represent areas of increased localized muscle tone.

A poor body alignment with a forward head posture and typical muscle imbalance is not only a predisposing but also a perpetuating factor, in chronic disorders, episodic pain, and/or chronic discomfort, and may lead to chronicity as well as to accidental decompensation and recurrent episodes of various acute pain syndromes.

In considering the role of muscles in the development of neck pain, the function of muscles of the shoulder as well as the neck merits a review.

The cervical spine is the most intricate region of the spine, and so are the muscles of this region. All movements of the arm, whether fast or slow, resisted or unresisted, require activation of the shoulder or neck musculature or both, in particular the upper trapezius, levator scapulae, and deep intrinsic muscles. Muscle recruitment will be more pronounced if the patient carries heavy loads or has developed poor motor habits.

Muscles of the neck and shoulder region always function as a unit, and there is no movement in the upper extremity that would not be reflected in the neck musculature. However, in some activities, this coordination can only be hypothesized, as it is very difficult to measure the activation of the deep intrinsic muscles. Because the coactivity of the neck and shoulder musculature is reflected in the mechanics of the entire shoulder–neck complex, it is often difficult to estimate whether the shoulder or neck was the primary source of a particular dysfunction or pathology. A detailed evaluation usually reveals changes in both areas.

Muscles of the head–neck–shoulder region can be divided into several groups:

1. A superficial spinohumeral layer attaching the shoulder girdle to the spine

2. (a) an intermediate spinocostal layer, which includes the serratus posterior superior and inferior; and (b) deep layers, incorporating the true muscles of the back

3. The anterior neck muscles

4. The hyoid muscles

5. The facial muscles

6. The masticatory muscles

Muscles and Central Nervous System Regulation

Muscles should be considered as lying at a functional crossroads, being strongly influenced by stimuli coming from both the central nervous system and the osteoarticular system.[6,7] In many ways the musculature should be understood as a sensitive, labile system that constantly reflects changes in all parts of the body, and not only in the motor system. This is so with respect to the neck muscles in particular.

Although this chapter is oriented toward clinical practice, a reference to relevant neurophysiologic factors provides a basis for understanding the presentations and assessments of disorders of the cervical and thoracic spine. Central nervous system mechanisms regulate the posture and position of the body in space, and this is reflected in adaptive reactions of the position of the head.[8,9] The latter are in turn reflected in the mechanics of the cervical joints and neck muscles, in particular. These reactions have to be taken into consideration, since they can play a hidden or unrecognized role in understanding a specific syndrome. If the central regulation is impaired, the dysfunction of the musculo-skeletal system becomes more apparent.

On the other hand, the compensatory reflex responses can be effectively used in treatment. For example, the compensatory eye movements may help to relax or inhibit, and/or facilitate specific neck muscle groups. This effect is widely used as a supportive factor in mobilization techniques involving the upper part of the body, and particularly in the post-isometric relaxation and proprioceptive neuromuscular facilitation (PNF) techniques.[10] According to clinical experience, a more pronounced relaxation of the neck muscles can be achieved while sitting with crossed legs than sitting with the legs parallel. This observation can be applied effectively in physical therapy to achieve a better relaxation of the neck muscles before a specific treatment. It could also be used to help the patient to relax at work when a constrained position creates discomfort in the neck muscles. Further, the brain stem reflexes commonly used in motor re-education in cases of upper motor neuron lesions can be effectively used in improving upper body control. It has to be borne in mind that the neck muscles not only have a motion and stabilization function, but are also strongly involved in the regulatory mechanism of posture. Indeed, this proprioceptive function of short, deep neck extensors is so strong that these muscles are often considered more as proprioceptive organs than as activators of movement.[11]

Neck muscles show a strong tendency to develop hypertonus and spasm, and not only for the reasons mentioned above. It has been shown[12] that afferent fibers constitute up to 80 percent of neck muscles, by comparison to most other striated muscles, which contain approximately 50 percent of such fibers. This may explain a greater sensitivity of the neck musculature to any situation that alters the proprioceptive input from cervical structures. Joint-motion restriction is such a situation.

The shoulder–neck muscle complex belongs to the part of the body that is strongly influenced by the functional status of the central nervous system, and particularly of the limbic system. This is reflected primarily in an increase in tone in terms of muscle spasm, and by a decreased ability to perform fine, economically coordinated movements.

The role of the limbic system in motor control and the quality of muscle tension has been a neglected area in physical therapy. The limbic system is a phylogenetically old part of the brain, and in humans is entirely covered by the more recently evolved neocortex. It comprises a number of structures with numerous connections to the frontal motor cortex, hypothalamus, and brain stem. The limbic system was originally and imprecisely named the rhinencephalon (olfactory brain).[8]

The limbic system regulates human emotions, and this control involves somatomotor, autonomic, and endocrine systems. It is closely associated with learning (including motor learning) and motor activation. It serves as a trigger to voluntary movements, and regulates pain perception and motivation.[8,13] All of these functions can substantially influence a physiotherapeutic result. The greatest influence of the limbic system is on the shoulder/neck area, and it is therefore not surprising that any function of the limbic system will be more evident here than in another part of the body.

Because the limbic system is very sensitive to stress,[13] it is not difficult to understand that its dysfunction, which influences numerous functions of the human body, can be reflected in an industrialized society by a gradually increasing number of disorders marked by musculoskeletal pain. This is particularly so with respect to various cervicocranial syndromes. An improved function of the limbic system, with a consequent improvement in the general regulatory system of the body, can be mistakenly explained as a positive result of a local physiotherapeutic procedure. This can be seen in the results of an unpublished study conducted by our group, in which a 4-week therapeutic stay in a spa facility, the main focus of which was treatment of chronic low back pain syndromes, produced the greatest improvement in cervicogenic syndromes, which were not specifically treated. It might be hypothesized that the calming environment of the spa influenced the function of the limbic system, which contributed significantly to the general therapeutic effect. This observation should be a reminder that evaluation of a particular therapeutic procedure, particularly one involving the neck area, should be done under conditions of careful control.

Of particular importance to conditions affecting the shoulder–neck muscle complex are the defense reflexes and defense behavior, which are closely associated with the limbic/hypothalamic system. These are expressions of anger and fear in humans. Besides the autonomic reactions, which are mainly associated with increased activity of the sympathetic system, there is a strong reaction in the head–neck–shoulder muscles, with their increased activation resulting in the adoption of a typical posture intended to protect the head. The head is poked forward and retracted between the elevated shoulders. This position is exactly the same as occurs in the upper crossed syndrome (see Fig. 10-1). Both the defense reaction and the muscle imbalance can thus potentiate the overstress of predicted segments, resulting in typical syndromes.

Although under physiologic conditions both the postural reflexes (tonic neck reflexes, deep tonic neck reflexes, righting reflexes) and the statokinetic

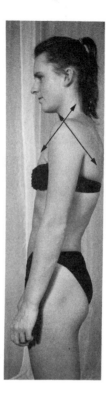

Fig. 10-1. The upper crossed syndrome.

reflexes are suppressed and inhibited (but not abolished), they influence the fine control of posture of the body and of the head in particular. This is associated especially with an increased activation of the neck and head extensors. Although these reflexes are difficult to measure under physiologic conditions in humans, their influence has to be presumed, and should be reflected in physical therapists' thinking.

Other important functional relationships also affect the shoulder–neck muscle complex, although the associated activity may often be remote. For example, the neck muscles are included in one of the most important life-preserving movement patterns—the prehension pattern—and because of this any movement of the upper extremity has to be associated with at least some activation of the neck muscles. This activation is initiated by the reflex mechanism and continued by biomechanical reaction. Therefore, as previously stated, any movement of the upper extremity has an influence on head and neck position.

The position of the head and cervical spine, and therefore the activation of muscles in these areas, adapts to any alteration of position of the lower part of the body, and particularly of the pelvis. Any scoliosis or scoliotic posture, or asymmetric position of the pelvis due to dysfunction of the pelvis itself or as a response, for example, to a leg-length asymmetry, will be reflected in the regulatory readjustment of the neck muscles to maintain equilibrium and an adequate position of the head. This regulatory control is primarily triggered reflexively, although it is potentiated by necessary biomechanical compensation.

The mutual influence of remote areas of the body on the neck muscles occurs, however, in even less obvious situations. In an unpublished electromyographic (EMG) study, we were able to demonstrate that even an unresisted but not well coordinated hip extension movement, performed in a prone position, is associated with an unwanted, increased activation of a majority of neck and shoulder muscles, resulting in a rotation and anterior tilt of the vertebrae of the lower cervical spine. Hyperextension of the hip joint is an essential part of the normal gait pattern. It can therefore be hypothesized that such a rotation and anterior tilt (which is no doubt the result of activation of the deep intrinsic neck muscles) will occur during each step of walking. This means that the lower cervical spine is exposed to repetitive, constrained additional and unwanted movements. This mechanism might help to explain the recurrence of neck syndromes or discomfort.

It should be kept in mind that the muscular response in such reflex mechanisms usually occurs early and distinctly.

The muscles of the upper part of the body have been studied electromyographically to a much lesser extent than those of the lower body. There are several reasons for this. A partial, obvious explanation is the larger size and greater accessibility of muscles of the lower part of the body. Further, the study of the upper body muscles requires more sophisticated EMG techniques; indeed, some muscles are accessible only under radiographic control.

The biomechanical function of the upper body muscles is also less well known, and more complex than that of the lower body muscles, and is a subject of controversy. This is true not only for the primary function of muscles or muscle groups, but also with respect to their synkinetic functions. For example, the explanation of the function of the accessory muscles of respiration has greatly changed[14,15]; the synkinetic movements of the head during chewing remain almost totally neglected; and the paradoxical function of the scaleni has not yet been analyzed. Particular attention should also be paid to the hyoid muscles. Although they may be a frequent source of headache[5] and other syndromes, they are not investigated as they should be. Neglecting them may lead to an incorrect diagnosis and disappointing results of therapy.

SIGNIFICANCE OF MUSCLE IMBALANCE AND ALTERED MOVEMENT PATTERNS

From the functional viewpoint, three basic dysfunctions should be considered in connection with disorders involving the muscles of the head and neck:

1. Muscle imbalance, characterized by the development of impaired relationships between muscles prone to tightness and those prone to inhibition and weakness.

2. Altered movement patterns, usually closely related to muscle imbalance.

3. Trigger points within muscles, and local and referred pain originating from these points.

Muscle imbalance describes the situation in which some muscles become inhibited and therefore weak while others become tight, losing their extensibility. Muscle tightness is generally a consequence of chronic overuse, and tight muscles therefore usually maintain their strength. However, in extreme and/ or long-lasting tightness, a decrease in muscle strength occurs. This phenomenon has been described as "tightness weakness."[16] Stretching of tight muscles may lead to recovery of their strength. Additionally, stretching of tight muscles results in improved activation of the antagonist (inhibited) muscles, probably mediated via Sherrington's law of reciprocal inhibition.

Muscle tightness (decreased flexibility or decreased extensibility, muscle stiffness, taughtness) should not be confused with other types of increased muscle tone, since each type is of different genesis and requires a different type of treatment. This confusion occurs particularly in relation to the scaleni, since inhibition and commonly spasm and/or trigger points in these muscles are mistakenly diagnosed as tightness. In the proximal part of the body, the following muscles tend to develop tightness: pectoralis major and minor, upper trapezius, levator scapulae, and sternocleidomastoid. While detailed analysis of the following muscles still remains to be undertaken, it is considered that the masseter, temporalis, digastric, and the small muscles connecting the occiput and cervical spine (the recti and obliques) also tend to become tight.

Muscles that tend to develop weakness and inhibition are the lower stabilizers of the scapula (serratus anterior, rhomboids, middle and lower trapezius), deep neck flexors, suprahyoid, and mylohyoid.

The reaction of the longus colli, longus capitis, rectus capitis anterior, subscapularis, supraspinatus, infraspinatus, and teres major and minor remains unclear. It should be emphasized that our knowledge of the function of the muscles of the neck region is inadequate, and that many current concepts relating to them may well undergo change.

The tendency of some muscles to develop inhibition or tightness is not random, but occurs as a systematic dysfunction associated with "muscle imbalance patterns."[6,7] The muscle imbalance does not remain limited to a certain part of the body, but gradually involves the entire muscle system. Since the muscle imbalance usually precedes the appearance of a pain syndrome, a thorough evaluation can be of substantial help in introducing measures to prevent this.

In adults, a muscle imbalance is usually more evident in the lower part of the body, and may precede the development of muscle imbalance in the upper part. The imbalance in the upper part of the body forms the "proximal or shoulder crossed syndrome." This is characterized by tightness and increased activation of the levator scapulae, upper trapezius, sternocleidomastoid, and pectoral muscles, and by weakness of the lower stabilizers of the scapula and the deep neck flexors. Topographically, when the weakened and shortened muscles are connected they form a cross (Fig. 10-1). This pattern of muscle imbalance produces typical changes in posture and motion. In standing, elevation and protraction of the shoulders are evident, as are also rotation and abduction of the scapulae, a variable degree of winging of the scapulae, and a forward head posture. This altered posture is likely to stress the cervicocranial and cervicothoracic junctions and the transitory segments at the level of C4 and C5. Further, the stability of the glenohumeral joint is decreased, owing to the altered angle of the glenoid fossa.

According to Basmajian,[17] almost no muscle activity is needed to keep the head of the humerus firmly in the glenoid fossa under normal conditions. In the proximal crossed syndrome, however, the biomechanical conditions change substantially. The plane of the glenoid fossa becomes more vertical because of the abduction, rotation, and winging of the scapula. Maintaining the humeral head in the glenoid fossa then provokes increased activity in the levator scapulae and trapezius. This occurs not only when the arm is used in vigorous movements, but also with the arm hanging by the side of the body. Such increased activity tends to lead to spasm and tightness in these muscles, which in turn augment the improper position of the scapula; thus a vicious cycle develops. It may be hypothesized that abnormalities in proprioceptive stimulation result and lead to dystrophic changes in the shoulder joint.

Muscle imbalance in children, in contrast to that in adults, usually starts in the upper part of the body. Why this development in children contrasts with that in adults has not been satisfactorily explained. It is presumed that the main reason for it has to do with the relatively large and heavy head of the child, which is supported by comparatively weak neck muscles, and with the fact that the center of gravity of the child's head is located forward, but is gradually shifted backward into a well balanced position during growth. In accord with the more evident muscle imbalance in the upper part of the body in children is the clinical observation that various syndromes originating in the neck, such as acute wry neck or "school headache," are common in children, whereas syndromes related to other segments of the spine are rare.

The muscles involved in the layer (stratification) syndrome[18] in the proximal part of the body are the same as those involved in the proximal (shoulder-neck) crossed syndrome.

EVALUATION OF MUSCLE IMBALANCE AND ALTERED MOVEMENT PATTERNS IN THE UPPER BODY

The assessment of muscle imbalance and altered movement patterns is undertaken in three stages: evaluation during standing, examination of muscle tightness, and examination of movement patterns. A great part of the assessment is based on visual observation. However, *deep palpation* helps to evaluate muscle tone, whether increased or decreased, and helps in estimating the type of increase in muscle tone. Limbic dysfunction in the upper part of the body will include hypertonicity of mimetic, masticatory, and hyoid muscles, as well as of the whole shoulder neck region, including the short neck extensors. The most obvious palpatory findings are in the area of the upper trapezius, levator scapulae, and deep short extensors of the neck. In this type of muscle hypertonicity, constant EMG activity at rest can generally be found.[19] At trigger points, increased tone and taut bands can be palpated, as described in detail by Travell and Simons.[5]

Analysis of Muscles in Standing

The analysis of the muscles of the lower part of the body in standing has been described elsewhere.[20] In this chapter, attention will be focused on analysis of the muscles in the upper part of the body, although the evaluations in the two regions cannot be separated. In addition, all other deviations of posture should be taken into consideration.

The patient is first observed from behind, noting particularly any changes in the interscapular space and in the position of the scapulae. Where there is weakness of the interscapular muscles (rhomboids, middle trapezius), the interscapular space will appear flattened (Fig. 10-2). In the case of a pronounced weakness already associated with some atrophy, a hollowing instead of a flattening may appear. In addition, the distance between the thoracic spinous processes and the medial border of the scapula is increased because of the rotation

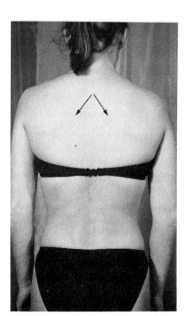

Fig. 10-2. Flattening of the interscapular space as a sign of weakness of the rhomboids and middle trapezius muscles.

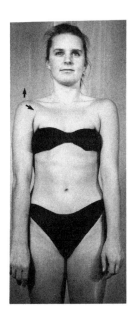

Fig. 10-3. Protracted, elevated, and medially rotated shoulders as a sign of a combined tightness of the pectoralis major, upper trapezius and latissimus dorsi muscles.

of the scapula. Improper fixation of the inferior angle to the rib cage and a winging scapula indicate weakness of the serratus anterior muscle.

Tightness of the upper trapezius and levator scapulae muscles, which almost invariably accompanies this weakness, can be seen in the neck–shoulder line. Where there is tightness of the trapezius only, the contour will straighten. If the tightness of the levator scapulae predominates, the contour of the neck line will appear as a double wave in the area of insertion of the muscle on the scapula. This straightening of the neck–shoulder line is sometimes described as "gothic" shoulders, since it is reminiscent of the form of a gothic church tower. In addition, there is an elevation of the shoulder girdle. Observation and palpation of the descending fibers of the trapezius along the cervical spine may reveal broadening and changed elasticity. Where there are tight pectoral muscles, there may be protraction of the shoulder girdle.

When observing the patient from the front, the belly of the pectoralis major should be observed first. The tighter (or stronger) the muscle, the more prominent it will be. Typical imbalance will lead to rounded and protracted shoulders and slight medial rotation of the arms (Fig. 10-3).

Much information can be obtained from observation of the anterior neck and throat. Normally, the sternocleidomastoid is just visible. Prominence of the insertion of the muscle, and particularly of its clavicular insertion, is a sign of tightness. A groove along this muscle is an early sign of weakness of the deep neck flexors (Fig. 10-4). The deep neck flexors tend to weaken and atrophy quickly, and, this sign, among others, has therefore been proposed as a reliable way in which to estimate biological age.[21] Straightening of the throat line is usually a sign of increased tone of the digastric muscle. Palpation frequently

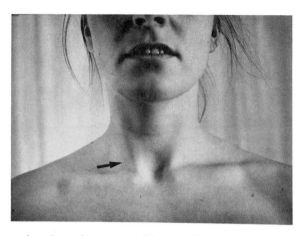

Fig. 10-4. Deepening along the sternocleidomastoid muscle as a sign of weak or atrophied deep neck flexors.

reveals trigger points. Careful examination of this muscle is extremely important, since pain referred from it is often misinterpreted.[5]

Head posture should also be observed. From the viewpoint of muscle analysis, a forward head posture is due to weakness of the deep neck flexors and dominance, or even tightness, of the sternocleidomastoid. During observation of the forward head posture, it is important to note the degree of cervical lordosis and the extent of the thoracic kyphosis.

Testing of Muscle Tightness (Flexibility, Extensibility, Stiffness, Tautness)

Although it is highly important, flexibility of the muscles of the upper part of the body is often ignored, in examination of the cervical and thoracic spine, and even worse, muscle tightness may be confused with increased activation of the particular muscle, with hypertonicity of various types,[19] and most frequently with trigger points. (Trigger points in muscles and myofascial pain in general are considered to be important components of pathologic changes in muscles. Physical therapists should be familiar with the palpatory techniques used in their assessment.[4,5]) Although a combination of signs can be found simultaneously in a single muscle, an exact differential diagnosis is the basic presumption for successful and rational treatment.

Because tight muscles influence movement patterns and, as clinical experience reveals, contribute substantially to inhibition of their antagonists, the evaluation of muscle tightness should precede the evaluation of movement patterns and of weakness. It can, however, be combined with palpation and the evaluation of muscle tone.

In the upper part of the body, the upper trapezius, levator scapulae, and pectoralis major are the principal muscles of concern. Other muscles, even the sternocleidomastoid, are difficult to evaluate because their range of movement is limited by joints and/or ligaments.

The extensibility of upper trapezius and levator scapulae is best examined with the patient in the supine position. For testing of the upper trapezius, the patient's head is passively inclined to the contralateral side and flexed, while the shoulder girdle is stabilized. From this position, the shoulder is moved distally (Fig. 10-5). Normally, there is free movement with a soft motion barrier. However, where tightness is present, the range of movement is restricted and the barrier hard. Testing of the levator is done in a similar manner, except that in addition, the head is rotated to the contralateral (i.e., non-tested) side (Fig. 10-6). If the muscle is tight, in addition to the movement restriction, a tender insertion of the levator can be palpated.

The pectoralis major is tested with the patient in the supine position with the arm moved passively into abduction. It is important that the trunk be stabilized before the arm is placed into abduction, since a twist of the trunk might suggest a normal range of movement. The arm should reach the horizontal (Fig. 10-7). To estimate the tightness of the clavicular portion, the arm is allowed to loosely hang down while the examiner moves the shoulder posteriorly (Fig. 10-8). Normally, only a slight barrier is felt, but where there is tightness this barrier is hard.

Evaluation of the sternocleidomastoid is difficult and imprecise, since this muscle spans too many motion segments.

The short deep posterior neck muscles (recti and obliques) can be palpated only while the upper cervical segments are passively flexed (Fig. 10-9). Resis-

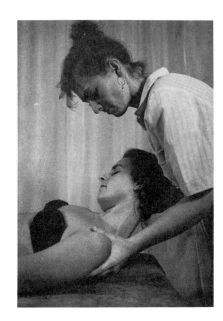

Fig. 10-5. Evaluation of the tightness of the upper trapezius.

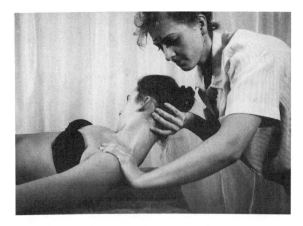

Fig. 10-6. Evaluation of tightness of the levator scapulae.

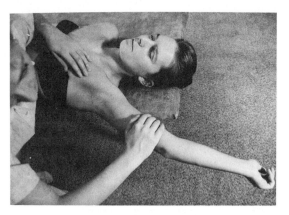

Fig. 10-7. Evaluation of tightness of the sternal portion of the pectoralis major.

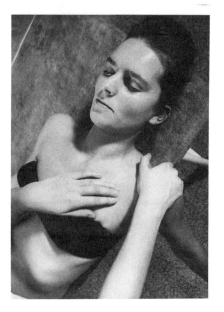

Fig. 10-8. Evaluation of the tightness of the clavicular portion of the pectoralis major.

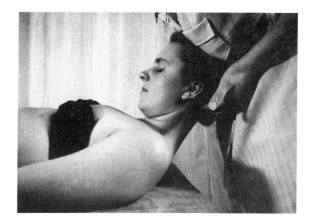

Fig. 10-9.   Evaluation of the deep short neck extensors.

tance felt upon palpation of the proximal segments of the cervical spine is, however, not necessarily indicative of tight musculature.

More specific details of tests of muscle flexibility may be found in texts devoted to this subject.[22,23]

Examination of Movement Patterns and Weakened Muscles

Testing of individual muscles may help to estimate muscle weakness and differentiate weakness due to a lower motor neuron lesion from weakness due to tightness, joint position (stretch), or trigger points, or weakness of arthrogenic origin. The detailed description of all individual muscle tests is beyond the scope of this chapter; such information can be found in other sources.[22–27]

In musculoskeletal disorders, evaluation of the basic movement patterns of different regions of the body is of paramount importance. In the upper part of the body, three movements are of particular value: the push up, head-forward bending, and abduction of the shoulder. An evaluation of movement patterns is usually more sensitive than testing of individual muscle groups, since it reveals minute changes in the coordination and programming of movements. These changes may often be more important for the diagnosis and treatment of a spinal disorder than a simple estimation of individual muscle strength. In other words, the therapist is more concerned with the degree of activation of all of the muscles recruited during a particular movement than with any single muscle, regardless of whether a particular muscle is or is not biomechanically capable of producing that movement.

Head flexion is tested in the supine position. The subject is asked to slowly raise the head in the habitual way. When the deep neck flexors are weak and the sternocleidomastoid strong, the jaw is seen to jut forward at the beginning of the movement, with hyperextension at the cervicocranial junction. An arc-

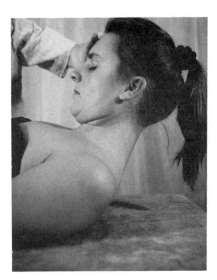

Fig. 10-10. Head flexion pattern, evaluation of weak deep neck flexors.

like flexion follows after approximately 10° of head elevation from the plinth has been achieved. If the pattern is unclear, slight resistance of about 2 to 4 g (one or two fingers pressure) against the forehead may be applied to make the hyperextension more evident. This test provides the therapist with information about the interplay between the deep neck flexors (which tend to become weak) and the sternocleidomastoids (which are usually strong and taut). If the test is performed by jutting the jaw forward, overstress of the cervicocranial junction is likely to exist (Figs. 10-10 and 10-11).

　　Push up from the prone position gives information about the quality of stabilization of the scapula. During push up, and particularly in the first phase of lowering the body from maximum push up, the scapula on the side on which stabilization is impaired glides over the thorax, shifting outward, and upward or rotating, or both (Fig. 10-12). If the serratus anterior does not function properly, winging of the scapula will result. The entire movement must be performed very slowly, or slight muscle weakness and incoordination may be missed. The

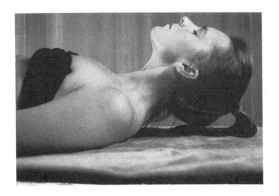

Fig. 10-11. Head flexion pattern; head "pushed forward" position as a sign of the predominance of the sternocleidomastoid muscle.

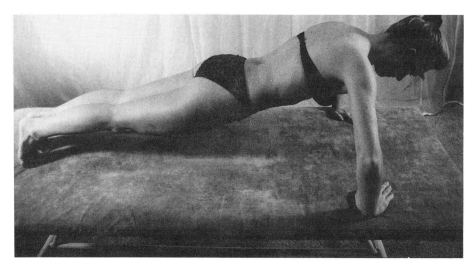

Fig. 10-12. The push up position for evaluation of weak lower stabilizers of the scapulae.

pathologic performance reveals that the movements of the upper extremity are somewhat impaired, and that increased stabilization of the cervical spine is needed.

Shoulder abduction is tested in sitting with the elbow flexed. Elbow flexion controls undesired humeral rotation. The subject slowly abducts the shoulder (Fig. 10-13). During this action, three components of the complex movement are evaluated: abduction at the glenohumeral joint, rotation of the scapula, and elevation of the whole shoulder girdle. Movement is stopped at the point at

Fig. 10-13. Evaluation of shoulder abduction pattern. Note: that three components are evaluated: abduction at the glenohumeral joint, rotation of the scapula, and elevation of the whole shoulder girdle.

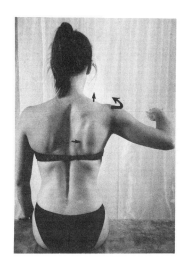

which shoulder girdle elevation commences. This usually occurs when 60° of abduction at the glenohumeral joint has been achieved. The therapist should not be misled by some activation of the trapezii at the start of shoulder abduction. This activity is necessary to stabilize the cervical spine and prevent lateral flexion of the head.

By itself, testing of the movement patterns provides only a basic clinical orientation to a patient's condition. In order to obtain comprehensive information, it is necessary to evaluate muscles and movements with multichannel electromyography. However, this method is unrealistic in a busy practice, since it is extremely time consuming as well as expensive.

HYPERMOBILITY

Muscles can be involved in many other afflictions. With regard to musculoskeletal syndromes, constitutional hypermobility should be considered.

Constitutional hypermobility is a vague, non-progressive clinical syndrome, and not strictly a disease. It is characterized by a general laxity of the connective tissue, ligaments, and muscles, although not to the same extent as in Ehlers–Danlos or Marfan syndromes. Its etiology is unknown, although a congenital insufficiency of mesenchymal tissue is postulated. While it has not been confirmed that "hypermobile" subjects are more prone to musculoskeletal pain syndromes, an instability of these subjects' joints may be evident. The muscles in general show decreased strength, and when subjected to a strength-training program, never develop the hypertrophy and strength of "normal" subjects' muscles. The muscle tone is decreased when assessed by palpation, and there is an increased range of joint movement.

Constitutional hypermobility involves the entire body, although its different parts may not be affected to the same extent, and a slight unilateral asymmetry can be observed. It is more frequent in women than men, and seems to involve the upper part of the body more commonly than the lower. In middle age the hypermobility decreases, in correspondence to the general decrease in range of movement that is seen with aging.

Muscle tightness may also develop in constitutional hypermobility, although this is not so obvious. In clinical practice, such a tightness is mainly considered to be an expression of a compensatory mechanism for improving the stability of the joints. Therefore, stretching should be performed carefully and gently, and should only be applied to key muscles. Stretching is indicated only in a limited number of cases, and should be only done after a thorough evaluation. Because the muscles in cases of constitutional hypermobility are generally weak, they may be easily overused, and trigger points may therefore develop easily in muscles and ligaments.

There is no effective treatment for the syndrome of constitutional hypermobility. However, reasonably prolonged strengthening and sensori-motor programs are usually helpful.

The identification of constitutional hypermobility requires a differential diagnosis since this clinical entity should not be confused with other possible sources of decreased muscle tone and increased range of motion. Among the most frequent errors in the diagnosis are confusion of constitutional hypermobility with the hypotonia in syndromes affecting the afferent nerve fibers, oligophrenia and cerebellar and extrapyramidal insufficiency.

Evaluation of Hypermobility in the Upper Part of the Body

The assessment of hypermobility is in principle based on the estimation of muscle tone and range of movement of the joints. In clinical practice, orientation tests are usually sufficient for such as assessment. In the upper body, the most useful tests are head rotation, the high-arm cross, touching of the hands behind the neck, crossing of the arms behind the neck, extension of the elbows, and hyperextension of the thumb.[23]

Head rotation is tested in sitting, with the patient first actively turning the head. At the end of this active range of motion phase, an attempt is made to increase the range passively. The normal range is about 80° to each side, and the ranges of active and passive movement are almost the same.

In the high arm cross, the patient, while standing or sitting, puts the arm around the neck from the front to the opposite side. Normally the elbow almost reaches the median plane of the body, and the fingers reach the spinous processes of the cervical spine.

Touching of the hands behind the neck is tested with the patient standing or sitting. The patient tries to bring both hands together behind the back. Normally the tips of the fingers can touch without any increase in the thoracic lordosis.

Crossing of the arms behind the neck is again tested in either the sitting or standing positions. The patient puts the arms across the neck with the fingers extended in the direction of the shoulder blades. Normally the fingertips can reach the spines of the scapulae.

Extension of the elbows is better tested in the sitting than in the standing position. The elbows and lower arms are pressed together in maximal flexion of the elbows. The patient then tries to extend the elbows without separating them. Normally the elbows can be extended approximately 110°.

In hyperextension of the thumb, the examiner performs a passive extension of the thumb and measures the degree of the achieved hyperextension. Normally it is up to 20° in the interphalangeal joint and almost 0° in the metacarpophalangeal joint.

IMPLICATIONS FOR TREATMENT

A number of points should be drawn together in concluding this chapter, and it must be emphasized that detailed controlled studies of various assessment and management techniques remain to be undertaken.

Muscle imbalance is an essential component of dysfunction syndromes of the musculoskeletal system. The overall treatment program for such syndromes includes techniques that depend upon recognizing factors that perpetuate the dysfunction, and methods directed toward its correction. This is true regardless of whether muscle imbalance is considered to cause joint dysfunction or to occur in parallel with it.

Since increased tone in a muscle that is in a functional relationship with a particular joint plays an important role in the production and perception of pain, it could be argued that the first goal of treatment should be to decrease this tone. The choice of a therapeutic technique for this may be less important than utilizing the approach in which the clinician is most skilled. Physiologically there is probably not a substantial difference between the effects of "classical" gentle mobilization and techniques based on post-facilitation inhibition. Clinically, however, techniques based on post-isometric relaxation (post-facilitation inhibition)[8,9,28] have been found to be most effective in treating musculoskeletal dysfunction. In conditions marked by acute pain, changes in muscle can be considered to be principally reflexive, and hard or vigorous stretching techniques are therefore not a treatment of choice. In chronic pain and/or in the painless period between acute attacks of pain, strong stretching is necessary.

Regardless of how effective they may be in decreasing muscle tone, the techniques selected for treatment must influence the basic impairment of central nervous system motor regulation and the concomitant muscle imbalance. In the long term, treatment of impaired muscle function has as its objective the restoration of muscle balance, with the achievement of optimum flexibility of muscles that are prone to tightness and improved strength in muscles prone to inhibition and weakness. This must be followed by the realization of a second objective: the establishment of sound and economic movement patterns for the patient. This approach is time consuming, and demands advanced skill on the part of the therapist and good cooperation on the part of the patient. In addition it is tiring, since it requires the total concentration of both the therapist and patient.

Moreover, because patients do not necessarily use "artificially " learned movement patterns in their everyday activities, the results of treatment are sometimes disappointing.

As a consequence, and based on some ideas of Freeman,[29,30] a program of "sensori-motor stimulation" has been developed.[31] Current knowledge stresses the important contribution of the cerebellum in the programming of primitive or simple movement patterns.[32] Consequently, a program of exercises has been developed to preferentially activate the spino-vestibulo-cerebellar and subcortical pathways and regulatory circuits, so as to increase proprioceptive flow from the peripheral parts of the musculoskeletal system. We believe that this makes it possible to include an inhibited muscle more easily and effectively in important movement patterns such as gait.[33] Since this is achieved more on a reflex, automatic basis, the technique requires less voluntary control by the patient. It is less tiring and can be satisfactorily realized as a home program. It is beyond the scope of this chapter to do more than briefly mention this approach.

No therapeutic approach is sufficient unless body posture generally is improved. Whatever the cause of the patient's problem, special attention should be given to it. Overall, improvement of posture is time consuming and not infrequently neglected, since both the therapist and the patient are often satisfied by the immediate alleviation of symptoms, and treatment is discontinued. However, an approach that is strongly prophylactic promises good long-term results and the prevention of recurrences of acute episodes of dysfunction.

Despite the very encouraging long term results of clinical treatment of muscle imbalance in patients with chronic pain syndromes, scientifically controlled studies of such treatment remain to be conducted. Enthusiastic but premature clinical claims may leave in their wake a tide of skepticism that may well prevent future progress in this important area.

ACKNOWLEDGMENT

I wish to thank Prof. Margaret Bullock and Dr. Joanne Bullock-Saxton for their willing assistance in preparing this chapter.

REFERENCES

1. Maigne R: Orthopaedic Medicine. Charles C Thomas, Springfield, IL, 1979
2. Bourdillon JF, Day EA, Bookhout MA: Spinal Manipulation, Butterworth–Heinemann, Edinburgh, 1992
2a. Lewit K: Manipulative Therapy in Rehabilitation of the Motor System. Butterworths, London, 1985
3. Frymoyer JW, Gordon SL (eds): New Perspectives in Low Back Pain. American Academy of Orthopaedic Surgeons, Park Ridge, IL, 1989
4. Kraus H: Diagnosis and Treatment of Muscle Pain. Quintessence, Chicago, 1988
5. Travell JG, Simons GD: Myofascial Pain and Dysfunction. The Trigger Point Manual. Williams & Wilkins, Baltimore, 1983
6. Janda V: Introduction to functional pathology of the motor system. p. 39. In Howell ML, Bullock MI (eds): Physiotherapy in Sports. University of Queensland, Brisbane, 3, 1982
7. Janda V: Muscles, central nervous motor regulation and back problems. In Korr IM (ed): The Neurobiologic Mechanisms in Manipulative Therapy. Plenum Press, New York, 1978
8. Schmidt RF: Fundamentals of Neurophysiology. Springer, New York, 1985
9. Fisher AG, Murray EA, Burdy AC: Sensory Integration. FA Davis, Philadelphia, 1991
10. Voss DE, Ionta MK, Myers BJ: Proprioceptive Neuromuscular Facilitation, Harper and Row, Philadelphia, 1985
11. Abrahams VC, Lynn B, Richmond FJR: Organization and sensory properties of small myelinated fibres in the dorsal cervical rami of the cat. J Physiol (Lond) 347: 177, 1984
12. Abrahams VC: The physiology of neck muscles; their role in head movement and maintenance of posture. Can J Physiol Pharmacol 55:332, 1977

13. Guyton AR: Basic Human Neurophysiology. Saunders, Philadelphia, 1981
14. Janda V: Some aspects of extracranial causes of facial pain. J Prosthet Dent 56: 484, 1986
15. Widmer CG: Evaluation of temporomandibular disorders, In Kraus SL (ed): TMJ Disorders. Churchill Livingstone, New York, 1988
16. Janda V: Muscle strength in relation to muscle length, pain and muscle imbalance. In Harms-Rindahl K (ed): Muscle Strength. Churchill Livingstone, New York, 1993
17. Basmajian JV: Muscles Alive. Williams & Wilkins, Baltimore, 1974
18. Janda V: Die muskulären Hauptsyndrome bei vertebragenen Beschwerden. In Neumann HD, Wolff HD (eds): Theoretische Fortschritte und Praktische Erfahrungen der Manuellen Medizin. Konkordia, Bühl, 1979
19. Janda V: Muscle spasm—a proposed procedure for differential diagnosis. J Manual Med 6:136, 1991
20. Jull G, Janda V: Muscles and motor control in low back pain. In Twomey LT, Taylor JR (eds): Physical Therapy for the Low Back. Clinics in Physical Therapy, Churchill Livingstone, New York, 1987
21. Bourliere F: The assessment of biological age in man. WHO, Public Health Papers 37, Geneva, 1979
22. Kendall HO, Kendall GP, Wadsworth GE: Muscles, Testing and Function. Williams & Wilkins, Baltimore, 1971
23. Janda V: Muscle Function Testing. Butterworth, London 1983
24. Daniels L, Worthingham C: Muscle Testing. Saunders, Philadelphia, 1986
25. Cole JH, Twomey LT: Muscles in Action. An Approach to Manual Muscle Testing, Churchill Livingstone, Melbourne, 1988
26. Clarkson HM, Gilewich GB: Musculoskeletal Assessment. Williams & Wilkins, Baltimore, 1989
27. Lâcote M, Chevelier AM, Miranda A, et al: Clinical Evaluation of Muscle Function, Churchill Livingstone, Edinburgh, 1987
28. Mitchell FL, Moran PS, Pruzzo NA: An Evaluation and Treatment Manual of Osteopathic Muscle Energy Procedures. Mitchell, Moran and Pruzzo Associates, Valley Park, East Lannsing, MI, 1979
29. Freeman MAR: Instability of the foot after injuries to the lateral ligament of the ankle. J Bone Joint Surg 47B:669, 1965
30. Freeman MAR, Dean MRE, Hanham IWF: The etiology and prevention of functional instability of the foot. J Bone Joint Surg 47B:678, 1965
31. Janda V, Vávrová M: Sensory Motor Stimulation. Video presented by J Bullock-Saxton. Body Control Videos, Box 730, Brisbane 4068, Australia
32. Lehmkukl LD, Smith LK: Brunnstrom's Clinical Kinesiology. FA Davis Co, Philadelphia, 1987
33. Bullock-Saxton JE, Janda V, Bullock MI: Reflex activation of gluteal muscles in walking. Spine 18:704, 1993

11 | The Upper Limb Tension Test Revisited

David S. Butler

In 1988, Kenneally et al.[1] made the apt description of the upper limb tension test (ULTT) as the "straight leg raise test of the arm." Although the straight leg raise (SLR) has clear surgical pathologic and imaging value for demonstrating an abnormal response, similar studies utilizing the ULTT are still lacking. However, since 1988, interest in the test as a neurodynamic diagnostic and treatment tool has grown. Within the area of physical therapy, interest in the ULTT has been shown in many fields, including orthopedics, neurology, and sports physiotherapy.

The neuroanatomy and neurobiomechanics relating to the ULTT have been well covered by Kenneally et al.[1] Readers new to the ULTT should consult this chapter. For further reading, Sunderland,[2] Breig,[3] Lundborg,[4] and Butler[5] have written useful texts.

This chapter aims to update the ULTT as a clinical test. It includes the relationship of the ULTT to neuropathology, and links it to current concepts of pain. The test is applied on the basis of clinical reasoning strategies, as outlined by Jones et al. (see Ch. 6). The discussion provided here includes pain patterns that warrant neural tension testing as a priority, variations on the ULTT, updated analyses of test results, and some broad guidelines for use of the ULTT in treatment. While the ULTT does stand alone as a test, this chapter also discusses tension testing as a concept, rather than in terms of a single particular test.

TERMINOLOGY

"Neural tension testing" is a term used frequently in physical therapy. It means physically testing the dynamics and associated sensitivity of the nervous system. Tension testing is based on the fact that neural tissue has elasticity and a movement relationship (such as glide and compression) with adjacent tissues. Consequently, the dynamics and associated sensitivity of the nervous system can be tested, just as can the dynamics and sensitivity of joint, muscle, and fascial tissues. Within the various systems of manual therapy this dynamic aspect of the nervous system has been overlooked in favor of features of joint and muscle tissue.

Pain and other symptoms may arise from mechanical or chemical stimulation of the peripheral terminals of the small-diameter, myelinated (A delta) fibers and the unmyelinated C fibers of the nervous system. This pain arises from the target tissues of the nervous system, such as muscles and joints, and is called nociceptive, somatic, or nerve-end pain. More complex neurophysiologic situations occur when symptoms arise from the tissues of the nervous system itself. These symptoms are referred to as neurogenic or, if a pathology can be demonstrated, neuropathic. Pain (or other symptoms) originating in the nervous system can be categorized by way of the tissues at fault (i.e., peripheral nerve, nerve root, spinal cord and brain). Symptoms arising from nerve roots are sometimes referred to as radicular. In seeking pain sources within the nervous system, consideration should also be given to the innervated connective-tissue supporting elements of neural tissue, such as epineurium and the dura mater, in addition to neural elements such as axons. However, to ascribe pain as a mere sensation requiring either a nociceptive stimulus or injury to the nervous system is a classic error in neuroanatomic reasoning, and misses the true significance of pain. Pain exists only as the individual perceives it. Those who attempt to analyze pain and other sensations must consider peripheral as well as central circuitry, ascending and descending control systems, and sensory and affective pathways, all of which are continually subject to adjustments in sensitivity. Therefore, to enable accurate analyses of neurogenic symptoms, physical therapists are urged to consider the mechanisms of symptoms as well as their sources. It is clinically useful to consider four mechanisms for neurogenic pain, all of which can be linked to particular patterns of signs and symptoms:

1. Peripherally evoked (from conducting and connective tissues of peripheral nerves and nerve roots and from the meninges, and therefore "outside" the dorsal horn or, in the case of facial pain, outside the cervico-trigeminal nucleus.

2. Centrally evoked (from altered dorsal horn gating or processing).

3. Autonomic involvement, particularly of the sympathetic nervous system.

4. Affective or emotional involvement.

These mechanisms utilize different pathways of the nervous system, yet all pain sensations will involve these mechanisms. It is when the tissues associated with a mechanism become pathologic that clinical patterns related to that mechanism and the involved tissues will emerge. Responses to the ULTT will differ according to the site of a neuropathy (e.g., median nerve entrapment in the carpal tunnel, compared to cervical nerve root fibrosis), and will also differ according to the mechanisms of symptoms (e.g., peripherally evoked as compared to centrally evoked).

NEURAL TISSUES INVOLVED IN THE ULTT

The test described by Kenneally et al.[1] was based on original work by Elvey.[6] This test, with a slight modification, is illustrated in Figure 11-1. The difference between the test as shown in Figure 11-1 and that described by

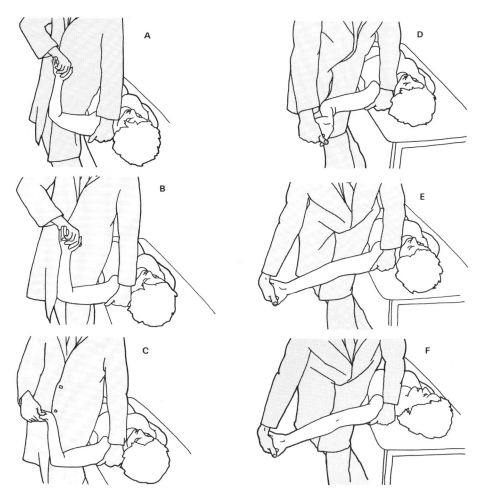

Fig. 11-1. Sequence of the ULTT1. (**A**) Starting position. (**B**) Glenohumeral abduction. (**C**) Forearm supination, wrist and finger extension. (**D**) Shoulder lateral rotation. (**E**) Elbow extension. (**F**) Contralateral lateral flexion. (From Butler,[5] with permission.)

Kenneally et al.[1] is that the component of elbow extension is added as a last component. This is simply because elbow extension is now seen to offer an easier and probably more accurate measure of range than wrist extension. Also, with the addition of elbow extension last, there is less provocation potential, since neural tissue is stronger at the elbow than at the wrist. The ULTT is regarded as a "base test,"[5] and because there are other ULTT base tests, the test as demonstrated in Figure 11-1 is referred to as the upper limb tension test 1 (ULTT1).

It is logical from the position of nerves relative to the moving joint axes, and the normal responses to the ULTT1 (Fig. 11-2), that the test is biased toward the median nerve, although some dynamics of all upper-limb nerves, particularly in the brachial plexus and nerve roots, will be tested. It is also clear that the test will load certain aspects of non-neural tissues, including the sensitivity and physical structures of muscle, tendon, joint, fascia, blood vessels, and skin. For example, the glenohumeral joint is taken toward an end range position, the biceps is stretched, and tension is applied to the subclavian artery,[7] and cervical contralateral lateral flexion produces some stretch on the zygapophyseal joints. Where the ULTT response is deficient, skill is needed in handling and analyzing the extent of involvement of the various tissues in the "sources of symptoms" hypothesis as outlined by Jones et al. (see Ch. 6).

If the test is taken to its full extent, it will include various tissues in the neural continuum, ranging from the end terminals of branches that may be

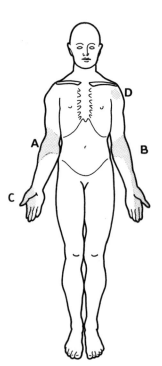

Fig. 11-2. Normal responses to the ULTT1 **(A)** Deep stretch or ache in the cubital fossa (in 99% of subjects). **(B)** Area A, extending into the radial aspect of the hand (80%). **(C)** Tingling in the thumb, index and middle fingers. **(D)** Occasionally a pull in the anterior shoulder. Cervical lateral flexion away from the side tested increases the response in approximately 90% of normal subjects. Cervical lateral flexion towards the side tested decreases the response in 70% of subjects. (Adapted from Kenneally et al.,[1] with permission.)

enclosed in tissues such as ligament, muscle, skin, and dura to peripheral nerve trunks and cords, cervical and upper thoracic nerve roots, aspects of meningeal and cord mechanics, and components of the sympathetic nervous system. The ULTT1 probably puts some stress on contralateral nerve roots and nerves as well.[1] The test therefore should not simply be considered a means of differentiating abnormalities arising in the neck from those arising in the shoulder, but as a physical test to display the mechanical sensitivity of any pathologic changes along the entire length of limb that is tested.

The ULTT is a dynamic test, used not only for evaluating aspects of the dynamics and sensitivity of the neural tissues during movement, but also placing them in differing movement relationships with non-neural tissues. Some of these relationships may be symptomatic.

The concept of the nervous system having mechanical features may be new to some readers. The nervous system is well designed for a role in movement, as can be observed from neuroanatomy and neurodynamics. For further information about this, the reader is directed to various anatomic studies.[3,4,8–11]

NEUROPATHOLOGY AND THE ULTT

A significant part of the professional province of physical therapists is the management of minor injury. Minor injury, and especially deeply located chronic injury creates a difficulty because clear pathologic evidence of the injury may not be available. For example, with a median nerve neuropathy postulated to be part of a painful arc syndrome of the shoulder, biopsy is impractical, nerve conduction tests are inaccurate with minor neuropathies,[12] target tissue function such as muscle strength may not have been measurably altered, and there are no reliable biochemistry tests. This highlights the need for physical therapists to apply careful clinical reasoning strategies. There should also be an awareness that the nervous system, despite its dynamic abilities, can be easily injured and its function altered. For example, the connective tissues of peripheral nerves react and inflame with slight rubbing,[4] the flow of axoplasm inside neurons will slow or stop with pressures below those in early stage carpal tunnel syndromes,[13,14] and changes in the dorsal horn response to a painful input are much more subtle and have more extensive implications than previously thought.[15]

The tissue constituents of the nervous system are normally mechanically sensitive to stretch, compression, and shear forces, particularly if chemically sensitized. The concept of links between altered neuromechanics and neurophysiology has only recently been proposed and examined.[2–5,12] Pathologic processes that may alter the sensitivity and dynamics of the ULTT may be located extraneurally (around the nervous system), intraneurally, or as is common with increasing chronicity, in both sites. Pathologic changes that might lead to the interpretation of a ULTT as being positive are discussed below.

EXTRANEURAL SITES OF ULTT COMPROMISE

Unaccustomed or excessive compromise by extraneural tissues and fluids may result in neural tissue rubbing on interfacing tissues, nerves "stuck" or irritated by blood or tissue fluid, impairment of feeder blood vessels, compression that is sufficient to mechanically damage axons or alter intraneural circulation, or irritated connective tissue that may ultimately involve outlying fascicles. Clinical manifestations are likely to be greater with compromise plus repetitive attempted use of the affected limb. No site in the nervous system can be exempt from injury, although the anatomy of certain extraneural tissues, such as the structures that form the carpal tunnel, may increase the risk to adjacent or enclosed neural tissue. Many texts are available on nerve and nerve root entrapment, including examples of the entrapments mentioned below.[2,4,12,16–18]

Muscle Tissue

Muscle tissue that is tight, weak, presents a fibrous edge to a nerve, exudes inflammatory mediators, or has an anomalous relation to a nerve may in various ways compromise neural tissues that pass through or are adjacent to it. Common sites of muscle compromise of the median nerve and its roots are the pronator teres, pectoralis minor, and scalene muscles. The radial sensory nerve may be involved in a pincer action between the tendons of the brachioradialis and extensor carpi radialis longus in the forearm, or may be entrapped by the supinator muscle in the arcade of Frohse or irritated by the fibrous edge of the extensor carpi radialis brevis and roots of this nerve compromised in altered or anomalous scalene muscles. The distal ulnar nerve may be entrapped or irritated in the cubital tunnel, and its roots are subject to a similar entrapment by the scalene muscles as are those of other nerves. Injury or alteration of the coracobrachialis may have an effect on the musculocutaneous nerve enclosed within it.

Joints

Abnormal joint mechanics and physiology, such as those associated with loss of tissue compliance, instability, and the development of osteophytes, callus, and arthritis may compromise neural tissue. The median nerve, for example, may be compromised by such alterations in the carpal bones, first rib, and C5-C6 segments. The radial nerve is anatomically adjacent to the radiohumeral joint and lateral radiocarpal complex, and may therefore be compromised by pathologic changes in and around these joints. The ulnar nerve is commonly compromised in the joint complexes of Guyon's canal, and at the cervicothoracic junction and in its sulcus at the elbow.

Other Compromising Forces

Pathologic changes in other than neural tissues, such as tissues of the blood vessels, fascia, and skin, may irritate or entrap nerves. External compressive forces, such as from crutches, prolonged unfavorable positioning of the arm on a hard surface (Saturday night palsy), and humeral fractures are particularly severe on the radial nerve. The ulnar nerve at the elbow is subject to external compressive forces, and is subject to such forces at the wrist in occupations such as motor mechanics, in which the hypothenar eminence may be used as a hammer.

INTRANEURAL SITES OF ULTT COMPROMISE

Neural Connective Tissues

The endoneurium, perineurium, and epineurium of peripheral nerves and nerve roots are innervated,[19] well vascularized,[4] and very reactive when rubbed excessively.[4] During a dynamic test such as the ULTT, these structures rub on and are compressed by many differing interfacing tissues. Given the extent of peripheral nerve excursion (up to 2 cm in relation to interfacing tissues in the upper arm[8]), these connective tissues are likely to be involved in friction trauma,[20] and are usually the first neural tissues to be injured in an extraneural compromise. With irritated or scarred connective tissues, it seems that stretch rather than compression would evoke more nociceptive responses from the nervi nervorum.

The ULTT will also stress the meninges, particularly with pretest posturing or cervical meningeal tensioning movements such as flexion or contralateral lateral flexion. The spinal dura mater and epidural tissue such as dural ligaments probably absorb most of the tension. The dura mater is tough, layered, and well innervated.[21–24] Because the sinuvertebral nerve enters the dura and forms an intradural network,[24] dural tearing, cutting, surgical debris, or posttraumatic scarring may lead to abnormal mechanical sensitivity of the dural tissue.

Dural ligaments connecting the dura mater to the anterior spinal canal are innervated,[25] and the mechanics of these ligaments are likely to be affected by trauma or exudate from disc trauma. Also innervated are the pia mater and arachnoid mater,[26] making them potential sources of symptoms.

Neural Tissue

For areas other than the impulse-generating terminal buttons, dorsal root ganglia, and neuronal pools in the spinal cord to become sources of persistent symptoms, there must be an abnormal impulse-generating site. Such sites may occur solely in neural tissue, but may also act in combination with damaged neural connective tissue. These sites are known as ectopic neural pacemakers.[27]

A neuroma is a common example of such a pacemaker. Neuromata may be located at the terminal end of a nerve or along the nerve trunk, and may be particularly mechanosensitive to tension tests[27] such as the ULTT. These pacemakers will also be sensitive to ischemia, anoxia, and inflammatory mediators.[28,29] Neuromata are usually a combination of neural and connective tissue, and may involve single axons, fascicles or whole nerves. Immature axons attempting to grow through scar are particularly mechanosensitive.[28] Other possible pain-provoking structures are chemical[30] and electrical[31] ephaptic (false) synapses between neurons, and sites of minor demyelination.[32]

Associated with the firing of ectopic pacemakers during tension tests must be the fact that normal peripheral nerve, when stretched by 8 percent,[33,34] will be deprived of enough blood to create an ectopic impulse. This 8 percent "critical level" will be reached earlier in the range of motion of a joint during neural tension maneuvers in which there is some pathomechanical factor, such as adhesions of nerves to adjacent tissues. However, despite being activated by stretch, ectopic pacemakers may not be detected during nerve conduction tests, since these tests cannot be specific to a single fascicle.[35]

The ULTT puts some mechanical stresses on the spinal cord, especially if the cervical spine is in flexion or in lateral flexion away from the test side. Neurons in the dorsal columns and dorsal horn run in a wavy pattern in the cord, and are stretched during tensioning maneuvers such as flexion and contralateral flexion.[3] Some cord-mediated responses may occur with the test if the cord is sufficiently compromised or sensitized.[3,36] The relationship between mechanical and chemical sensitization, evident in peripheral nerves, may be less appreciated by physical therapists when considering the spinal cord.

Double and Multiple Crush

The double crush hypothesis[37] states that a proximal source of nerve compression or stretch would make the distal nerve more susceptible to compression. This clinically based hypothesis came from observations of the coexistence of cervical discogenic disease with carpal tunnel syndrome. This concept, recently reviewed by Mackinnon,[38] has experimental verification in primate and rodent models. Other reported examples of double crush include relationships between the cubital tunnel and cervical spine[36] and "reversed double crush,"[4,39] in which a distal compression leads to a more proximal compression and compromise. Approximately 32 percent of all carpal tunnel syndromes are bilateral, and many are linked to cervical arthritis.[40] Double or indeed multiple crush[12] thinking could be applied here, although with bilaterality of symptoms some thought must be given to the possible role of altered spinal cord processing.

Mackinnon[38] emphasizes the importance of dynamic compression. Patients may be asymptomatic at rest, and only particular combinations of movements or activities may distort the nervous system enough to provoke their symptoms.

Because the ULTT is a dynamic test of neural tissue extending from terminals to the central nervous system, and can be adapted to an individual patient, it is well suited for clarifying double crush-type symptoms and for helping to identify multiple sites of compromise, either intraneural, extraneural, or both.

THE ULTT AND CURRENT CONCEPTS OF PAIN

Before a ULTT is performed on any patient, hypotheses should be calculated, on the basis of patient questioning, of probable neurogenic sources of pain, and even of pathologic changes such as nerve entrapment or dural tethering. Hypotheses should also be calculated about the mechanisms of symptoms of which the patient complains and which could be produced during testing [i.e., the peripheral, central, autonomic, and affective (emotional) contributions to symptoms]. Pain should not be considered a primary sensation, such as hearing or taste, but one that is subject to complex chemical and electrical gating in the dorsal horn, brain stem, and higher neurons.

Neurogenic sensations are complex, especially when pathologic in origin. The peripherally evoked pain of simple entrapment or neuritis may be quite familiar and understandable,[2,4,5] but Devor and Rappaport[41] have pointed out what many physical therapists already know: "that the association of positive symptoms including pain with injury or disease in a particular nerve or nerve root does not necessarily mean that the neural processes reside in that nerve or root." Physical therapists must consider contributions of central and autonomic neurons to symptoms. Affective or emotional mechanisms associated with pain are beyond the scope of this chapter, and the reader is referred to Fields[29] and relevant chapters in Wall and Melzack[42] for discussions of these mechanisms. Patterns of neurogenic pain can be differentiated into those that are peripherally and centrally evoked and those of which the autonomic nervous system becomes the dominant mechanistic source. Overlap, however, is inevitable.

Some symptom patterns occur with injury to the target tissues of the nervous system, such as muscles and joints (i.e., nociceptive or nerve-end patterns of symptoms). These are well covered by the relevant chapters in this book. The following sections relate to patterns that occur with injury or alteration of various neurogenic tissues related to the pain experience.

PERIPHERALLY EVOKED PATTERN

The symptom patterns realized when peripheral nerves, nerve roots, and the meninges are injured are perhaps the most familiar patterns to physical therapists. Often, and perhaps confusingly in the clinic, these neurogenic patterns are likely to coexist with patterns originating in non-neural tissue. Thus, for example, cervical disc trauma compromising a nerve root may be marked by radicular symptoms from the nerve root and nociceptive symptoms from the disc.

Features of a symptom pattern that may strengthen hypotheses for its peripheral evocation include:

1. Symptoms existing in a clear neuroanatomic pattern, such as in a peripheral nerve or nerve root innervation field, or in "lines" along a peripheral nerve.

2. Extrasegmental symptoms. Cyriax[43] advised readers to "suspect the dura mater when symptoms have no localising value." His advice is excellent and should be extended to suspecting the nervous system when symptoms do not fit familiar non-neural tissue patterns for pain. The meninges are capable of non-dermatomal referral patterns, and so, probably, are peripheral nerves.

3. Symptoms related to vulnerable neuroanatomic sites. Neural tissue is more vulnerable to injury at sites such as tunnels (carpal tunnel, intervertebral foramen, scalenes), branches (deep and superficial branch of the radial nerve above the elbow), hard interfaces (brachial plexus on the first rib), and locations in which it is located superficially (radial sensory nerve on the lower radius).

4. Linked symptoms. The mechanism of "double crush," whereby a neuropathy (e.g., entrapment) makes other areas of nerve more vulnerable to injury, provides an explanation for the common onset of symptoms and/or local injury above or below the site of an initial injury. Symptoms may be linked historically, behaviorally (occurring together or one without the other), or anatomically (e.g., along the same nerve trunk).

5. The patient's vocabulary in describing symptoms includes terms like "pulling," "burning," "tingling," and "electrical." In peripheral nerves and nerve roots, symptoms associated with the innervated connective tissues are more likely to be familiar, whereas those associated with conducting tissues may be more unfamiliar and elicit a wider descriptive vocabulary.[44] The patient may complain of night symptoms, probably related to sustained nocturnal postures, and a decrease in blood pressure at night, and inflammatory responses elicited by repetitive irritation at the site of compromise.

6. Symptoms associated with stretch of neural tissue. In general, pain due predominantly to peripheral mechanisms has clear aggravating and easing patterns. These may include gross movements such as stretching of the arms in hanging out wash, or a very specific activity such as playing a musical instrument or using a computer keyboard. Antalgic neural postures, such as holding an arm above the head to alleviate symptoms caused by mid- to low cervical nerve root compromise, may be evident.

The ULTT response in patients in whom the pain from a neuropathy is evoked peripherally is linked behaviorally to mechanical stimuli (i.e., there is usually a link between symptom provocation and activity or test movements). Symptoms related to the test are easily reproducible and similar on retesting. Latency is not usually a feature of such symptoms. Even in the case of a minor neuropathy, once a provocative position is found (perhaps with a modified ULTT or a painful position that the patient has "found"), it should be similar on retesting. Further details of peripherally evoked symptom patterns are available.[5]

CENTRAL MECHANISMS AND PATTERNS

As Wall has noted,[15] there are pain-free as well as painful neuropathies, and a variable relationship of pathology to pain. Clinicians familiar with the use of the ULTT or indeed with any tension test will have noted the variations in test responses among patients with presumed neuropathic pain. Some clinicians may have prematurely dismissed a neurogenic component of a disorder because their analysis of the findings in a test was based solely on knowledge of pain from target tissues or on peripherally evoked neurogenic pain. Much of the variability in patterns of neuropathic pain is probably due to the nature of the neurons of the central nervous system (CNS). These neurons have plasticity and spatially extensive receptive fields (perhaps an entire limb), receive convergent input from nociceptive and non-nociceptive primary afferent nerve fibers, and are subject to peripheral and central inhibitory influences over short and long time frames.

The dorsal horn of the spinal cord, and the cervico-trigeminal nucleus in the case of facial pain, are the sites at which arriving neural impulses are initially processed. Changes in the dorsal horn may be generated by a prolonged afferent barrage, especially along unmyelinated afferents. The initial neuronal excitability is due to neuropeptide release,[45] but if this state is maintained, morphologic changes are known to occur in cells of the dorsal horn.[46,47] This maintains hypersensitivity and allows situations such as the firing of nociceptive-specific cells with innocuous stimuli such as touch or contralateral input.[48,49] Changes in the central nervous system may also result from abnormal concentrations of neuropeptides such as substance P, carried by axonal transport and deposited in the dorsal horn.[50] These changes could be maintained simply by a trickle of abnormal afferent inputs.[51] In addition, the descending pain-control mechanisms mediated by the mid-brain, reticular formation, and dorsolateral funiculus may be impaired by injury or psychological status (e.g., depression). Further reading on these issues is available.[15,29,42]

Central Pain Patterns

Patterns of pain associated with abnormal neural processing in the dorsal horn have been identified.[15,42,52] Most central pain patterns encountered by physical therapists in orthopedic manual therapy will be secondary to persistent ectopic input from the periphery, or perhaps associated with trauma such as whiplash. There may not be any measurable motor deficits. Severe neurologic trauma, such as stroke, or disease such as multiple sclerosis, may also provoke pain of primary central origin.

Features of central pain patterns are:

1. Unpatterned symptoms that may be little influenced by peripheral stimuli (such as palpation of nerves and the ULTT), and which are spontaneous and frequently described as stabbing.

2. Allodynia (a painful response to a stimulus that would not normally hurt) and hyperalgesia (an exaggerated response to a stimulus that would normally be painful). The patient may exhibit mechanical allodynia (e.g., pain when a shirt collar rubs or pain on small movements) or thermal allodynia (e.g., an extreme pain reaction to warmth).

3. Provoked pain may require summation (e.g., cutting sandwiches, keyboard operation), and there may be a latent response (10 to 20 seconds) after an activity. This may relate to the "wind-up" feature of neurons in the dorsal horn that have a wide dynamic range, which requires repeated afferent impulses for the central cell to fire and continue to fire.

4. Sensory deficits are non-dermatomal and are usually dispersed over a greater area than the area of symptoms.

5. Associated motor deficits, such as heightened sympathetic reflexes, spasm, and hypertonus. The complaint of tiredness may relate to continual minor hypertonus.

6. Symptoms may begin very early after injury or some months later. In the first instance the mechanism is probably impulse generated. In cases in which there is a slower onset of symptoms, the mechanism may be related to abnormalities in the quality of axoplasm reaching the dorsal horn.[15]

7. Associated with possible minor injury to the central nervous system, such as whiplash and multiple surgery, especially when the spinal canal is invaded.

8. Frequent linkage to an altered psychological status.

The main feature of centrally evoked neurogenic pain is that the pain is manifested pathologically, rather than necessarily displaying the more familiar and more easily reproducible pattern of occurrence of most peripherally activated pains. Tension-test responses will show great variation. With pain evoked entirely by central mechanisms it may be difficult to reproduce symptoms with the ULTT; the symptoms on each retesting may be variable, and there may be latency and hints of abnormal mechanics in all major nerves. Although the ULTT may yield a seemingly full-range result, repeating the test a number of times may provoke constant symptoms. The pattern will not be as clear as in nociceptive pain or peripherally evoked neurogenic pain, and the patient may not be able to clearly describe activities that aggravate and ease the pain.

AUTONOMIC MECHANISMS AND PATTERNS

The autonomic nervous system is continually active and will respond to all pain states regardless of their severity. In some pain states the sympathetic nervous system appears to acquire an extraordinary role in pain generation and maintenance. Because the sympathetic supply to the limbs and trunk is efferent, the mode of effect in such pain states is most likely via alterations in blood flow and sensitization of noradrenaline-sensitive target tissues. The sympathetically maintained pain syndrome (SMPS) has been defined as consisting of "pain (that is) dependent on the sympathetic innervation of the area afflicted by the pain."[53] There is a wide spectrum of SMPS, ranging from the severe reflex sympathetic dystrophies (RSD) to the more minor manifestations, in which there may be only one or two features of sympathetic stress.

Sympathetic Pain Patterns

Some of the clinical features suggesting that the sympathetic nervous system plays more than a physiologic role in a particular disorder are as follows:

1.   Altered blood flow, reflected in skin color (red, white, or mottled), temperature changes, and cutaneous capillary vasodilatation.
2.   Altered sweating (either increased, decreased, or occurring in patches).
3.   Swelling or sensations of swelling, often in the extremities and around the neck.
4.   Trophic changes, such as glossy skin or cracking nails.
5.   Abdominal bloating and undiagnosed "organ disease" despite multiple tests.
6.   Pain and stiffness in the thoracic region, often associated with neck or limb pain.
7.   Thoracic postures, such as the forward head posture and upper thoracic segmental lordosis.
8.   Patient complaints may be restricted only to pain or stiffness, without any of the other signs or symptoms listed above.

The above list represents features of a minor sympathetically maintained pain state. More severe states, such as reflex sympathetic dystrophy, may feature marked mechanical allodynia and hyperalgesia.

The responses to the ULTT will often depend on the involvement of the sympathetic nervous system in the patient's disorder. Many clinicians will have observed that techniques that mobilize the thoracic spine or depress the sympathetic nervous system, such as interferential currents, often lead to improved ULTT responses.

Patients whose symptom complex includes features of sympathetic stress often have positive tension signs, including those found on the ULTT. Tension signs can be quite marked in patients with RSD, and less so in patients with milder manifestations. Most of the neurons in the sympathetic trunk are preganglionic, and any compromise of these neurons may mean abnormal sympathetic contributions to all nerves, yielding positive results in a number or all of the base tests. Examination of the sympathetic trunk is discussed in Chapter 15.

VARIATIONS AND ANALYSIS OF THE ULTT

The ULTT1 as outlined in Figure 11-1 will not be the optimum test for all patients. Pathologic changes may affect nerves other than the median nerve, and in the clinic this test often cannot be taken to its full extent, owing to

Table 11–1. The Base Upper Limb Tension Tests

Test	Main Sensitizing Components	Nerve Bias
ULTT1	Shoulder abduction Elbow extension	Median
ULTT2A	Shoulder girdle depression Shoulder external rotation	Median
ULTT2B	Shoulder girdle depression Shoulder internal rotation	Radial
ULTT3	Elbow flexion Shoulder abduction	Ulnar

neural and/or non-neural pathology and associated irritability. Because of the continuum of the nervous system, the need to perform a ULTT, may in many patients, be accompanied by the need to perform another tension test such as a passive neck flexion, straight leg raise, or slump test.[5]

As Kenneally et al.[1] suggested, the ULTT can be directed at any nerve. Butler[5] has encouraged clinicians to employ a "base test" system of four tests, each of which employs neural sensitizing movements and biases toward particular nerve trunks (Table 11-1). The pattern of a patient's symptoms may dictate which test is a priority. For example, with "tennis elbow"-type symptoms, the ULTT2B, in which the bias is toward the radial nerve, would be a suitable test. From these base tests the clinician can explore the patient's range of movement and vary the test, utilizing information obtained from the patient about aggravating and easing activities and enhanced by a knowledge of neuroanatomy.

In many situations there is no need for a full test. For example, in a patient with a "frozen shoulder," the shoulder can be taken to its limit (for example, 60° abduction), with the test then being performed from that position. Only parts of the test should be undertaken, and great care should be exercised when examining patients with an acute nerve root lesion or following whiplash trauma.

NEW BASE TESTS

ULTT2A (Median Nerve Bias)

The main sensitizing maneuver in the ULTT2A test (Fig. 11-3) is shoulder girdle depression. It appears worthwhile both in the clinic and experimentally[54] to utilize base tests that employ shoulder girdle depression as well as tests using shoulder girdle abduction. To the author's knowledge there have been no normative studies performed for the ULTT2A test.

ULTT2B (Radial Nerve Bias)

Because the ULTT2B test is biased to the radial nerve and its roots, it is applicable to disorders such as "tennis elbow," de Quervain's disease, and mid- to lower cervical nerve root syndromes. Note that a key to the test (Fig.

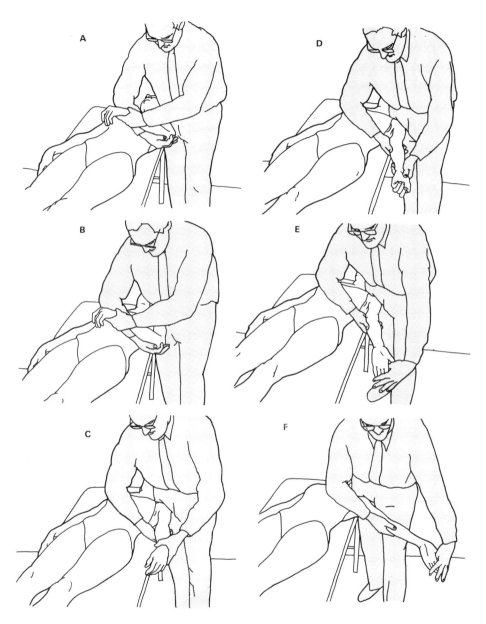

Fig. 11-3. ULTT2A (median nerve bias). (**A**) Starting position. (**B**) Shoulder girdle depression. (**C**) Elbow extension. (**D**) Lateral rotation of the shoulder. (**E**) Wrist and thumb extension. (**F**) Abduction of the shoulder. (From Butler,[5] with permission.)

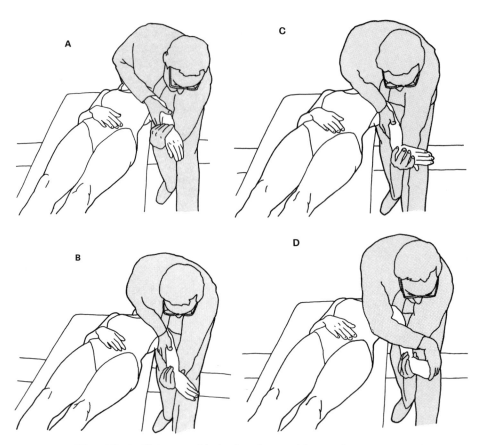

Fig. 11-4. ULTT2B (radial nerve bias). Starting position as for ULTT2A. Shoulder abduction may also be used as a sensitizing maneuver. **(A)** Medial rotation of the shoulder. **(B)** Examiner's elbow "locks" patient's elbow into extension. **(C)** Wrist and finger flexion. **(D)** Alternative method of wrist and finger extension. (From Butler,[5] with permission.)

11-4) is to maintain internal rotation of the shoulder with the clinician's elbow. Yaxley and Jull[54] reported on the normal responses in this test among 40 asymptomatic young subjects (Fig. 11-5). Other reports[12] indicate that similar tests can reproduce the symptoms of de Quervain's tenosynovitis, which must question the normally accepted concept of a tendon and tendon-sheath origin of this disorder.

ULTT3

Because all of the base tests described above employ elbow extension, neuropathies related to the ulnar nerve may be missed. Therefore, the ULTT3, utilizing elbow flexion, is suggested. Examples of syndromes that would neces-

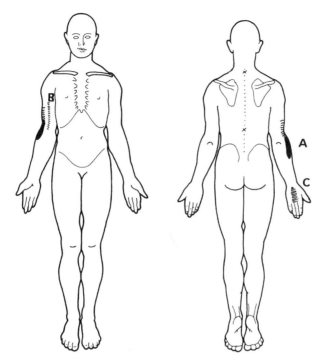

Fig. 11-5.   Normal responses to the ULTT2B. **(A)** Strong painful stretch over the radial aspect of the proximal forearm (in 84% of normal subjects). **(B)** Strong stretch in the biceps. **(C)** Occasionally a stretch over the dorsal aspect of the third, fourth, and fifth fingers (approximately 12% of normal subjects). (From Yaxley, et al.,[54] with permission.)

sitate such a test are ''golfers elbow'' and C7 to T1 nerve root disorders. This test is illustrated in Figure 11-6. Normal responses to this test have been established.[55]

OTHER TESTS

In some cases the symptoms and history of a disorder point to a neuropathy residing in a particular nerve other than the radial, median, or ulnar. In the upper limb, particular notice should be given to the musculocutaneous, axillary, and suprascapular nerves.[16]

Musculocutaneous Nerve

As with any nerve, injury is possible anywhere along the length of the musculocutaneous nerve. This nerve may be compromised at the dorsolateral aspect of the wrist,[12] under the coracobrachialis muscle,[20] and at the elbow,

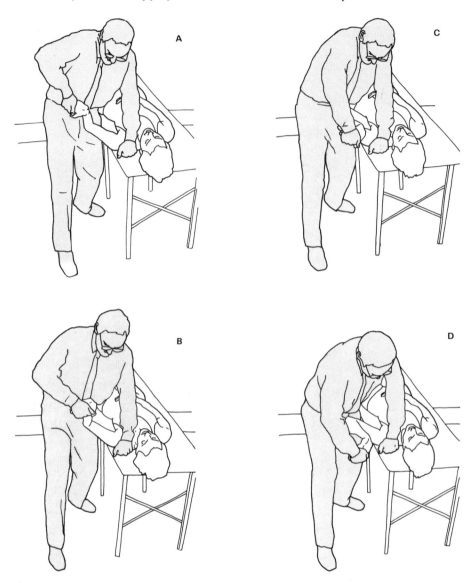

Fig. 11-6.   The ULTT3. **(A)** Starting position. **(B)** Wrist extension, forearm supination (or pronation may be more sensitive). **(C)** Elbow flexion. **(D)** Shoulder depression plus lateral rotation. *(Figure continues.)*

where it emerges between the brachialis and biceps muscles. To test the mechanics of the nerve, shoulder girdle depression, glenohumeral extension, elbow extension, and wrist ulnar deviation are suggested. The starting position may be the same as used in the ULTT2 maneuvers, and the glenohumeral extension appears to be a potent sensitizer.

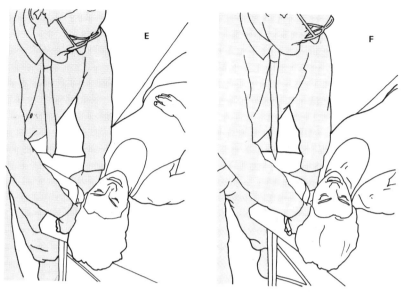

Fig. 11-6. *(Continued).* **(E)** Shoulder abduction. **(F)** Shoulder lateral flexion away from the test side. (From Butler,[5] with permission.)

Axillary Nerve

The common orthopedic event of shoulder dislocation has drawn attention to the vulnerability of the axillary nerve at the shoulder.[2,16,17] In addition to being caused by overstretch, a considerable number of axillary neuropathies must result from the immobilizing consequences of the local inflammatory exudate. To test the mechanics responsible for an axillary neuropathy, glenohumeral internal rotation, contralateral cervical lateral flexion, and shoulder girdle depression, plus some shoulder abduction to approximately 40 degrees, are suggested.

Suprascapular Nerve

Because the subscapular nerve has to slide through the scapular notch, the shoulder girdle protraction and retraction movement required by some sports (e.g., basketball), or occupations (e.g., computer keyboard operation) may put the nerve at risk. The neurodynamic sequence suggested to test this nerve is shoulder girdle protraction with the arm in internal rotation, cross-body adduction, cervical lateral flexion away, and shoulder girdle depression. Compression syndromes about the shoulder have recently been reviewed by Narakas.[56]

GUIDELINES TO ANALYSIS OF TENSION TESTS

With practice and guidance, the ULTTs are not difficult to perform. However, any responses to these tests will require a careful analysis that is tailored to the individual patient.

Positivity

Concepts of positivity in which a measurement in degrees is given to the joint component of a tension test are not relevant. More important is the relevance of the response to hypotheses formulated about the mechanisms of symptoms, the structures at fault, and the relationship between these structural sources of symptoms, such as muscles, joints, and nerves and other relevant factors (see Ch. 6). A measurement in degrees should be used only as part of the reassessment of the efficacy of treatment.

During testing, physical therapists should be seeking pain and movement responses that differ from those on the other side of the body and also differ from what is known to be normal. Neural/non-neural structural differentiation can be employed. "Structural differentiation" is a clinical strategy employed to confirm or challenge a hypothesis that posits an alteration in nervous system dynamics in a particular patient. For example, if a "trapezius" length test provokes symptoms, and these symptoms are then altered by elbow (Fig. 11-7), or hand movements, the inference is that something is mechanically amiss with the nervous system or its adjacent tissues. Many clinicians already use structural differentiation in the lower limbs. For example if the addition of ankle dorsiflexion worsens SLR-evoked lumbar symptoms, then neural origin for

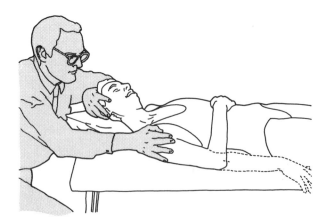

Fig. 11-7. Structural differentiation. If symptoms provoked by a "trapezius stretch" are altered by elbow movements, the inference is that the symptoms evoked are related to pathologic changes in the nervous system.

these symptoms is usually inferred. In general, structural differentiation will be clearer with nerve-end pain and peripherally evoked neuropathic pain than with central or autonomically related pain.

A Suggested Categorization of Responses

For comprehension of neuropathies, a categorization of responses to tension tests has been suggested,[5] comprising physiologic, clinical physiologic, and neurogenic responses.

A *physiologic* response may be considered the normal response to a tension test or any movement. Symptoms may be evoked from any tissue, and it would be expected that symptoms would be commonplace during some sequence of the ULTT, even in asymptomatic subjects.[1]

A *clinical physiologic* response is one that differs from the response on the other side of the body or what is known to be normal. This may mean that some symptoms (not necessarily those of which the patient complains) are reproduced at unexpected points in the range of movement and are different from the test responses in the contralateral arm. For example, in a patient with a chronic left-sided cervical nerve root irritation producing symptoms of an episodic nature, the ULTTs may not reproduce the symptoms. However, the response to a ULTT performed on the left arm may differ from that on the right in such a way as to indicate that something is amiss.

Neurodynamics are complex, and it may take considerable test sequencing and sensitizing to reproduce the symptoms of a patient's condition, if this can be done at all, but in the clinic this may not be necessary if consideration is given to clinical physiologic symptoms.

A *neurogenic* response can be inferred by structural differentiation. For example, if a physiologic or clinical physiologic response is produced at the elbow during ULTT2A, and neck movements alter this response, then a neurogenic origin of symptoms can be suspected. The inference of a neurogenic origin will be strengthened by other data, such as associated neurogenic symptoms including tingling, burning, or a positive nerve conduction test. Note that a neurogenic response can be a normal response to a particular combination of movements.

The Role of Non-Neural Tissue

The mechanics of the nervous system cannot be examined in isolation. All tissues interfacing with the involved nerve trunk(s), roots, meninges, and autonomic supply need examination. For example, in a patient with lateral elbow pain, tissues interfacing with the radial nerve, such as the structures on the radial aspect of the wrist, lateral forearm tendons, supinator muscle, shoulder joint, pectoralis minor muscle, middle and lower cervical intervertebral segments, and thoracic spine to the T9 level need examination for mechanical hyperalgesia.

The possibility of the injured nervous system maintaining a hyperalgesic state in target tissues by releasing abnormal concentrations of vasoactive neuropeptides such as substance P and calcitonin gene-related peptide from nociceptive endings must be considered.[42,57] These peptides help maintain abnormal concentrations of non-neurogenic pain mediators such as histamine[58] at the injury site. Thus, the ULTT may reveal a neuropathy that is contributing to continued target tissue sensitization, and in a vicious cycle of events, the target tissue may be chemically, and later mechanically, maintaining the neuropathy. It is very difficult to ascribe this solely to the nervous system; unistructural disorders must be extremely rare if they exist at all.

Sequence of Additions

Altering the sequence in which the components of a ULTT are applied is an extremely useful variation of the test. For example, the ULTTs can be performed from the distal end of the arm, starting from the fingers and wrist rather than from the shoulder. This can be useful for the structural differentiation of peripheral disorders such as carpal tunnel syndrome. In general, the best access to the nervous system will come from taking up the affected component at a site of abnormal tension and progressively increasing the tension.[59] For example, with a carpal tunnel syndrome, wrist extension can be the starting position, with proximal median nerve tension added later. If a C8 nerve root compromise is suspected, cervical lateral flexion and flexion may be the starting position, with ulnar nerve tension added progressively.

Component sequencing can be invaluable when deciding how to examine a patient with an easily irritated pain state. Thus, for a patient who appears to have an easily provoked pain in the shoulder area, it would be best to begin a ULTT from the distal end of the arm.

TREATMENT UTILIZING THE ULTT

The aim of treatment of painful neurogenic syndromes involving the arm, neck, or both is to restore the normal mechanics and sensitivity of the nervous system with the minimum of force. This usually means utilizing both non-neural and neural based techniques and both passive and active techniques. There are as yet no studies affirming or denying the efficacy of treatment via the ULTT, although one study has shown the value of neural mobilization via the slump positions for hamstring tears.[60] At this stage, clinical reasoning provides a strategy, and a reassessment of the subjective and physical responses to treatment is therefore essential. If a particular line of treatment does not work at a rate appropriate to the patient's presumed pathology, it should be abandoned. Treatment utilizing the ULTTs is described in greater detail elsewhere.[5,61,62]

GUIDELINES

General

With all passive and active arm and neck movements, the nervous system will be loaded and will respond mechanically by a combination of stretching and sliding along interfacing tissues. For example, shoulder quadrant techniques,[63] while directed at joint tissues, inevitably mobilize the brachial plexus, nerve roots, and upper limb peripheral nerves. Perhaps some of the past beneficial responses to such tests may have been due to the mobilization of neural structures.

Signs of upper limb tension may alter with the treatment of non-neural tissues, including mobilization, electrotherapy, and postural awareness. All that may be required during treatment is a reassessment to ensure that the signs of tension are improving.

If a pathologic process limiting a ULTT is extraneural, occurring in tissues surrounding the neural tissue such as joint and muscle, then the technique of choice would be one directed at the extraneural tissue. In addition, large-amplitude movements of the neural tissue (i.e., sliding of the neural tissue through its normal range of motion) may be warranted. Nearly all disorders involve a number of structures; in the case of "tennis elbow" type complaints, for example, restricted ranges of movement in the cervical, thoracic, and elbow joints are common, as are mechanical hyperalgesia and allodynia about the elbow. In such cases, treating the extraneural tissues to investigate the effect on the neural tissues may be a safe and instructive way for a physical therapist to commence mobilization of the nervous system.

Mobilization via the ULTTs

Some guidelines for physical therapists attempting to mobilize the nervous system are to:

1.   Think of mobilization rather than stretch. Mobilization as most physical therapists know it implies the use of such aspects of treatment as gentle and firm movements, through-range and end-range mobilization, and use of active and passive mobilization with respect for the individual patient's symptoms.

2.   Use the continuum of the nervous system. This means that a treatment does not have to be directed at the anatomic component that is the site of adverse neural mechanics. When a cervical nerve root disorder is easing, for example, either arm can be put into some tension and the movements of the elbow utilized to perform the treatment.

3.   Consider the extent of the pathophysiology and pathomechanics of the

Table 11-2. The Relationship Between Irritability and Pathology

(Acute) Irritable	(Subacute) Moderately Irritable	(Chronic) Non-irritable
←——— Decreasing dominance of the pathophysiologic response ←———		
———→ Increasing dominance of the pathomechanical response ←———		

(Adapted from Butler and Gifford,[62] with permission.)

disorder[62] (Table 11-2). When, for example, pathophysiology (or prevalence of acuteness, pain, and irritability) is dominant, as in the early postoperative period or following whiplash trauma, mobilization may be done non-provocatively or with great respect for the patient's symptoms, using through range movements, avoidance of resistance or spasm, awareness of the response to treatment, and movement of a part distal or proximal to the main site of the disorder. However, where pathomechanics (or prevalence of chronicity, loss of range of movement, or non-irritability) is the dominant feature of a disorder, such as in a "frozen shoulder" or an old and stable nerve root syndrome, mobilization may involve techniques involving resistance, the provocation of some symptoms, treatment of extraneural tissues, and mobilization in a position of tension. For example, in a patient with an old and stable cervical nerve root syndrome, a suitable technique may be to place the patient in a position of upper limb tension and then to mobilize the cervical spine.

4. Self mobilization of the nervous system is appropriate once the response to repeated movements in the clinic is ascertained.[5] Analysis of the pathophysiologic and pathomechanical components of the patient's disorder will again assist in exercise prescription.

Precautions in Treatment

Most physical therapists have developed a feel for altered compliance in joint and muscle tissue. The quality of the altered compliance that occurs when the nervous system is loaded via the ULTTs may be a new sensation for some clinicians, and the techniques for eliciting it therefore require great care. There are some situations in which the ULTTs should not be used or should be used with extreme care. Remember that in most assessment and treatment situations the test will not need to be taken to its limit. Situations requiring very great care are as follows:

1. Worsening neurologic signs, which are a contraindication to tension testing.
2. Injury or disease of extraneural structures, such as a dislocating shoulder, cervical instability, or osteoporosis.

3. Following neurosurgery, such as nerve repair, and after acute injury, such as whiplash.

4. Diseases affecting the mechanical integrity of the nervous system, such as diabetes, acquired immune deficiency syndrome (AIDS), and rheumatoid arthritis.

5. Inflammatory and infective disorders.

6. Undiagnosed pain syndromes.

SUMMARY

In association with clinical reasoning strategies, the ULTT is anecdotally a useful clinical diagnostic and treatment tool. Unlike the SLR, the ULTT is still a new test and the handling it requires is more difficult. This update, in which the aim has been to make the concept of upper limb tension testing more clinically applicable, has urged continued clinical experimentation and attempts at experimental validation of tension testing. It is likely that with a greater focus on neuropathies and a greater understanding of pain mechanisms, the ULTT will grow as a diagnostic and clinical tool, and in the next revision of this text will be presented with greater experimental support and clinical validity.

REFERENCES

1. Kenneally M, Rubenach H, Elvey R: The upper limb tension test: the SLR test of the arm. In Grant R (ed): Physical Therapy of the Cervical and Thoracic Spine. Clinics in Physical Therapy. Churchill Livingstone, New York, 1988
2. Sunderland S: Nerves and Nerve Injuries. 2nd Ed. Churchill Livingstone, Melbourne, 1978
3. Breig A: Adverse Mechanical Tension in the Central Nervous System. Almqvist & Wiksell, Stockholm, 1978
4. Lundborg G: Nerve Injuries and Repair: Churchill Livingstone, Edinburgh, 1988
5. Butler DS: Mobilisation of the Nervous System. Churchill Livingstone, Melbourne, 1991
6. Elvey RL: Brachial plexus tension tests and the pathoanatomical origin of arm pain. In Idczack RM (ed): Aspects of Manipulative Therapy. Lincoln Institute of Health Sciences, Carlton, Australia, 1981
7. Wilson S, Selvaratnam P, Briggs C: Strain at the subclavian artery during the brachial plexus tension test. Proceedings of the Seventh Biennial Conference of the Manipulative Physiotherapists Association of Australia, Sydney, Australia, November 27–30, 1991
8. McLellan DC, Swash M: Longitudinal sliding of the median nerve during movements of the upper limb. J Neurol Neurosurg Psychiatry 39:556, 1976
9. Millesi H: The nerve gap. Hand Clin 2:651, 1986

10. Wilgis EFS, Murphy R: The significance of longitudinal excursion in peripheral nerves. Hand Clin 2:761, 1986
11. Pechan J, Julis F: The pressure measurement in the ulnar nerve: a contribution to the pathophysiology of cubital tunnel syndrome. J Biomech 8:75, 1975
12. Mackinnon SE, Dellon AL: Surgery of the Peripheral Nerve. Thieme, New York, 1988
13. Rydevik B, Maclean WG, Sjostrand J, Lundborg G: Blockage of axonal transport induced by acute graded compression of the rabbit vagus nerve. J Neurol Neurosurg Psychiatry 43:690, 1980
14. Dahlin LB, McLean WG: Effects of graded experimental compression on slow and fast axonal transport in rabbit vagus nerve. J Neurol Sci 72:19, 1986
15. Wall PD: Neuropathic pain and injured nerve: Central mechanisms. Br Med Bull 47:631, 1991
16. Mumenthaler M, Schliack H (eds): Peripheral Nerve Lesions. Thieme, New York, 1990
17. Szabo RM (ed): Nerve Compression Syndromes. Slack, Thorofare, NJ, 1989
18. Dawson DM, Hallett M, Millender LH: Entrapment Neuropathies. Little Brown, Boston, 1983
19. Hromada J: On the nerve supply of the connective tissues of some peripheral nervous system components. Acta Anat 55:343, 1963
20. Sunderland S: Nerve Injuries and Their Repair. Churchill Livingstone, Melbourne, 1991
21. Edgar MA, Nundy S: Innervation of the spinal dura mater. J Neurol Neurosurg Psychiatry 29:530, 1966
22. Bogduk N: The innervation of the lumbar spine. Spine 8:286, 1983
23. Cuatico W, Parker JC, Pappert E, Pilsl S: An anatomical and clinical investigation of spinal and meningeal nerves. Acta Neurochir 90:139, 1988
24. Groen CJ, Baljet B, Drukker J: The innervation of the spinal dura mater: Anatomy and clinical considerations. Acta Neurochirur 92:39, 1988
25. Parke WW, Watanabe R: Adhesions of the ventral dura mater. Spine 15:300, 1990
26. Janig W, Koltzenburg M: Receptive properties of pial afferents. Pain 45:77, 1991
27. Devor M: Neuropathic pain and injured nerve: peripheral mechanisms. Br Med Bull 47:609, 1991
28. Wall PD, Gutnick M: Ongoing activity in peripheral nerves: the physiology and pharmacology of impulse originating from a neuroma. Exp Neurol 43:580, 1974
29. Fields HL: Pain. McGraw-Hill, New York, 1987
30. McMahon SB: Mechanisms of sympathetic pain. Br Med Bull, 47:584, 1991
31. Granit R, Skoglund CR: Facilitation, inhibition and depression at the artificial synapse formed by the cut end of a mammalian nerve. J Physiol 103:435, 1945
32. Calvin WH, Devor M, Howe JF: Can neuralgias arise from minor demyelination? Spontaneous firing, mechanosensitivity and afterdischarge from conducting axons. Exp Neurol 75;755, 1972
33. Lundborg G, Rydevik BL: Effects of stretching the tibial nerve of the rabbit. A preliminary study of the intraneural circulation and the barrier function of the perineurium. J Bone Joint Surg 55B:390, 1973
34. Ogata K, Naito M: Blood flow of peripheral nerve, effects of dissection, stretching and compression. J Hand Surg 11B:11, 1986
35. Mackinnon SE, Dellon AL: Experimental study of chronic nerve compression. Clinical implications. Hand Clin 2:639, 1986

36. Smith KJ, McDonald: Spontaneous and mechanically evoked activity due to central demyelinating lesion. Nature 286:154, 1980

37. Upton ARM, McComas AJ: The double crush in nerve entrapment syndromes. Lancet 2:359, 1973

38. Mackinnon SE: Double and multiple "crush" syndromes. Hand Clin 8:369, 1992

39. Cherington M: Proximal pain in carpal tunnel syndrome. Arch Surg 108:69, 1974

40. Hurst LC, Weissberg D, Carroll RE: The relationship of double crush to carpal tunnel syndrome. J Hand Surg 10B:202, 1985

41. Devor M, Rappaport ZH: Pain and the physiology of damaged nerve. In Fields HL (ed): Pain Syndromes in Neurology. Butterworth–Heineman, Oxford, 1990

42. Wall PD, Melzack R (eds): Textbook of Pain. 2nd Ed. Churchill Livingstone, Edinburgh, 1989

43. Cyriax J: Textbook of Orthopaedic Medicine. 8th Ed. Ballierre Tindall, London, 1982

44. Asbury K, Fields HL: Pain due to peripheral nerve damage: an hypothesis. Neurology (Cleveland) 34:1587, 1984

45. Coderre RJ, Katz J, Vaccarino AL, Melzack R: Contribution of central neuroplasticity to pathological pain: review of clinical and experimental evidence. Pain 52:259, 1993

46. Cook AJ, Woolf CJ, Wall PD, McMahon SB: Expansion of cutaneous receptive fields of dorsal horn neurones following C primary afferent fibre inputs. Nature 325: 151, 1987

47. Susimoto T, Bennet GJ, Kajander KC: Transynaptic degeneration in the superficial dorsal horn afer sciatic nerve injury, effects of chronic constriction injury, transection and strychnine. Pain: 42:205, 1990

48. Woolf CJ: Recent advances in the pathophysiology of acute pain. Br J Anaesth 63: 139, 1989

49. Cook AF, Woolf CJ, Wall PD, McMahon SB: Expansion of cutaneous receptive fields of dorsal horn neurones following C primary afferent fibre inputs. Nature 325: 151, 1987

50. Fitzgerald M: The course and termination of primary afferent fibres: In Wall PD, Melzack R (eds): Textbook of Pain. 2nd Ed. Churchill Livingstone, Edinburgh, 1989

51. Wall PD: The biological function and dysfunction of different pain mechanisms. Adv Pain Res Ther 20:19, 1992

52. Bowsher D: Neurogenic pain syndromes and their management. Br Med Bull 47: 644, 1991

53. Campbell JN, Meyer RA, Davis KD, Raja SN: Sympathetically maintained pain: A unifying hypothesis. In: Willis WD (ed): Hyperalgesia and Allodynia. Raven Press, New York, 1992

54. Yaxley GA, Jull GA: A modified upper limb tension test: an investigation of responses in normal subjects. Aust J Physiother 37:143, 1991

55. Flanagan M, Bell A: Normative responses to the ulnar nerve bias tension test. Aust J Physiother (in press)

56. Narakas A: Compression syndromes about the shoulder including brachial plexus. In Szabo RM (ed): Nerve Compression Syndromes. Slack, Thorofare, NJ, 1989

57. Chahl LA, Ladd RJ: Local oedema and general excitation of cutaneous sensory receptors produced by electrical stimulation of the saphenous nerve in the rat. Pain 2:25, 1976

58. Lembeck F: Sir Thomas Lewis' nocifensor system, histamine and substance P containing primary afferent nerves. Trends Neurosci 6:106, 1983
59. Slater H, Shacklock MO, Butler DS: The dynamic central nervous system—examination and assessment using tension tests. In Boyling J, Palastanga N (eds): Grieve's Modern Manual Therapy of the Vertebral Column. 2nd Ed. Churchill Livingstone, Edinburgh (in press)
60. Kornberg C, Lew P: The effect of stretching neural structures on Grade 1 hamstring injuries. J Sports Phys Ther, June, 481, 1989
61. Elvey RL: Treatment of arm pain associated with abnormal brachial plexus tension. Aust J Physiother 32:225, 1986
62. Butler DS, Gifford LS: The concept of adverse mechanical tension in the nervous system. II: Examination and treatment. Physiotherapy 75:629, 1989
63. Maitland GD: Peripheral Manipulation. 3rd Ed. Butterworths, London, 1991

12 | Examination and Treatment By Passive Movement

Helen Jones
Mark Jones
Geoffrey D. Maitland

Passive movement is used by physical therapists in the evaluation and treatment of patients with orthopedic, neurologic, and cardiorespiratory problems. The principles outlined in this chapter are discussed in relation to the orthopedic patient, but the underlying clinical reasoning and suggested applications of passive movement are relevant to all three types of patient named above. The Maitland Concept[1] forms the basis of this discussion of evaluation and treatment by passive movement. The Maitland Concept entails a thorough evaluation and a continual attempt to relate treatment to a patient's symptoms, history, and signs, and to the biomedical sciences (e.g., pathology, neurophysiology, and biomechanics).

An understanding of evaluation and treatment by passive movement requires consideration of the therapist's clinical reasoning. That is, clinical decisions regarding how, what, and how much to evaluate and treat should always be related to the therapist's evolving interpretation(s) of the individual patient's presentation[2] (see also Ch. 6). The physical examination should be considered an extension of the subjective examination. Hypotheses will have been formed and modified throughout the subjective examination, culminating in decisions about the mechanisms of the symptoms evoked, the sources of the symptoms, contributing factors, precautions, contraindications to physical examination and treatment, appropriate management, and prognosis (see Ch. 6, 7, and 15).

The therapist should make a preliminary judgement about each of these hypothesis categories before commencing the physical examination. Mechanisms of symptoms will assist in determining the breadth of examination that is relevant, while sources and contributing factors highlight structures that require specific examination. A hypothesis about precautions and contraindications is then crucial to guide the safe extent of physical examination and treatment.

THE PHYSICAL EXAMINATION: WHAT TO EXAMINE AND WHY

With the aim of testing hypotheses about the mechanisms by which the symptoms in a particular case are evoked, the structures involved, and precautions and management options, the physical examination, including examination by passive movement, should test all potential sources (structures) and contributing factors, including:

Structures (e.g., joints, muscles, soft tissues, nerves) that underlie the areas in which symptoms occur.
Structures that can refer to the areas of symptoms.
Structures that can mechanically, chemically, and/or neurophysiologically affect (e.g., alter normal equilibrium through changing stresses, tension, loads, chemical/fluid flows, impulse transmission) adjacent and remote structures contributing to symptom production.

Two major sources of information are available to assist therapists in selecting examination and treatment options. Maitland[3] has portrayed these sources of information in his "permeable brick wall," in which both clinical presentation and theoretical knowledge are suggested guides to examination and treatment. The first source of information is the patient's signs and symptoms, recognizing that multiple presentations are possible within the same diagnostic category. For example, although a patient may present with medial scapular pain stemming from the costovertebral/transverse articulations, this source of symptoms can have a wide range of clinical presentations. Variability in presentation occurs partly because syndromes such as the costospinal syndrome can present in isolation or in combination with pathologic components from other sources (e.g., adjacent zygapophyseal articulations and the autonomic nervous system) or with other contributing factors (e.g., postural weakness and respiratory disorders). Further variation in the clinical presentation of this particular diagnostic category can take the form of symptoms ranging from those of the acutely irritable stage, requiring gentle examination and treatment, to those of the chronic, non-irritable stage, requiring extended examination and more vigorous treatment. When these sources of variability are considered along with environmental, neurologic, and physiologic effects on the patient's behavior and psyche, it is no wonder that no two patient presentations are the same. Examination and management should be tailored to the individual patient. This requires clinical reasoning rather than the mere application of clinical routines.

The second source of potentially helpful information in guiding the therapist's examination and treatment is the therapist's biomedical knowledge. The signs and symptoms of a condition can be interpreted as they relate to this biomedical knowledge, which will broaden the examination and treatment options available. In the example given above, posture may be the factor responsible for the symptoms arising from the costospinal articulation. Biomedical knowledge, such as a knowledge of regional anatomy, biomechanics, and pathophysiology will direct the physical therapist to further examine aspects of spinal mobility, muscle length, and muscle function that are not directly implicated by a consideration of symptoms alone.

Biomedical knowledge should also direct the physical therapist to examine other structures remote from the presenting symptoms but which are capable of mechanically, chemically, and/or neurophysiologically affecting the source of the symptoms. In the example given above, the dorsal scapular nerve could also be a source of the medial scapular pain. In this case, biomedical knowledge of regional anatomy and pathophysiology should direct the therapist to examine the nervous system as a whole, including the tissues interfacing with the dorsal scapular nerve, such as the scalenus medius muscle, which this nerve pierces.

It is biomedical knowledge that enables the therapist to develop a structural diagnosis. Structural differentiation, in which selective tissue assessment implies the involvement of specific structures in a patient's condition, is probably valid in peripherally evoked nociception. However, interpretation of the findings in a structural assessment must change when a centrally evoked nociceptive pattern is suspected. For further discussion of nociceptive patterns and the validity of structural differentiation, the reader is referred to Chapter 15 by Butler and to Zusman.[4]

EXAMINATION BY PASSIVE MOVEMENT

Passive movement is only a single part of the examination of the patient. Other components of the physical examination include the assessment of posture, of the position or movement that functionally aggravates the patient's condition, and of active physiologic movements, the nervous system, and the vascular system, as well as soft tissue palpation including the viscera, and an assessment of muscle function. All soft-tissue structures are potentially stressed and can therefore be evaluated and treated by passive movement, including muscle, ligament, cartilage, fascia, viscera, and the nervous system. A number of passive movement techniques are directed at evaluating the involvement of specific soft-tissue structures. However, a passive movement technique that is directed at a particular structure will also have an effect on other soft-tissue structures. Issues relating to examination and treatment by passive movement will be discussed with the joint as a focus, although this is not meant to indicate that joint dysfunction is the only or most important factor in symptom presentation.

Passive Movements Used

Assessment of the patient's functional aggravating activity or posture is a useful component of the physical examination. It provides a degree of structural differentiation and provides an evaluation that is meaningful to the patient. The patient is asked to demonstrate an activity or position that reproduces his or her symptoms. (The word "pain" occurs throughout this chapter only as an example of a symptom elicited with passive movement. The points discussed are applicable to any symptom). For example, the patient may report neck pain when turning around to steer a car in reverse. In this example, the movements involved would include cervical rotation with some degree of extension and lateral flexion, as well as a combined thoracic movement. More remote body segments may also contribute to producing symptoms, through mechanical or neural tension created, for example, by the position of the arms, lumbar spine, and lower extremities.

To do a physical differentiation in the position that reproduces the patient's symptoms, the therapist must selectively alter the various components of the painful position while maintaining the position. Thus, if the patient demonstrates a cervical pain on rotation to the right, with the right arm resting on the back of the front passenger's seat (in a left-hand-drive car), the therapist might maintain the painful cervical/thoracic position and alter wrist flexion and extension to assess the possibility of a neural component. Similarly, the cervical position could be maintained while thoracic or lumbar movements are altered. The cervical position could also be divided into its component movements to further stress rotation, extension, and lateral flexion. While the later example does not implicate a specific structure, it does incriminate the most significant movement component, which can then be correlated with the findings in a more localized passive movement examination.

The passive joint movement tests available include physiologic movements, accessory movements, combined physiologic movements, combined accessory movements, and combined physiologic and accessory movements. In the cervical and thoracic regions specifically, passive movement testing of the joints includes physiologic movements; passive accessory intervertebral movements (PAIVMs); physiologic intervertebral movements; accessory movements of rib and costal articulations (costotransverse, costovertebral, sternocostal, costochondral, and intercostal), and the passive assessment of relevant peripheral joints. Passive movement tests for the cervical and thoracic spine are discussed in detail by Maitland[5] and in Chapters 7 and 9. Additional specialized passive movement tests for the cervicothoracic region include tests of vascular involvement and vertebral instability. These tests are described in Chapters 7 and 8, respectively.

Maitland regards the assessment of PAIVMs as providing the most useful information about the status of the spinal joint and surrounding tissues. PAIVMs incriminate the intervertebral level and component of the motion segment (e.g., intervertebral body, interlaminar, zygapophyseal joint) that are responsible for symptoms. The unique accessibility of the cervical spine allows PAIVMs to be assessed from the posteroanterior, anteroposterior, and transverse directions. In the cervical and thoracic spine, PAIVMs can be angled medially, laterally, cephalad, and caudad. These angles can also be combined and a PAIVM performed with the spine in any physiologic position.

When performing passive movement tests, the therapist should not only obtain information about range of movement, but should also ascertain the quality of resistance and provocation of symptoms. For spinal movement to be classified as "normal," it must cover the full physiologic and intervertebral range that would be expected in the context of the patient's age and somatotype. Normal spinal movement should provoke the same degree of sensation or discomfort with the application of overpressure as movement to the opposite side. Even minimal abnormality detected in a range of movement, quality of resistance, or in the provocation of symptoms makes the passive movement test potentially relevant.

The relationship between perceived resistance and the provocation of symptoms is useful in determining the significance of a passive movement test and how the movement involved in the test could be used in treatment. Maitland[3] has proposed the use of movement diagrams to portray this relationship between resistance, passive movement, and symptoms. A movement diagram is a graph of the nature and intensity of symptoms (e.g., local and/or referred pain, dizziness) and nature and degree of signs (e.g., resistance, spasm) occurring in the range of passive movement being assessed. Representation of the various components on the diagram permits a visual analysis of their interrelationship (e.g., whether pain or resistance occurs first in the range of movement, and their relative proportion at any point in that range). Clinically, therapists should think in terms of movement diagrams whenever they assess passive movement. For a detailed discussion of movement diagrams, the reader is referred to Magarey[6] and Maitland.[3]

Examination by passive movement requires continual communication with the patient to monitor the symptoms being experienced while simultaneously relating these to the quality of passive movement perceived by the therapist. The accuracy of the therapist's perception of movement quality is influenced by his/her manual handling skills. Strategic positioning of the patient and therapist, along with supportive hand positions, provides the control needed to optimally perceive abnormalities in passive movement.

The significance of a passive movement test can be interpreted from two perspectives. First, a movement test that stresses a specific structure can be used to judge the involvement of that structure in a diagnostic sense. For example, passive intervertebral movement of a zygapophyseal joint may be considered abnormal (and hence a source of and/or factor contributing to symptoms) if, upon testing, hypomobility is perceived and/or pain is provoked. Similarly, neural involvement may be present if a neural tension test, such as the upper limb tension test (ULTT), is limited and/or reproduces symptoms (see Ch. 11). Second, the relationship of resistance to symptoms assists in revealing the movement and direction of movement most limited by resistance and/or pain, without necessarily requiring any change in the diagnostic interpretation. To think only in structural terms limits the value of passive movement testing. For example, altering the angle at which a PAIVM is directed is unlikely to change the structure implicated. However, a change in the relationship of resistance to symptoms, evident in the varied angle of pressure, can be extremely useful in revealing the direction of movement most involved in the symptoms. This in turn will greatly assist the selection and efficacy of treatment. The combination of these two perspectives will often lead to the most effective treatment technique for a particular condition. For example, if the most symptomatic passive movement follows a specific direction of cervical zygaphophyseal joint movement, and passive testing also suggests involvement of neural tissues, the therapist's biomedical knowledge would lead to the exploration of a combination of PAIVMs in a position of neural tension as a treatment of choice. (Some of these considerations are illustrated in the case studies in Chapter 14).

Decisions about the choice of passive movement tests for a particular patient, about how many of these can be employed at the first consultation, and about the extent to which each passive movement test can be taken depend on the individual patient presentation. Standard routines of passive movement testing exist, but these should be tailored to each patient. Clues to the structures that should be examined, the extent of the examination, and the precautions required will arise throughout the subjective examination. To illustrate the reasoning involved in these important decisions in planning the passive movement examination, the following discussion divides patients into the two broad categories of those undergoing a limited and those having a full examination.

Limited Examination

A limited examination implies that examination procedures, including passive movement tests, can be taken to the point at which symptoms are produced or begin to increase. The number of passive tests may have to be limited, and standard test positions may need to be altered for patient comfort (e.g., posterior cervical palpation in the supine rather than prone position). The decision to limit the physical examination is based on the following information obtained in the subjective examination:

Severity of the disorder.
Irritability of the disorder.
A worsening disorder.
Stability (variability and predictability) of the disorder.
Unknown behavior of symptoms (e.g., immediately after trauma, surgery, or casting).
Unpredictable behavior of symptoms.

Known pathology (e.g., rheumatoid arthritis, osteoporosis, instability, recent onset or worsening of neurologic signs).

Indications of more sinister or impending pathologic processes (e.g., unexplained weight loss, bowel and bladder dysfunction, spinal cord involvement, vertebrobasilar insufficiency).

Usage or a history of usage of medication that may have an adverse effect (e.g., corticosteroids, anticoagulants).

For further discussion of these concepts the reader is referred to Chapter 7 and Maitland.[3] The need for caution in the physical examination and treatment procedure is not determined by a single factor; the factors that prompt it exist as a continuum (e.g., irritability presents in degrees), and all of them must be taken into consideration. Thus, for example, a non-irritable disorder in a patient with rheumatoid arthritis will require caution in handling of the patient.

Similarly, there is no easy formula for determining the extent of physical examination once the need for caution has been recognized. In some patients it is appropriate to obtain relevant information about each area and structure involved, by careful testing (active, passive, and resistive) to the point of onset of symptoms. Thus, for example, some disorders are irritable to specific movements, while still enabling everyday function. Consider the case of a woman who, with the occurrence of mild symptoms, can continue packing shelves at a supermarket provided she does not pack the shelves above a certain height and thereby extend her neck. If, on the other hand, the combination of arm activity and cervical extension is maintained for more than a minute, cervical pain is provoked for 2 hours. Here it should be possible to perform a relatively extensive examination of the patient to the point of onset of symptoms, taking particular care when using maneuvers that involve cervical extension. In doing this, an attempt is made to gauge the amount and direction of activity involved in the patient's account of the behavior of her symptoms, so as to provide a guide to the extent and direction of the activity that may be undertaken in the physical examination. In other situations the extent of such an examination might only serve to aggravate the disorder. Thus, for example, in a disorder in which symptoms are constant and most movements are painful, as with an active inflammatory process, nothing is gained by testing all possible movements, and doing so may indeed cause harm. At this stage of the disorder, structural differentiation is difficult, and if undertaken becomes counterproductive, since the patient's symptoms are likely to be aggravated. In this instance the examination should be centered on identifying the most effective pain-relieving position and movement pattern for the patient. Being able to examine the patient without aggravating the patient's symptoms enables the therapist to treat a disorder effectively even at this stage of its presentation. Clearly, as the symptoms resolve, further examination can be performed, allowing a more specific structural analysis (e.g., including hypotheses about sources and contributing factors).

Full Examination

A full examination implies that examination procedures including passive movement testing can be taken to their full extent, including the addition of passive overpressure to all primary and combined movements. Passive movement tests can be taken to their full extent without the risk of aggravating symptoms if a disorder is non-irritable and not severe, and if its nature, history, stability, and progression do not dictate the need for caution. A full examination enables the therapist to obtain a much more complete clinical picture. By weighing the presenting signs of an abnormality, the therapist can determine the relative contribution made by different potential sources and contributing factors, as well as the most appropriate treatment. As with the passive movement testing described in a limited examination, the relationship between range of movement, quality of movement (e.g., resistance), and provocation of symptoms should be noted.

As an illustration of a full examination, consider a right-handed tennis player complaining of an ache in the right upper thoracic area that becomes apparent only after four or five service games. The ache does not stop him from finishing a match, but he feels that it inhibits him from applying his full service power. He does not feel that the ache affects any other of his tennis strokes, nor does he feel it during or after any other activities. The ache is relieved after half an hour of rest from serving. There was no trauma initiating the symptoms, which have now been present for 6 months, and the history indicates a stable disorder. In order to reproduce by passive movement a symptom that in everyday life is aggravated only by considerable mechanical force or activity, it will be necessary to take the passive movement examination to its full extent. Since any physical abnormality is likely to be minimal, strong overpressure can and may have to be applied to all physiologic, accessory, and combined movements to reproduce the symptoms. Routine passive movements are unlikely to provide sufficient information on which to base treatment, even with the use of strong overpressure. Combined passive movements of the upper limb, spine, or both, as well as combinations of passive movements directed at specific structures (e.g., passive spinal lateral flexion combined with the ULTT to simulate the tennis serving position), passive movement under compression, and sustained spinal movements simulating the serving posture may be necessary to reveal relevant signs. An assessment of neural tension may need to be taken beyond the base test. This assessment would include maneuvers to test the nervous system both longitudinally (e.g., with the slump test) and transversely (e.g., with ULTTs), with consideration also given to tension testing of the autonomic nervous system (see Ch. 15). Presensitizing the structures at fault, (i.e., examining the patient after he has been playing tennis) would provide valuable information. With this more minor presentation the patient's ache may not necessarily be reproduced. The therapist must therefore be attuned to the more subtle abnormalities present on movement testing, including changes in end-feel and more than normal discomfort on overpressure.

To group all patients into two categories is clearly an oversimplification. In reality there is a continuum from the presentation in which extreme care is needed to avoid an exacerbation of the patient's symptoms to the presentation in which additional test procedures incorporating increased loads or repetitive movement are required. The complexity of these decisions is illustrated in the patient with severe pain that is moderately irritable but who has symptoms that are stable and chronic. While care must still be taken, particularly in progressing the vigor of treatment, the therapist may determine that treatment will need to be strongly applied and that the aggravation of symptoms that ensues is acceptable even if it lasts for several days.

TREATMENT BY PASSIVE MOVEMENT

Management considerations are not left until the end of the examination. Clues that elicit a range of management options will have emerged throughout the subjective and physical examination of the patient. Within the broader management plan, specific options for passive treatment will also be drawn from patient data as the latter accumulates. As stated before, there are two major sources of information to assist therapists in selecting examination and treatment options. These are the patient's signs and symptoms and the therapist's biomedical knowledge. Attention to each of these sources leads to complementary and sometimes different treatment considerations, and the combination of these two sources results in a greater range of treatment options.

Biomedical knowledge is essential as a basis for determining which structures are potential sources of a patient's symptoms (i.e., capable of producing those symptoms or contributing to their production and maintenance). The knowledge that a cervical disc disorder may refer symptoms to the thoracic spine is a case in point. This may necessitate examination and treatment of the cervical spine. For example, central PAIVMs on the C4 spinous process may reveal restrictions of accessory movement and reproduce a patient's medial scapular pain. When this sign is combined with findings from the entire subjective and physical examination, the therapist may suspect a cervical discogenic basis for the patient's pain. Clearly this judgement is based on past experience and biomedical knowledge. However, the specific technique used in treating the patient will depend more heavily on the signs and symptoms elicited when the symptomatic spinal levels are thoroughly examined by passive movement. If the most relevant finding was a restriction of PAIVMs applied just lateral to the spinous process and over the C4-C5 articular pillar, restoration of this movement would be instrumental in resolving the patient's symptoms.

In other circumstances, biomedical knowledge will take a greater role in the selection of treatment. For example, knowledge of the varying angles of cervical and thoracic facet planes is a prerequisite to the correct positioning of a patient for a localized manipulation. In other circumstances treatment is based on biomedical knowledge in the absence of signs and symptoms, usually as a preventive measure. An example of a choice of treatment based more on biomedical knowledge than on signs or symptoms is direct neural mobilization to prevent recurrence of a carpal tunnel lesion during a subsequent pregnancy.

The art of treatment by passive movement will be enhanced when the precise mechanisms by which pain is relieved by passive movement are known. Many proposed neurophysiologic effects of passive movement may contribute to pain relief, including the inhibition of reflex muscle spasm; conduction block of sensitized nociceptors by stimulation of large- and small-diameter afferents; stimulation of endogenous opioids; soft-tissue elongation reducing afferent discharge; improvement in axoplasmic flow enhancing neural function; and psychological effects. For details of the current research status of these proposed mechanisms, the reader is referred to Austin et al.[7]

The decision about whether a passive movement technique needs to be performed gently or more firmly is based on the therapist's hypothesis about the need for caution as determined from the subjective examination, as well as on the relationship between the quality of movement and the symptoms produced during the performance of the particular passive movement. As discussed earlier, the recognition that caution is needed is based on the patient's presenting behavior and history of symptoms, as well as on the nature of any known disorder (e.g., rheumatoid arthritis, instability).

Maitland[3,5] has suggested principles of treatment by passive movement, based on the relationship between quality of movement and symptoms. These principles require analysis of the relationship of pain to resistance, and of which factor—pain or resistance—is limiting the passive movement. To illustrate this principle very simply, patients will be divided into two extreme categories that are similar to the categories used earlier to illustrate the extent of examination. It is likely that patients who require a limited examination will have signs elicited by passive movement that are markedly limited by pain, while patients who require an extended examination will have signs that are limited by tissue resistance.

Techniques of passive movement have been graded for use in different clinical presentations. A brief review of the grades of movement proposed by Maitland[3,5] is necessary to the further discussion of treatment by passive movement. A grade of movement is defined by two parameters, the relationship of the passive movement to resistance and the amplitude of the movement (see Fig. 12-1).

The grades of passive movement are as follows:

Grade I: A small-amplitude movement performed at the beginning of the range.
Grade II: A large-amplitude movement in a resistance-free part of the range.
Grade III: A large-amplitude movement performed to the point of approximately 50% of the resistance.
Grade IV: A small-amplitude movement performed to the point of approximately 50% of the resistance.

In situations in which it is inappropriate to assess the end-range resistance in order to determine whether it is equivalent to a Grade III or IV movement (e.g., in a moderately irritable disorder), 50% of the resistance is estimated.

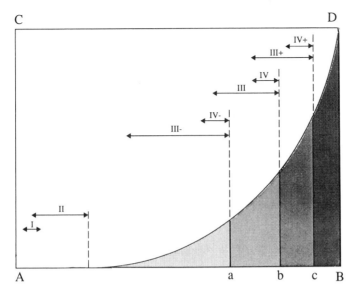

Fig. 12-1. Grades of movement. *(A–B)* Range of movement. *(A–C)* Degree of resistance. *(a)* Point in range of 25 percent total resistance. *(b)* Point in range of 50 percent total resistance. *(c)* Point in range of 75 percent total resistance.

Pluses (+) and minuses (−) are also used to describe the variations possible within the four defin¦tions given above. A plus or minus added to a Grade I and II refers to an increase or decrease in the amplitude (and hence range) of the respective passive movement. For example, a II + is a larger amplitude movement than a II, and therefore extends further into the range of movement without resistance. Large (III) and small amplitude (IV) passive movements are also subclassified according to degrees of resistance.

The variations in the grades of passive movement are as follows:

Grade III − − and IV − −: Movement taken to the point at which resistance is first perceived (R1).
Grade III − and IV −: Movement taken to 25% or less of the point of resistance.
Grade III + and IV +: Movement taken to approximately 75% of the point of resistance.
Grade III + + and IV + +: Movement taken to the maximum resistance or limit of the joint range.

Pain Is the Only Factor Limiting Movement

In some patient presentations, pain is the only factor limiting a passive movement. The pain is likely to be felt early in the range of passive movement, and it is the nature of the pain (e.g., severe or irritable) that causes the therapist to stop further movement before any resistance may be perceived. An example of such a pain-limiting situation is an acute discogenic wry neck, in which pain limits many passive movements (accessory and physiologic). Options for the initial treatment of this condition by passive movement include the use of either accessory or physiologic movements performed through the greatest range of movement that is possible without provoking symptoms (e.g., Grade I or II). In this example, the neck would be supported in its position of comfort or deformity. The passive movement most likely to ease the presentation would be a physiologic or accessory movement further in the direction of deformity.

Continual communication with the patient is essential to ensure that the treatment technique being used remains pain-free, and to enable the therapist to modify the technique in accordance with the patient's response. An increase in symptoms during the technique would require modification of the amplitude or perhaps the direction of the technique, while an easing of symptoms may encourage the therapist to progress the technique.

Patient comfort in the treatment position, and the therapist's handling skills, are essential prerequisites for the successful treatment of a pain-limiting presentation with passive movement. While this may seem obvious, poor results, particularly with the gentler techniques, are often the result of therapist error. Failing to ensure the most comfortable patient position from which to commence the technique, and lack of a smooth, supportive mobilization technique will provoke muscle guarding and jeopardize the success of treatment.

Progression of treatment is then based on findings in the subjective and physical reassessment. A full discussion of the importance and various types of reassessment is beyond the scope of this chapter, and the reader is referred to Maitland.[1,3] for a detailed discussion of this topic. If the reassessment is favorable, passive movement treatments can be progressed by:

Increasing the amplitude, speed, and sharpness of change of the movement technique.

Performing the same technique with the patient in a different position.

Progressing the passive movement technique to the provocation of some pain.

Tissue Resistance is the Only Factor Limiting Movement

In some patient presentations, tissue resistance is the only factor limiting movement. In these presentations, passive movement testing (physiologic or accessory) will reveal abnormal resistance throughout a particular movement, and a reduction in the range of movement as the result of resistance. However, passive movements are unlikely to cause significant pain. Instead, the patient will typically experience only a degree of abnormal discomfort or pressure at the limit of movement. An example of such a presentation is stiffness as a sole complaint when turning the head to drive a car in reverse. Treatment in this presentation, in which increased tissue resistance is the prominent feature, involves firm mobilization directed at the most severely limited passive movements. The treatment will have to be multidirectional and applied to all involved spinal levels. Alternating mobilization of accessory and physiologic movements is suggested.

Passive treatment techniques that should be considered in the example given above include physiologic movements in the most severely restricted direction (cardinal planes or movement combinations), accessory movements from neutral to various combined physiologic positions, localized manipulation, and techniques employing combined cervical and thoracic positions. Passive movement techniques that incorporate other structures could also be considered, including joint mobilization in positions in which the nervous system is longitudinally and/or transversely pre-tensioned. If the treatment creates soreness, the latter can be eased by using the same passive movement but in a large amplitude and to a point of slightly less resistance.

Most patient profiles do not belong within either of the two categories described above, but somewhere in between. That is, passive movement testing elicits both pain and abnormal resistance in varying proportions.

Pain and Resistance Limit Movement

When pain and resistance are both present on passive movement testing, selecting the firmness of treatment depends on which factor (pain or resistance) is limiting the movement, and on the relationship between the pain and resistance throughout the available range of movement. If pain is the limiting factor, treatment should be begun and progressed as outlined in the "pain only" presentation above. The earlier the pain is reported during the performance of the passive movement, and the greater the difference between the point of onset of pain (P1) and the point at which resistance is first perceived (R1), the greater the need to utilize patient positions of maximal comfort. Gentle passive movement techniques performed in the comfortable part of the range can reduce the patient's pain and therefore permit a greater active range of movement. As the pain improves, the resistance factor may also show signs of improvement. However, when resistance fails to further improve with the use of gentle techniques to alleviate pain, progression into resistance should be undertaken so as to more directly address the reduction in movement. The techniques used for this should initially employ slow, small-amplitude movements (e.g., IV−) done with respect for pain, with progression into greater degrees of pain and tissue resistance during subsequent treatment sessions.

When pain is the factor limiting a particular passive movement, it may be possible to use movement of the joint in another direction, or to alter the position of the patient so that the passive movement involves a smaller proportion of pain to resistance[8] (see Ch. 9 and 14). Both treatment employing the most painful direction of movement and treatment using a less symptomatic but still painfully restricted movement have merit and should be tried.

When pain and resistance are both present and resistance is the limiting factor to movement, the grade of mobilization will depend upon the severity, quality, and behavior of the pain associated with the resistance. This movement restriction may be treated from the beginning with accessory, physiologic, or combined accessory and physiologic movement techniques. The discomfort felt during the technique should be in rhythm with the technique, and should lessen or at least remain unchanged with treatment. The pain must not be allowed to worsen, and initially, any mobilizing technique employed should not reproduce a patient's referred pain.

When an assessment by passive movement reveals a rapid increase in pain through the movement, small amplitude movements into resistance and with respect for pain are indicated. Stronger techniques (e.g., IV, IV+, IV++) with movements into greater resistance and pain can then be progressively used. With improvement, one would expect pain to occur later in the range of movement, and the intensity of the pain to decrease. Again, with improvement resistance will start later in the range of movement, with a decrease in the degree of resistance perceived through the movement and an increase in the total range of movement. When significant tissue resistance is present through the range of movement, large-amplitude techniques are indicated.

A unique presentation of this pain and resistance category is "momentary pain." Such pain is typically experienced as severe pain of short duration, which is usually elicited only at the extreme of a particular movement or position (e.g., thoracic pain felt only at the extreme of a ball toss when serving in tennis). Momentary pain may also occur when the involved structure is subjected to a load, as with an anterior chest pain (e.g., costosternal) that is experienced only when lifting weights. In presentations involving a peripheral joint, such as the carpometacarpal joint of the thumb, the patient may report dropping objects even in the absence of pain. This momentary "giving way" or weakness may result from a pain-induced inhibition that can be treated in a manner similar to momentary pain. When examining a patient who has momentary pain, it is essential to identify the sign that is most comparable with the patient's symptoms. If the joint proves to be the source of the patient's symptoms, this sign will usually be a combined accessory and physiologic movement. For example, in the case of the tennis serve that elicits thoracic pain, a unilateral PAIVM on a thoracic zygapophyseal joint in a position of combined extension and rotation may be an effective treatment technique. Success requires finding the physical examination sign that reproduces the momentary pain, and then provoking that pain with the treatment technique.

A presentation that is difficult to categorize because of the absence of resistance in its passive movement assessment is an intra-articular disorder. An intra-articular disorder is characterized by the provocation of pain when joint surfaces are compressed during passive movement. When an intra-articular component is suspected and pain is dominant in the disorder, physiologic movements can be used in conjunction with distraction techniques in a position of maximum comfort. At the other extreme, when strong techniques have been judged necessary, passive movement techniques may have to include compression of joint surfaces with the aim of reproducing the patient's symptoms.

This overview of treatment principles based on the factors of pain and tissue resistance has been quite basic. Other signs, such as spasm and crepitus, must also be considered. For a discussion of more complex presentations, the reader is referred to Magarey.[6]

SUMMARY

It is hoped that the specific principles and techniques discussed in this chapter will be seen as an extension of the therapist's clinical reasoning. The chosen focus has been on joint mobilization, but it is recognized that the joint is but one of a number of structures that contribute to symptom production. It is also recognized that passive movement will affect multiple structures simultaneously. Nevertheless, the principles outlined in this chapter are equally applicable to the passive movement of other structures. Maitland[3] has called any physiotherapy technique the "brainchild of ingenuity." This provides an appropriate point of closure. A good knowledge base of both the biomedical sciences and the clinical principles of selecting and progressing treatment provide a logical foundation for clinical reasoning. It is only by openmindedness and logical and creative thinking that new treatment techniques will emerge.

REFERENCES

1. Maitland GD: The Maitland Concept. In Twomey LT, Taylor JR (eds): Physical Therapy of the Low Back. Churchill Livingstone, New York, 1987
2. Jones MA: Clinical reasoning in manual therapy. Phys Ther 72:875, 1992
3. Maitland GD: Peripheral Manipulation. 3rd Ed. Butterworth-Heinemann, London, 1991
4. Zusman M: Central nervous system contribution to mechanically produced motor and sensory responses. Aust J Physiother 38:245, 1992
5. Maitland GD: Vertebral Manipulation. 5th Ed. Butterworths, London, 1986
6. Magarey ME: Examination and assessment in spinal joint dysfunction. In Grieve GP (ed): Modern Manual Therapy of the Vertebral Column. Churchill Livingstone, Edinburgh, 1986
7. Austin L, Maitland GD, Magarey ME: Manual therapy: what, when and why? In Australian Physiotherapy Association (Victorian Branch) (eds): Sports Physiotherapy: Applied Science and Practice. Churchill Livingstone, Melbourne (in press)
8. Edwards BC: Manual of Combined Movements. Churchill Livingstone, Edinburgh, 1992

13 | Headaches of Cervical Origin

Gwendolen A. Jull

Cervical headaches are headaches whose causes are found in painful dysfunction of the structures of the cervical spine, particularly those innervated by the upper three cervical nerves.[1-3] A relationship has been established between headache symptoms and cervical joint trauma, arthropathy, and segmental hypo- and hypermobility.[2-9]

The cervical spine can be the primary cause of headache. Its role becomes less straightforward and differential diagnosis more complex when cervical dysfunction contributes to combined headache forms, headache continua, or seems to be in part responsible for the intensity of pain and frequency of attack in some migraines.[10-12] Knowledge is indeed incomplete when cervical structures act as a mechanical trigger for some vascular and neurogenic headaches,[12-14] or when injury to the neck precipitates a true migraine.[15]

The clinical physical therapist, when consulted by the patient with headache, especially on a first contact basis, must decide whether cervical dysfunction is a primary cause, a partial cause in a headache continuum, is enhancing symptoms of other forms of headache, or has no role in the patient's headache. On this basis, decisions are made to treat, trial treat, or refer the patient for appropriate medical management. These clinical decisions must be made with the realization that the causes of headache are many and varied,[16] and that chronic benign headache often represents a difficult diagnostic area.

The characterization of headache is not always an easy task. At present, there are a lack of laboratory tests and radiologic examinations that can assist in the positive medical diagnosis of many benign chronic forms of headache.[16,17] Diagnosis is largely based on the nature, characteristics, and temporal pattern of a headache. The difficulty is that there can be marked symptomatic overlap between common forms of chronic headache such as migraine without aura, tension headache, and headache associated with craniomandibular dysfunction and cervical headache. Nevertheless, accurate differential diagnosis is essential to successful treatment.

When examining the headache patient, the physical therapist should be cognizant of the various forms of headache and should identify a symptomatic pattern suggestive of a cervical cause. Physical examination must reveal signs of cervical dysfunction that are compatible with the patient's headache complaint. Both subjective and physical criteria need to be present to rationalize physical therapy of the cervical spine as the primary management approach for a particular headache patient.

SYMPTOMATIC CHARACTERIZATION OF CERVICAL HEADACHE

The subjective examination of the headache patient is helped by adopting a consistent approach to history taking, in an attempt to elicit a pattern that may characterize a particular type of headache.[18] As there is overlap between symptoms of different headaches, especially those of a chronic nature, reliance cannot be placed on any one feature (e.g., associated neck pain) as indicating a cervical origin for the headache. Rather, to make an informed decision, the clinician must evaluate characteristics that both suggest and dismiss cervical headache.

Length of History and Temporal Pattern

The length of the history and the temporal pattern of a headache (i.e., its frequency and duration) are established during the first meeting with a patient.[18] This gives the clinician an overall perspective on the headache and provides important diagnostic indicators before specific details are sought.

Cervical headaches may present in acute, subacute, or commonly, chronic forms of many months or years duration.[6,8,19,20] The pattern of headache can be variable. In an acute form of cervical headache following a neck injury, the headache may be almost constant but fluctuant in its intensity. In other situations a cervical headache may be episodic, lasting from a few hours to several days. A bout of such headaches may last for some weeks and then resolve, to return at a later time. When the cervical headache becomes chronic, it may be semicontinuous or follow a pattern of at least two to three headaches per week.[2,3,19-22]

These patterns, which are well documented for cervical headache, are also shared by some other forms of chronic headache. These include tension headaches, headaches associated with craniomandibular dysfunction, frequent migraine without aura (common migraine), and even some less common forms of headache, such as hemicrania continua.[16,18,23-26] Therefore, the temporal pattern of cervical headache is not uniquely characteristic.

The temporal patterns of some chronic forms of headache can, however, be diagnostic. The essential qualities of migraine are its episodic nature, its reasonably consistent duration for a particular individual, and its termination within a specified period, usually less than 24 hours.[17,18] The periods between headaches are classically pain free. Cluster headaches are characterized by attacks of pain of short duration occurring at variable intervals within a day or week. The bouts last up to 1 or 2 months. The patient will then have a remission period that ranges from 6 months to 2 years.[18,27,28] Such attacks also affect persons with chronic paroxysmal hemicrania, but this chronic form of headache differs from cluster headache in that it lacks remission periods.[27-29] When the patient relates such typical temporal patterns, the clinician begins to exclude a primary cervical cause of headache.

Temporal patterns may be more difficult to define when patients experience continua of headache or mixed headache syndromes.[18,30] If patients suffer two or more types of headache the clinician attempts to obtain a clear definition and pattern of each. In such situations the physical therapist may be able to help alleviate one component of the patient's headache syndrome.

Area of Symptoms

The area of pain of headache has limited diagnostic significance. Similar areas of pain are documented for many chronic forms of headache.[17,24,27,28,31] This is not surprising, since whatever its cause, headache will be associated with nociceptive activity in the trigemino-cervical nucleus.[32-35] The more common sites documented for cervical headache are frontal, retro-orbital, temporal, and occipital, with the head pain being associated with suboccipital and neck pain.[2,3,19,20,36] These areas of pain probably reflect the stronger projections of the opthalmic division of the trigeminal nerve into the C1 to C3 cord segments.[32]

Neck or suboccipital pain associated with the head pain is considered a characteristic feature of cervical headache, its presence being reported in almost all subjects in studies of cervical headache.[3,5,19,20] However, neck pain or aching is not exclusive to cervical headache, and therefore cannot be diagnostic of it. What seems to be of greater significance is the area of onset of pain. Sjaastad et al.,[37] in studying groups of patients with migraine and cervical headache, found that although both groups reported neck and head pain, the onset of pain was more frequently in the head in the subjects with migraine, with subsequent spread to the neck. In contrast, the focal onset of pain in the patients with cervical headache was in the neck, with spread to the head. This head pain often becomes the maximal area of cervical headache.[22] Solomon et al.[14] found that while 70 percent of their group of 100 cluster headache patients suffered concurrent neck pain, the origin of pain was in the neck in only 10 percent. Neck pain in all of their patients was always minor in comparison with the intense pain in the retroorbital or frontal areas. These studies suggest that careful questioning about the area of onset of pain and its spread, in conjunction with questioning about areas of greater intensity, may have more diagnostic significance than the area of headache alone.

Some headaches, such as migraine and cluster headaches, chronic paroxysmal hemicrania, and occipital neuralgia are typically unilateral in distribution, while tension and muscle-contraction headache are classified as bilateral.[16,37] There is some difficulty in characterizing cervical headache in these terms. Even though Sjaastad et al.[2] first characterized cervical headache as strictly unilateral, subsequent studies have shown that the headache can be unilateral, unilateral with spread, or bilateral.[3,19,22]

There is no side preponderance for cervical headache,[6] but there is side consistency. Cervical headaches do not change sides,[2,20] as may migraine with aura and occasionally cluster headaches.[27,28,38] The clinician's suspicion of a cervical origin of headache should be aroused if patients report such side alternation.

Quality of Symptoms

Cervical headache is most commonly of an aching or deep boring quality, but descriptions such as throbbing or pulsing have been recorded.[3,6,19,36] Such descriptions are not unique to cervical headache. However, while cervical headache may be of moderate to severe intensity, it never reaches the excruciating levels of pain experienced in, for example, a cluster headache,[27] nor presents with the lancinating pains of true neuralgia. Moreover, cervical headaches can be variable in their intensity. Patients often report that at different times their headaches can be mild, moderate, or sometimes severe.[21] In contrast, migraine, if not controlled, inevitably builds to a severe and often disabling level with each attack.

Associated Symptoms

Many and varied symptoms can occur in association with a cervical headache. Those most commonly reported include nausea, visual disturbances, dizziness, or lightheadedness.[6,19–21] Such symptoms do not characterize cervical headache, since they are reported in many types of headache.[39] However, it is of interest that when symptoms such as visual ones are unilateral in cervical headache, they are ipsilateral.[2] In contrast, in migraine with aura, there is no clear correlation between the side of headache and the focal neurologic features.[17] These symptoms may present opposite to the side of pain.

Neurologic Symptoms

Symptoms commensurate with irritation or compression of an upper cervical nerve are rare in the patient with cervical headache, indicating that their headache is more typically a referred pain.[40] There are occasional reports of a slight sensory deficit in the distribution of the C2 and C3 nerves.[20] Cases of true compression of the C2 roots have been reported, and these are usually associated with instability at the atlantoaxial articulations.[41-43]

Time and Mode of Onset

The cervical headache is often present on waking or, alternatively, may come on during the day, in relation to activity.[2,4,19,40] There may be a warning of onset of headache via a pain or stiffness in the neck before build up of the headache.[20] A diagnosis of cervical headache can be dismissed when patients report a warning of focal neurologic symptoms that typify migraine with aura.[17] Premonitory symptoms such as hunger or euphoria occurring up to 24 hours before the headache also typify migraine. Additionally, the clinician doubts a cervical origin of headache when patients report the headache as an attack of head pain, such as occurs with the cluster type of headache.[27]

Precipitating and Relieving Factors

Cervical headaches are typically precipitated or aggravated by sustained neck postures, movements, and stress situations.[2,16,19,44] The headaches usually have a mechanical trigger, but it is not uncommon for patients to be unable to identify a precipitating factor. That stress can provoke headache does not necessarily imply that the patient suffers from tension headache, since stress can precipitate many forms of headache.[17]

Patients with cervical headache often have difficulty in identifying factors that relieve their headache. Some may gain relief with a change of posture or lying down, but many cannot find strategies for relief.[19] Simple analgesics may help in the early stages of the condition, but once the headache is chronic and of sufficient intensity, these often offer little relief.[45,46] Cervical headache patients do not benefit from drugs used to treat migraine.[20,47,48]

General Medical History

A thorough medical appraisal of current and past general health and a careful screen of each body system are necessary in the differential diagnosis of headache.[18] The cervical headache patient usually has no related medical history, although some may have a past or current history of migraine.[6] There is no familial tendency in cervical headache, such as can be present in migraine.[6,17] While headaches such as migraine and cluster have a typical age span of onset,[17,27] the onset of cervical headache is independent of age, ranging from childhood to old age.

History of Onset

Patients will present with cervical headache of weeks, months, or quite commonly, several years duration.[8,19,20] The two common provocative causes are degenerative joint disease and trauma.[4,20,29] Studies have shown that at least 50 percent of cervical headache patients will relate the onset of headache to neck or head trauma, or will have a past history of relevant neck injury.[6,20,49,50] Accumulation of microtrauma from poor postural, movement, or work habits must also be considered.[51-53]

While the history of onset of headache may be quite precise, the situation becomes more complex when patients suffer a headache continuum, combined headaches, or transitional forms of headache. In these cases the clinician must take careful note of the behavior and history of each component headache in order to try to differentiate a possible cervical origin for part of the headache complex.

PHYSICAL CHARACTERIZATION OF CERVICAL HEADACHE

The physical examination of the neck and upper functional kinetic chain assumes considerable importance in the diagnosis of cervical headache. As already seen, reliance cannot be placed on subjective data alone, since there is considerable overlap in the symptomatology of several forms of headache. Indeed, aching of the neck and muscle soreness can accompany many types of headache.[14,54-57] Additionally, the objective medical diagnostic methods that can positively confirm cervical involvement in headache are not in widespread use clinically, and are only used on selected patients, often on a research basis. These methods include specific cervical nerve or joint blocks[3,6,58,59] and computer-based radiographic techniques to plot the axis of motion of cervical joints.[46,60] It is unfortunate that such commonly used diagnostic methods as plain radiography, qualitative analysis of motion radiographs, and computed tomographic (CT) scans have proven insensitive for assisting the diagnosis of cervical headache. They are not reliable in discriminating the relevant pathology, in accurately detecting motion abnormalities, or indeed even in detecting significant cervical structural damage after neck trauma.[6,59-62]

The lack of sensitivity of these methods emphasizes the importance of an accurate and discriminatory physical examination. The term "discriminatory" has been used because as neck soreness or stiffness can accompany many different forms of headache, palpable tenderness of cervical structures does not automatically indicate a cervical cause of headache.[12,35,55,57,63,64]

The physical examination must be comprehensive. It is on the basis of the physical findings, together with the subjective information gained, that the clinician decides that the cervical structures are the cause of headache or a partial cause in a headache syndrome, or that headache is unrelated to cervical dysfunction. This is not always an easy task. There is the need to establish the type of physical dysfunction that must be present in the cervical neuro-muscular-articular structures to make these decisions.

There is a growing scientific base and clinical understanding of the nature of the neuro-muscular-articular dysfunction associated with cervical conditions and with headaches of cervical origin. The cause, effect, and extent of the dysfunction can be complex and, while the understanding of such dysfunction is increasing, knowledge about it is still incomplete. On an uncomplicated neuroanatomic basis, structures supplied by the fourth to eighth cervical nerves have pain distributions to the neck, shoulder region, and upper limb.[65,66] Those receiving innervation from the upper three cervical nerves can refer pain to the head.[1,66-68] These include the atlanto-occipital, atlantoaxial, and the C2-3 articulations and their associated ligaments. Muscles receiving innervation from the upper three cervical nerves include the deep anterior and posterior suboccipital muscles, the upper trapezius and sternocleidomastoid, and the occipital and suboccipital portions of all cervical extensors.[69] Additionally, the dura mater of the upper spinal cord and posterior cranial fossa, and the upper portion of the vertebral artery also receive innervation from the upper cervical nerves.

This anatomic substrate gives reason to examine these articular, muscular, and neural structures as immediate sources of head pain. However, such simple anatomic deductions do not reflect the postural, movement, muscle, and motor-control factors that must be examined to gain the comprehensive understanding of cervical dysfunction that is necessary not only for the physical diagnosis but also for the successful management of cervical headache needed to achieve beneficial long-term treatment outcomes.

Articular Dysfunction

One diagnostic criterion that has been established for cervical headache is the presence of symptomatic articular dysfunction manifested as a painful abnormality of motion at a relevant segment in the cervical spine.[16] A primary diagnosis of cervical headache is consistent with an abnormality within the upper cervical joints (occiput to C3).[3-8,12,33,46] The link between the upper three cervical joints and referred head pain does not, however, intimate that patients will not have problems at other segments. Not unexpectedly, associated motion abnormalities have been demonstrated at the mid- and lower cervical levels as well as in upper thoracic segments.[50,59,70] Instances of headache relief have been reported with surgical management of the C5-6 or C6-7 segments.[71,72] A direct link between these lower levels and headache is more difficult to prove anatomically, and with the current state of knowledge, the causal association is thought to be muscle spasm.[72]

There is no single pathology of the upper cervical joints that is pathogenic of cervical headache. Rather, it is the associated symptomatic abnormality of motion that characterizes the headache.[2,7,16,60,73] The motion abnormality may result from direct joint trauma, chronic strain, degenerative joint disease, or inflammatory joint disease.[4,41,44,49,70,73] The motion abnormality may present as symptomatic joint hypomobility, hypermobility, or instability.[19,41,46,51,60,74]

The cervical joints are assessed in the physical examination through tests of active movement and manual examination of motion at the segmental level. To support a diagnosis of cervical headache, symptomatic abnormalities of motion must be elicited at comparable segments in the cervical spine.

Active Movement Testing

In testing for cervical headache through active movement, the primary physiologic movements are examined in each plane. The active movements should be guided to their full available range by the physical therapist, through the application of passive overpressure.[75] Dvorak et al.[76] have shown that the application of this gentle passive force at the end of the range of movement more truly defines the motion status of the joints in a particular plane than do the patient's active attempts alone. The upper cervical joints are more specifically examined with the movements of craniocervical flexion and extension (occiput-C1, C1-2), head rotation with the mid- and lower cervical segments fully flexed (C1-2), and head rotation with the upper cervical segments held in flexion (C2-3).[75,77] The examination can be progressed to test movements in combination so as to provide more information about the nature of the patient's movement restriction, which will assist in the selection of treatment techniques.[78]

Various studies indicate that patients with cervical headache generally present with some pain and restriction of neck motion in one or more directions.[2,3,8,20] The restriction of gross motion may be subtle. Persons with cervical headache do not seem to have a common pattern of movement restriction[2,3] that would reflect the origin of the headache from any of the upper cervical structures. However, crepitus with neck motion is commonly reported.[2,6]

Craniocervical Ligament Testing

When the onset of cervical headache is related to substantial trauma, consideration must be given to the integrity of the craniocervical ligamentous complex. In a postmortem study of cervical spine injuries associated with skull fractures after traffic accidents, Jonsson et al.[62] determined that of the 22 cases studied, 13 had a total of 44 ruptures of joint capsules and ligaments in the upper cervical region. Ligamentous ruptures were variously observed in the alar, apical, and cruciate ligaments, as well as in the tectorial membrane.

There is a growing awareness and recognition of upper cervical ligament injury resulting from motor vehicle accidents, with a forced flexion and rotation injury being advocated as a mechanism for damage to the alar ligament and tectorial membrane.[79–81] Stress radiographs of upper cervical rotation and lateral flexion have been used to investigate damage to the alar ligament.[82,83]

In clinical testing of this region, lateral flexion stress tests are also principally advocated for the alar ligaments, while a localized craniovertebral axial distraction is considered to give an indication of the integrity of the tectorial membrane.[74,84] The sensitivity and specificity of the clinical tests used in the upper cervical region have yet to be established, although an initial case study has shown concordance between the results of clinical and radiologic testing of the alar ligaments.[74] Awareness and recognition of the possibility of such ligamentous damage are vital to the plan of treatment for the patient with a post-traumatic cervical headache.

Manual Examination of Intersegmental Motion

Relevant, symptomatic abnormalities of segmental motion are among the most important differential diagnostic criteria for cervical headache. The physical therapist's skill in the manual examination of segmental motion assumes considerable importance in the diagnosis of cervical headache, especially when it is recognized that the only other method with reliability in such diagnosis is sophisticated functional radiography.

Manual examination encompasses an assessment of bony alignment, soft tissue texture, and motion at the segments from the occiput to the mid-thoracic region. Positional anomalies of a rotatory nature of the atlas and axis have been noted in some headache subjects.[8,12] Caution should be exercised when interpreting the pathologic relevance of these positional deviations, since they have also been detected in normal, asymptomatic subjects.[12,19] Their presence is probably of more significance when associated with a symptomatic abnormality of motion.[85]

Changes in texture of the soft tissues are sought, such as increased muscle tone and thickening around the articular processes, interspinous spaces, and muscle attachments. Trigger points in muscles supplied by the C1 to C3 nerves may be found in the headache patient.[8,86] Muscle tissue in vivo is very pliable and, with care, a deep palpation can be performed and spasm found in segmental muscles overlying the involved joint. Spasm in the C2-3 segmental multifidus is a notable example of this.

The accessory or translatory movements and all physiologic directions of movement are examined at each intevertebral segment[5,87–89] (Fig. 13-1). Abnormalities are sought in the perception of the stiffness properties of individual joints (i.e., the relationship between the perceived passive displacement and resistance to displacement in each direction). Some restriction of motion alone is not necessarily pathognomonic for cervical headache, and may be an asymptomatic effect of aging.[85] Those physical features that have been found to reliably identify a symptomatic joint are altered displacement, an abnormal quality of physical resistance to motion of the joint, and provocation of pain (local or referred) by the testing procedure.[7]

A careful evaluation is made of the relationship between the joint signs found on manual examination and the symptomatic and historical features of the patient's headache. As the symptomatic pattern of headache alone is not

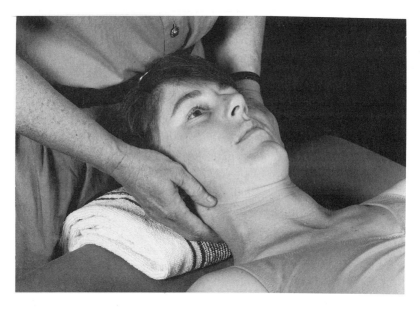

Fig. 13-1.   Manual examination of anteroposterior glide of the (R) C2-3 zygapophyseal joint.

always diagnostic, such an evaluation is one of the key components in deciding whether the cervical spine is the major cause, a partial cause, or has no part in the patient's headache. For a diagnosis of cervical headache, the joint involvement should be at an appropriate level in the cervical spine, and the magnitude of dysfunction and soft-tissue reactivity should be comparable to the patient's headache symptomatology.

Vertebral Artery

Symptoms of dizziness or lightheadedness may accompany the headache of cervical origin. Frequently, these symptoms are provoked by irritation of upper cervical somatic structures.[58,90] However, headache can be a symptom of vertebrobasilar insufficiency (VBI), and the clinical screening tests for VBI should be conducted on patients complaining of dizziness and headache.[91,92]

The earlier contention that a migraine-like headache was caused by cervical pathology irritating the vertebral nerve and thus causing vasoconstriction of the vertebral artery[93,94] has been disproven.[95] Terms such as "migraine cervicale" are considered misleading and should be abandoned.[2]

Neural Tissues

Cervical headache is more commonly a referred pain, but incidences of C2 or C3 nerve root irritation or compression have been reported.[20,41,43] Recent years have seen an increasing clinical interest in the concept of adverse tension in the nervous system as a source of pain.[96] The dura mater of the upper spinal cord and posterior cranial fossa receives innervation from branches of the upper three cervical nerves, and could therefore be a source of pain in cervical headache if its free movement or extensibility is compromised. There is surgical evidence of some cases of cervical headache being associated with fibrosis of the C2 nerve and of the occipital nerve in its course before its perforation through the tendinous lamina of the upper trapezius muscle.[47,97]

Conditions affecting the cervical spine may present with dysfunction in all components of the highly integrated neuromuscular articular system, and adverse tension in the nervous system should be considered routinely as a possible source of pain in the examination of patients with cervical headache. Clinical testing procedures for this purpose have been described,[96] with upper cervical flexion being a key sensitizing movement for the upper-limb and spinal-canal neural tension tests in the headache patient. Testing should always proceed with due care and in a progressive manner, since compromised neural tissues often show considerable reactivity. Head pain can be easily provoked.

Currently there is considerable clinical belief in the role of adverse neural tissue tension in states of musculoskeletal pain. Case histories of the involvement of such tension in patients with neck-induced headache have been presented.[96,98] However, it must be appreciated that at this time, clinical theory and practice are in advance of any proven research base for such a concept. Even incidence data are lacking. Furthermore, the findings of Hildebrandt and Jansen[99] and Jansen et al.[97] serve as a cautionary note. These investigators presented the findings in 16 patients with a chronic cluster-like headache, who had surgically confirmed compression of the C2(10), C3(3), and C4(3) nerve roots as the cause of their headache. In six cases the compression was due to spondylitic changes or scar tissue around the roots, which would be in accord with the clinical theory of adverse neural tension. In nine other cases, however, there was a vascular compression of the root, with surgery revealing "varicose" like veins densely interwoven around the nerve. While it could be postulated that these latter patients may have presented with positive signs in neural tissue tension tests, treatment by passive mobilization of the nervous system would be inappropriate in such cases.

Muscle Dysfunction and Postural Form

Considerable clinical knowledge and theory exists about the nature of the muscle dysfunction and postural change in the neck and upper functional kinetic chain that can occur with painful dysfunction of the craniocervical and cervical regions as well as of the craniomandibular complex.[52,83,100–103] The dysfunction in the muscle system appears to be related to disproportionate activity levels between different muscles, which may be provocative of, or reactive to, painful musculoskeletal dysfunction. It is thought that this imbalanced muscle activity may arise from inherently poor sensorimotor integration, or may be acquired through the effects on the muscle system of motor patterns used in lifestyle activities or acquired from the effects of trauma and pain on articular and soft tissues.[52,104,105]

This imbalanced activity can result in postural change and poor patterns of movement in the neck–shoulder complex. The articular tissues often fail to receive sufficient active, protective support from muscles having a prime stabilization role, with resulting altered mechanics and an altered load distribution on articular and soft tissues. The cervical tissues are subjected to adverse stress and chronic strain, with resultant pain.

In the neck–shoulder girdle region, the muscles that can become overactive in posture and movement include the upper trapezius, levator scapulae, sterno-cleidomastoid, scalenes, and pectorals. Those that have a tendency toward inhibition or weakness include muscles with an important stabilizing role for the neck and girdle, such as the deep cervical flexors and mid- and lower trapezius. Therefore, imbalances between muscles that are overactive and underactive can occur in muscles with an agonist–antagonist relationship (e.g., the upper and lower trapezius) and between synergistic muscles (e.g., sternocleidomas-toid, deep cervical flexors). Length-associated changes may accompany this imbalanced activity, with overactive muscles having a tendency to tighten and inhibited muscles a tendency to lengthen. Some muscles seem to deviate from these patterns. For example, the deep suboccipital extensors do not seem to become overactive (with the exception of reactive spasm), yet they can shorten. This could be a secondary reaction to acquired postural positions or even to tight neural tissue.

Research into this intricate area of muscle and postural dysfunction in relation to the development of pain states is difficult, and especially so in the cervical area, where many of the important deep muscles are not readily accessi-ble. Such research is in its infancy, but some data are beginning to emerge.

A forward head posture is the most commonly reported postural anomaly in patients with either cervical or craniomandibular dysfunction.[106–111] The presence of this postural anomaly in cervical headache patients was confirmed by Watson and Trott[111] in a comparative study with normal controls. Weakness in the neck flexors has been identified in patients with cervical pain.[112,113] More specifically, Watson and Trott[111] found that patients with cervical headache exhibited less strength and endurance in the upper cervical flexors than did the control group. In relation to the important role of stabilization of these muscles, a poorer endurance capacity of these deep cervical flexors was related to the magnitude of the forward head posture. Proprioceptive deficits have also been identified in patients with neck pain. Revel et al.[114] determined that head–neck kinesthetic sensibility was significantly poorer in a group of patients with neck pain than in controls. These findings are beginning to confirm the complexity of the problem of muscle and postural dysfunction and give directions for the re-education of posture, muscle control, and proprioception.

The clinical assessment of postural and muscle dysfunction in the headache patient needs to be conducted with care and precision. Several assessment techniques can be used. The observation of posture and muscle form provides initial information about the status of the muscle system and the presence of overactive as well as underactive superficial muscles.[52,53,101] The muscles are tested specifically for length by standard tests,[115,116] and a differentiation is made between hypertonicity and true muscle shortening. The presence of muscle inhibition and weakness and the patient's motor program can be assessed by examining the timing, sequencing, and level of activation of particular muscles during certain designated tasks. For accuracy, multichannel electromyoraphy (EMG) is required for this examination. However, this can become impractical in the clinical setting, and additionally, surface EMG cannot be used to examine the important relationship between the superficial and deep neck flexors. Janda[52] describes the normal and abnormal movement patterns in three tests that can be used clinically for the cervical spine–shoulder complex. These include head and neck flexion, shoulder abduction, and a push up from the prone position to detect problems in the deep neck flexors and scapular stabilizing muscles.

An additional and more specific method has been developed to examine those muscles that have an important stabilizing role for the neck–shoulder girdle complex. This method assesses the muscles' ability to hold and control joint positions replicating their functional, postural role, which demands holding a submaximal contraction over a prolonged period.[117] The precision of the classic muscle test positions for a Grade III low load test[118] provides the basis for testing the inner-range isometric holding capacity of the shoulder girdle muscles. A more precise test is required for the deep neck flexors. Their action must be isolated so that any deficit in these muscles is not masked by the action of the more superficial flexors such as the sternocleidomastoid or scalenes. The test for the deep cervical flexors is a gentle upper cervical flexion (or chin tuck) action in the supine position, with the head resting on a support so that the weight of the head does not offer resistance or a load to the test. To improve the precision of the test and to have some objective measure of performance (as well as feedback for the patient), an inflatable pressure sensor (Stabilizer, Chattanooga, Australia) is used to monitor the control of neck position with this action (Fig. 13-2). The time for which this submaximal contraction can be held is used as the objective test.[119] Timing ceases when there is either a change in pressure (indicative of loss of control or substitution by the sternocleidomastoid or scalenes), or when phasic erratic movement occurs (indicative of fatigue). These clinical tests have proved very useful in detecting functional deficits in these supporting muscles when substitution is controlled.

There is a critical need for more research in this area of muscle, movement, and postural dysfunction, not only so as to define the problems inherent in such dysfunction, but to have quantifiable measures of them. In relation to the differential diagnosis of cervical headache, evidence exists for the diagnostic feature of upper cervical joint dysfunction. However, it is believed that the coexistence of significant articular, muscular, and perhaps neural tissue dysfunction is what may ultimately truly characterize cervical headache and differentiate it from headache of other causes.

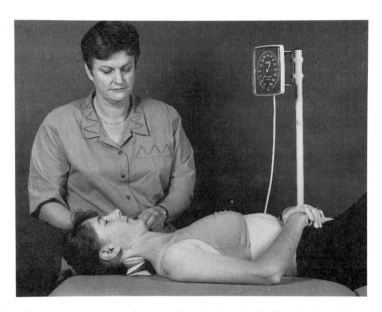

Fig. 13-2. Pressure sensor used to monitor the level of effort in the chin-tuck action for the deep neck flexors. The pressure sensor is inflated to fill the space between the neck and examination bed (approximately 30 mmHg). Once the physical therapist has taught and tested the correct action, the patient may use the pressure increase as a guide for future precise exercise. Often a pressure increase of 10 mmHg is noted with the correct action.

TREATING THE HEADACHE PATIENT

On completion of the subjective and physical examination, the first clinical decision to be made is whether or not to offer treatment to the patient. The cervical spine can be a primary cause of headache, and there is the opinion that the frequency of its involvement is considerably underestimated, especially in the differential diagnosis of chronic forms of headache.[46] Nevertheless, there is symptomatic overlap between various forms of chronic headache. A decision that the headache is of cervical origin and amenable to physical therapy must be based on the presence of a painful motion abnormality in the upper cervical joints, accompanied by other physical signs of muscle and movement dysfunction. The absence of such signs indicates that the headache has another cause. Not only is a rational basis lacking for the treatment of such patients, but such treatment can also be counterproductive. Such patients must be referred for other appropriate investigations.

Decision making is more difficult when it is suspected that the cervical spine is either a partial cause of a patient's headache syndrome or is enhancing the symptoms of other types of headache (e.g., migraine). In such cases a trial of treatment is warranted, with the nature of the trial and the expectations of it being carefully explained to the patient. The efficacy of treatment must be stringently evaluated and treatment ceased if no improvement is achieved or if the improvement reaches a plateau. The chronic headache patient is vulnerable and often eager to pay any amount for a promised "cure."

Treatment of the cervical headache patient requires a comprehensive approach, since the patient's problem invariably has many components. In principle, initial treatment is directed toward the pain-provoking structures. This is usually the articular dysfunction, but there can also be very relevant and interdependent involvement of neural structures. The muscle and postural dysfunction must be addressed as early in the treatment program as possible, since it is believed that sustained and long-term improvement will not be achieved without the return of adequate muscle control and support. This rehabilitation may begin as early as the first or second treatment session, since the initial exercises involved in it are very precise and of low load, and do not overload articular structures. However, if there is any provocation of pain (as can occur when neural structures are involved), the introduction of exercise is delayed, since pain can inhibit muscle activation and render exercise counterproductive.

Treatment of the articular dysfunction is guided by the findings in the manual examination. The findings encompass the segments involved, the direction of motion loss, the nature of tissue resistance (spasm, tissue fibrosis), and the intensity of pain. Techniques of manual therapy and their progressive application are well described in many physical therapy texts.[75,78,88,120] However, a worthy reminder is that the cervical condition causing headache is often irritable, and headache is easily provoked. Handling skills and techniques should be such that treatment evokes minimal local discomfort, and the production of head pain is avoided. It may take two to three treatment sessions to appreciate the extent of treatment that the joints can tolerate. When indications exist for manipulative thrust techniques, such techniques are undertaken with due caution and care, and only after negative premanipulative screening tests for VBI.[91,92]

Joint motion gained with passive treatment is reinforced with active mobilization. Exercises must be precise and localized as fully as possible to the dysfunctional joints. Patients are taught to use their own fingers or hand to assist in this localization. Precision is emphasized, not only for its benefits on joint motion, but also to assist in proprioceptive retraining.

The results of tests for adverse tension or lack of free movement of the structures of the nervous system, as part of the headache patient's physical dysfunction, can direct specific approaches to treatment. The lack of free movement of neural tissues may resolve with treatment of the patient's painful articular structures. However, there are indications for introducing techniques that directly move or apply tension to neural structures. These include situations in which the restoration of normal neural movement or extensibility is slow or fails to occur, or when tension on neural tissue structures remains directly provocative of pain. The tension or movement imparted to neural structures is applied in a very gradual and progressive manner. Descriptions of treatment approaches in such cases are provided by Butler.[96] In relation to the cervical headache patient, the limb or body position and/or movement used in treatment is guided by the findings on examination of whether the tension is more closely related to neural structures of the spinal canal or upper limb. An initial approach to treatment could involve the mobilization of articular structures, with neural tissues subjected to progressively increasing tension. For example, if the neural tension is related to neural structures of the upper limb, it may be necessary to apply anteroposterior gliding mobilization to the dysfunctional C2-3 joint (Fig. 13-1), with progressively increasing angles of shoulder abduction and external rotation. The treatment may need to be progressed to a direct mobilization of neural structures in the upper cervical region, using either upper cervical flexion or upper limb, girdle movement. Treatment involving the mobilization of neural tissues must always be progressed with care. Once the response to treatment is established, patients can be given a home program of mobilization based on the procedures used in formal treatment.

Several problems often need to be addressed simultaneously when rehabilitating a patient's muscle and postural dysfunction. Clinical testing often reveals a poor capacity of muscles important for active stabilization, particularly the deep neck flexors and the mid- and lower trapezius. Activating these muscles and improving their holding ability becomes a priority in helping to restore postural control and joint support.

Retaining begins under low load conditions, so that muscle activation can be as isolated and precise as possible. Training against load or resistance necessarily recruits many muscles to resist the applied force, and they may substitute for the action of the weak target muscle. Activation of the deep neck flexors may be trained with the patient in the supine position (Fig. 13-2). The emphasis is on accuracy. Neither forceful movements or attempts to lift the head are permitted, and the therapist monitors for any substitution by the superficial neck flexors. The pressure sensor is used to monitor performance and provide feedback and incentive to the patient. Patients who cannot activate the relevant muscles in the supine position practice while sitting against a wall to utilize the assistance of gravity. Gentle manual facilitatory resistance can be applied to the chin.

Not infrequently, the mid- and lower trapezius are initially trained in sitting to relieve arm loading of the exercise in the prone position. Facilitatory resistance can be applied through the inferior angle of the scapula, or the patient may assist the setting of these muscles with slight compression through the hands and arms in the sitting position.

Once the patient can consciously set the muscles, the holding time of the contraction is increased. At first, the patient trains to achieve ten, 5-second holds. Fatigue should be avoided, since it often encourages muscle substitution patterns.

When a localized contraction of the deep cervical flexors is achieved, they are coactivated with the mid- and lower trapezius to encourage co-contraction of the stability muscles. This muscle coactivation is incorporated into the re-education of postural control (Fig. 13-3). In a home program, the patient practices the ten repetitions of the muscle setting on the hour, and increases the

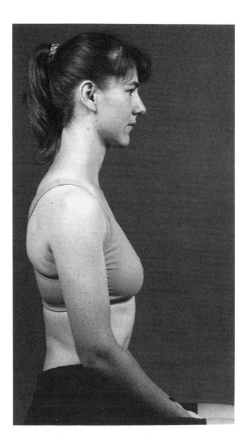

Fig. 13-3. Re-education of postural control, with emphasis on submaximal activation of the mid- and lower trapezius and the deep neck flexors.

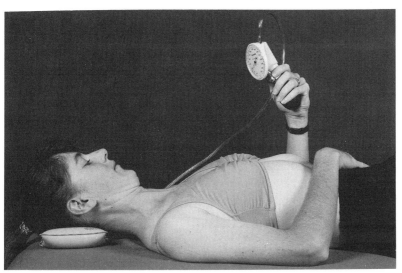

Fig. 13-4. The pressure sensor placed under the head provides a method for progressively grading head loading during strength training of the neck flexor synergy.

holding time to 10-second periods. This repeated practice and retraining are incorporated into daily activities. Reactivation of the supporting muscles in conjunction with postural control is often commensurate with patient reports of pain control.

Introduction of this muscle retraining program is delayed if the setting actions reproduce neck pain or headache. This can be due to the patient's joint condition, but the actions of upper cervical flexion and scapular retraction and depression may also irritate sensitive neural tissue. For the same reasons, care may be required with the introduction of muscle-lengthening procedures.

The retraining program is progressed to increase the isometric strength and endurance of the neck and shoulder girdle muscles. For the neck flexors, head weight is added. The aim is to achieve a balanced interaction between the deep and superficial muscles. The patient consciously controls the upper

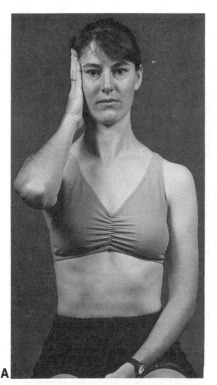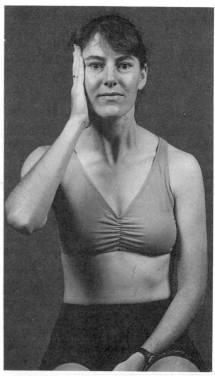

Fig. 13-5. **(A)** Isometric exercise using a self-applied submaximal rotatory resistance. Better clinical results are achieved by presetting the deep neck flexors and scapular stabilizers and maintaining postural control prior to adding resistance. **(B)** Poor exercise posture and technique may emphasize incorrect muscle patterns.

cervical flexion position as head weight is taken, and simultaneously coactivates the scapular stabilizing muscles. Progressive increments of head load are used. Exercises may begin in the supported reclined sitting position, and may be progressed to the supine position to increase the gravitational load. The pressure sensor is used to grade the increments of head weight in these positions (Fig. 13-4). Again, control is emphasized and the exercises ceased if chin position is lost, if the shoulders lift forward, or if phasic erratic movements occur. The coactivation of the neck flexors and extensors can be trained with techniques such as rhythmical stabilizations or alternating isometrics[121] (Fig. 13-5). Progressive load is also added to the lower scapular stabilizers. Arm load in the prone position is often sufficient (Fig. 13-6), gradually increasing the level to an above-head position.

The patient also learns control during movements of the neck and shoulder girdle. Formal patterns can be practiced, but attention is also directed to occupational and sporting activities. Advice is particularly given for sedentary activities, but correct lifting and carrying techniques are as important for the neck-pain patient as for patients with back complaints. At all stages of the re-education process, the patient is given a program for home practice. Most importantly, as a prophylactic measure, the patient should be provided with a simple, ongoing program for maintaining muscle control once formal treatment has ceased.

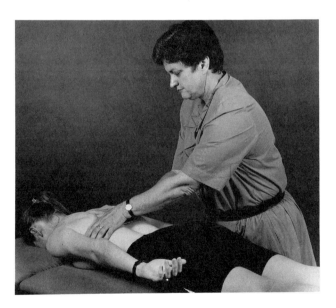

Fig. 13-6. Training of the mid- and lower trapezius using arm loading.

SUMMARY

The patient with chronic headache presents a challenge to the professions of medicine and physical therapy, both in differential diagnosis and management. Good examination and clinical decision-making skills will determine whether the cervical spine has a primary, contributory, or no role in a patient's headache syndrome.

The problems in the neuro-muscular-articular system of the cervical headache patient are often multiple. A well-planned treatment program is needed to address each component of these problems. Special emphasis must be placed on the correction of muscle, movement, and postural dysfunction to achieve a successful outcome with respect to long-term results and the prevention of recurrent dysfunction.

The pattern of headache is often variable, and temporary relief of pain is not difficult to achieve. The efficacy of treatment can be evaluated only by a long-term follow-up of the patient.

REFERENCES

1. Kerr FWL: Structural relation of the trigeminal spinal tract to upper cervical roots and the solitary nucleus in the cat. Exp Neurol 4:134, 1961
2. Sjaastad O, Saunte C, Hovdal H et al: "Cervicogenic" headache. An hypothesis. Cephalalgia 3:249, 1983
3. Bogduk N, Marsland A: On the concept of third occipital headache. J Neurol Neurosurg Psychiatry 9:775, 1986.
4. Trevor-Jones R: Osteoarthritis of the paravertebral joints of the second and third cervical vertebrae as a cause of occipital headache. S Afr Med J 38:392, 1964
5. Ehni G, Benner B: Occipital neuralgia and C_1–C_2 arthrosis syndrome. J Neurosurg 61:961, 1984
6. Pfaffenrath V, Dandekar R, Pollman W: Cervicogenic headache. The clinical picture, radiological findings and hypothesis on its pathophysiology. Headache 27:495, 1987
7. Jull GA, Bogduk N, Marsland A: The accuracy of manual diagnosis for cervical zygapophysial joint pain syndromes. Med J Aust 148:233, 1988
8. Jaeger B: Are "cervicogenic" headaches due to myofascial pain and cervical spine dysfunction. Cephalalgia 9:157, 1989
9. Lamer TJ: Ear pain due to cervical spine arthritis: Treatment with cervical facet injection. Headache 31:682, 1991
10. Parker GB, Tupling H, Pryor DS: A controlled trial of cervical manipulation for migraine. Aust NZ Med J 8:589, 1978
11. Parker GB, Pryor DS, Tupling H: Why does migraine improve during a clinical trial? Further results from a trial of cervical migraine. Aust NZ Med J 10:192, 1980
12. Boquet J, Boismare F, Payenneville G, et al: Lateralisation of headache: Possible role of an upper cervical trigger point. Cephalalgia 9:15, 1989
13. Sjaastad O, Saunte C, Graham JR: Chronic paroxysmal hemicrania VII. Mechanical precipitation of attacks: new cases and localisation of trigger points. Cephalalgia 4:113, 1984

14. Solomon S, Lipton RB, Newman L: Nucal features of cluster headaches. Cephalalgia 9, suppl. 10:201, 1989
15. Winston KR: Whiplash and its relationship to migraine. Headache 27:452, 1987
16. Headache Classification Committee of the International Headache Society: Classification and diagnostic criteria for headache disorders, cranial neuralgias and facial pain. Cephalalgia 8, suppl. 7:1, 1988
17. Rose FC: Clinical characterisation of migraine. p. 3. In Olesen J, Edvinsson L (eds): Basic Mechanisms of Headache. Elsevier, Amsterdam, 1988
18. Lance JW: Mechanisms and Management of Headache. 4th Ed. Butterworths, London, 1982
19. Jull GA: Headaches associated with the cervical spine—A clinical review. p. 322. In Grieve GP (ed): Modern Manual Therapy of the Vertebral Column. Churchill Livingstone, Edinburgh, 1986
20. Fredriksen TA, Hovdal H, Sjaastad O: "Cervicogenic headache": Clinical manifestations. Cephalalgia 7, suppl. 6: 147, 1987
21. Edeling J: Manual Therapy for Cervical Headache. Butterworths, London, 1988
22. Sjaastad O, Fredriksen TA, Pfaffenrath V: Cervicogenic headache: Diagnostic criteria. Headache 30:725, 1990
23. Reade PC, Steidler NE: Temporomandibular joint pain—dysfunction syndrome: a common form of headache. Patient Management 8:56, 1984
24. Langemark M, Olesen J, Poulse DL, Bech P: Clinical characteristics of patients with chronic tension headache. Headache 28:590, 1988
25. Olesen J: Clinical characterisation of tension headache p. 9. In Olesen J, Edvinsson L (eds): Basic Mechanisms of Headache. Elsevier, Amsterdam, 1988
26. Bordini C, Antonaci F, Stovner L et al: Hemicrania continua—a clinical review. Headache 31:20, 1991
27. Russell D: Clinical characterisation of the cluster headache syndrome. p. 15. In Olesen J, Edvinsson L (eds): Basic Mechanisms of Headache. Elsevier, Amsterdam, 1988
28. Sjaastad O: Cluster headache syndromes. Neurol Clin 7:387, 1988
29. Sjaastad O, Dale I: Evidence for a new (?) treatable headache entity. Headache 14:105, 1974
30. Saper JR: The mixed headache syndrome: a new perspective. Headache 22:284, 1982
31. Gelb H, Bernstein I: Clinical evaluation of two hundred patients with temporomandibular dysfunction. J Prosthet Dent 49:234, 1983
32. Bogduk N: The anatomy of headache. p. 1. In Dalton M (ed): Proceedings of Headache and Face Pain Symposium. Manipulative Physiotherapists Association of Australia, Brisbane, 1989
33. Bogduk N: Cervical causes of headache. Cephalalgia 9, suppl. 10:172, 1989
34. Angus-Leppan H, Lambert GA, Boers P et al: The cervical spinal cord is a relay centre for the central nervous system processing of input from the cranial vasculature. Cephalalgia 9, suppl. 10:137, 1989
35. Gawl M, Rothbart P: Occipital nerve block in the management of headache and cervical pain. Cephalalgia 12:9, 1992
36. Fredriksen TA, Sjaastad O: Cervicogenic headache. A clinical entity. Cephalalgia 7, suppl. 6:171, 1987
37. Sjaastad O, Fredriksen TA, Sand T: The localization of the initial pain attack. A comparison between classic migraine and cervicogenic headache. Funct Neurol 4: 73, 1989

38. Sjaastad O, Fredriksen TA, Sand T, Antonaci F: Unilaterality of headache in classic migraine. Cephalalgia 9:71, 1989
39. Ziegler DK, Stephenson-Hassanein R, Couch JR: Headache syndromes suggested by statistical analysis of headache symptoms. Cephalalgia 2:125, 1982
40. Bogduk N: Greater occipital neuralgia. p. 175. In Long D (ed): Current Therapy in Neurosurgery. Marcel Dekker, Toronto, 1985
41. Dugan MC, Locke S, Gallagher JR: Occipital neuralgia in adolescents and young adults. N Engl J Med 267:1163, 1962
42. Lance JW, Anthony M: Neck-tongue syndrome on sudden turning of the head. J Neurol Neurosurg Psychiatry 43:97, 1980
43. Bertoft ES, Westerberg C: Further observations on the neck-tongue syndrome. Cephalalgia 5, suppl. 3:312, 1985
44. Edmeads J: Headache and head pain associated with diseases of the cervical spine. Med Clin North Am 62:533, 1978
45. Edeling JS: The true cervical headache. S Afr Med J 62:531, 1982
46. Mayer E, Herrmann G, Pfaffenrath V et al: Functional radiographs of the craniocervical region and the cervical spine. A new computer-aided technique. Cephalalgia 5:237, 1985
47. Sjaastad O, Fredriksen TA, Stolt-Nielsen A: Cervicogenic headache, C_2 rhizopathy and occipital neuralgia: A connection? Cephalalgia 6:113, 1986
48. Anthony M: Occipital neuralgia. Cephalalgia 9, suppl. 10:174, 1989
49. Braaf MM, Rosner S: Trauma of the cervical spine as the cause of headache. J Trauma 15:441, 1975
50. Jensen OK, Justesen T, Nielsen FF, Brixen K: Functional radiographic examination of the cervical spine in patients with post-traumatic headache. Cephalalgia 10:295, 1990
51. Lewit K: Ligament pain and anteflexion headache. Eur Neurol 5:365, 1971
52. Janda V: Muscles and cervicogenic pain syndromes. p. 153. In Grant R (ed): Physical Therapy of the Cervical and Thoracic Spine. Churchill Livingstone, New York, 1988
53. Sahrmann S: Postural applications in the child and adult. Neurodevelopmental aspects. p. 295. In Kraus SL (ed): TMJ Disorders. Management of the Craniomandibular Complex. Churchill Livingstone, New York, 1988
54. Clark GT, Green EM, Dornan MR, Flack VF: Craniocervical dysfunction levels in a patient sample from a temporomandibular joint clinic. J Am Dent Assoc 115:251, 1987
55. Drummond PD: Scalp tenderness and sensitivity to pain in migraine and tension headache. Headache 27:45, 1987
56. Henry P, Dartigues JF, Puymirat E et al: The association of cervicalgia-headaches: An epidemiologic study. Cephalalgia 7, suppl. 6:189, 1987
57. Saadah H, Taylor FB: Sustained headache syndrome associated with tender occipital nerve zones. Headache 27:201, 1987
58. Bogduk N: Local anaesthetic blocks of the second cervical ganglion: A technique with application in occipital headache. Cephalagia 1:41, 1981
59. Sluijter ME, Rohof OJ, Vervest AC: Cervical headache. Diagnosis with the aid of computerised analysis of cervical mobility. Cephalalgia 9, suppl. 10:199, 1989
60. Pfaffenrath V, Dandekar R, Mayer E Th et al: Cervicogenic headache: Results of computer-based measurements of cervical spine mobility in 15 patients. Cephalalgia 8:45, 1988
61. Fredriksen TA, Fougner R, Tangerud A, Sjaastad O: Cervicogenic headache. Radiographic investigations concerning head/neck. Cephalalgia 9:139, 1989

62. Jonsson H, Bring G, Rauschning W, Saalstedt B: Hidden cervical spine injuries in traffic accident victims with skull fractures. J Spinal Disord 4:251, 1991
63. Langemark M, Jensen K: Myofascial mechanisms of pain. p. 332. In Olesen J, Edvinsson L (eds): Basic Mechanisms of Headache. Elsevier, Amsterdam, 1988
64. Aprill C, Dwyer A, Bogduk N: Cervical zygapophyseal joint pain patterns. II: A clinical evaluation. Spine 15:458, 1990
65. Dwyer A, Aprill C, Bogduk N: Cervical zygapophyseal joint pain syndromes. I: A study in normal volunteers. Spine 15:453, 1990
66. Campbell DG, Parsons CM: Referred head pain and its concomittants. J Nerv Ment Dis 99:544, 1944
67. Feinstein B, Langton JNK, Jameson RM et al: Experiments on pain referred from deep somatic tissues. J Bone Joint Surg 36Λ:81, 1954
68. Bogduk N: Cervical causes of headache and dizziness. p. 289. In Grieve G (ed): Modern Manual Therapy of the Vertebral Column. Churchill Livingstone, Edinburgh, 1986
69. Williams PL, Warwick R, Dyson M, Bennister LA (eds): Gray's Anatomy. 37th Ed. Churchill Livingstone, Edinburgh, 1989
70. Jensen OK, Nielsen FF, Vosmar L: An open study comparing manual therapy with the use of cold packs in the treatment of post-traumatic headache. Cephalalgia 10:241, 1990
71. Chirls M: Retrospective study of cervical spondylosis treated by anterior interbody fusion (in 505 patients performed by the Cloward technique). Bull Hosp Jt Dis Orthop Inst 39:74, 1978
72. Michler RP, Bovim G, Sjaastad O: Disorders in the lower cervical spine. A cause of unilateral headache? Headache 31:550, 1991
73. Bogduk N, Corrigan B, Kelly P et al: Cervical headache. Med J Aust 143:202, 1985
74. Derrick LJ, Chesworth BM: Post-motor vehicle accident alar ligament laxity. Journal of Orthopaedic and Sports Physical Therapy 16:6, 1992
75. Maitland GD: Vertebral Manipulation. 5th Ed. Butterworths, London, 1986
76. Dvorak J, Froehlich D, Penning L, et al: Functional radiographic diagnosis of the cervical spine. Flexion/extension. Spine 13:748, 1988
77. Dvorak J, Dvorak V: Manual Medicine, Diagnostics. Georg Thieme-Verlag, Stuttgart, New York, 1984
78. Edwards BC: Manual of Combined Movements. Churchill Livingstone, Edinburgh, 1992
79. Dvorak J, Panjabi M, Gerber M, Wichmann W: CT—functional diagnostics of the rotatory instability of upper cervical spine. 1. An experimental study on cadavers. Spine 12:19, 1987
80. Panjabi M, Dvorak J, Crisco J et al: Effects of alar ligament transection on upper cervical spine rotation. J Orthop Res 9:584, 1991
81. Oda T, Panjabi M, Crisco J et al: Role of tectorial membrane in the stability of the upper cervical spine. Clin Biomech 7:201, 1992
82. Reich C, Dvorak J: The functional evaluation of craniocervical ligaments in side flexion using X-Rays. J Manual Med 2:108, 1986
83. Dvorak J, Hayek J, Zehnder R: CT—functional diagnostics of the rotatory instability of the upper cervical spine. 2. An evaluation on healthy adults and patients with suspected instability. Spine 12:726, 1987
84. Aspinall W: Clinical testing for the craniovertebral hypermobility syndrome. Journal of Orthopaedic and Sports Physical Therapy 12:47, 1990

85. Jull GA: Clinical observatons of upper cervical mobility. p. 315. In Grieve G (ed): Modern Manual Therapy of the Vertebral Column. Churchill Livingstone, Edinburgh, 1986
86. Travell JG, Simons DG: Myofascial Pain and Dysfunction. The Trigger Point Manual. Williams & Wilkins, Baltimore, 1983
87. Schneider G, Pardoe M: Translation of the facets during coupled motion in the cervical spine. A pilot study. Aust J Physiother 31:39, 1985
88. Grieve GP: Common Vertebral Joint Problems. 2nd Ed. Churchill Livingstone, Edinburgh, 1988
89. Bourdillon JF, Day EA, Bookhout MR: Spinal Manipulation. 5th Ed. Butterworth–Heinemann, Oxford, 1992
90. de Jong P, de Jong JM, Cohen B et al: Ataxia and nystagmus induced by injection of local anaesthetics in the neck. Ann Neurol 1:240, 1977
91. Grant R: Dizziness testing and manipulation of the cervical spine. p. 111. In Grant R (ed): Physical Therapy of the Cervical and Thoracic Spine. Churchill Livingstone, New York, 1988
92. Aspinall W: Clinical testing for cervical mechanical disorders which produce ischaemic vertigo. Journal of Orthopaedic and Sports Physical Therapy 11:176, 1989
93. Gayral L, Neuwirth E: Oto-neuro-ophthalmologic manifestations of cervical origin. Posterior cervical sympathetic syndrome of Barre-Lieou. NY State J Med 54:1920, 1954
94. Stewart DY: Current concepts of "Barre Syndrome" or the "posterior cervical sympathetic syndrome." Clin Orthop 24:40, 1962
95. Duckworth JW, Lambert GA, Bogduk N et al; Effects of humoral agents and sympathetic stimulation on vertebral blood flow in the monkey (abstract). Proc Aust Physiol Pharm Soc 10:158, 1979
96. Butler DS: Mobilisation of the Nervous System. Churchill Livingstone, Melbourne, 1991
97. Jansen J, Markakis E, Rama B, Hildebrandt J: Hemicranial attacks or permanent hemicrania—a sequel of upper cervical root compression. Cephalalgia 9:123, 1989
98. Rumore AJ: Slump examination and treatment in a patient suffering headache. Aust J Physiother 35:262, 1989
99. Hildebrandt J, Jansen J: Vascular compression of the C_2 and C_3 roots—yet another cause of chronic intermittent hemicrania. Cephalalgia 4:167, 1984
100. Kendall HO, Kendall FP, Boyton DA: Posture and pain. Williams & Wilkins, Baltimore, 1952
101. Kendall FP, McCreary EK: Muscles, Testing and Function. 3rd Ed. Williams & Wilkins, Baltimore, 1983
102. Janda V: Some aspects of extracranial causes of facial pain. J Prosthet Dent 56:484, 1986
103. Richardson CA: Rehabilitation of muscular dysfunction. p. 94. In Dalton M (ed): Proceedings of headache and face pain symposium. Manipulative Physiotherapists Association of Australia, Brisbane, 1989
104. Janda V: Muscles, motor regulation and back problems. p. 27. In Korr IM (ed): The Neurobiologic Mechanisms in Manipulative Therapy. Plenum, New York, 1978
105. Richardson CA: Muscle performance assessment: the case for specific antigravity muscle testing procedures. (Submitted for publication, 1994)
106. Gelb H, Bernstein I: Clinical evaluation of two hundred patients with temporomandibular dysfunction. J Prosthet Dent 49:234, 1983

107. Ayub E, Glasheen-Wray M, Kraus S: Head posture: a case study of the rest position of the mandible. JOSPT 5:179, 1984
108. Sakuta M, Sakuta Y: Drooping head syndrome: significance of flexed posture and neck instability as a cause of muscle contraction headache. Cephalalgia 9, suppl. 10:119, 1989
109. Braun B: Postural differences between asymptoamtic men and women and craniofacial pain patients. Arch Phys Med Rehabil 72:653, 1991
110. Mannheimer JS, Rosenthal RM: Acute and chronic postural abnormalities as related to craniofacial pain and TMJ disorders. Dent Clin North Am 35:185, 1991
111. Watson D, Trott P: Cervical headache. An investigation of natural head posture and upper cervical flexor muscle performance. Cephalalgia 13:272, 1993
112. Krout RM, Anderson TP: Role of anterior cervical muscles in production of neck pain. Arch Phys Med Rehabil 69:603, 1966
113. Silverman J, Rodriquez A, Agre J: Quantitative cervical flexor strength in healthy subjects and in subjects with mechanical neck pain. Arch Phys Med Rehabil 72: 679, 1991
114. Revel M, Andre-Deshays C, Mineuet M: Cervicocephalic kinesthetic sensibility in patients with cervical pain. Arch Phys Med Rehabil 72:288, 1991
115. Evjenth O, Hamberg J: Muscle Stretching in Manual Therapy. A Clinical Manual. Alfta Rehab, Alfta, Sweden, 1984
116. Janda V: Muscle Function Testing. Butterworths, London, 1983
117. Richardson C, Comerford M, Jull G: Pressure biofeedback: A focus on testing and rehabilitation of muscle stabilization function. 67th Annual Conference, American Physical Therapy Association, Denver, June 16, 1992
118. Daniels D, Worthingham C: Muscle Testing: Techniques of Manual Examination. WB Saunders, Philadelphia, 1986
119. Richardson C, Jull G, Comerford M: The stabilizer (pressure biofeedback): New dimensions in muscle control and stabilization. Tutorial video, Chattanooga, Australia, 1992
120. Kaltenborn F: Mobilisation of the Spinal Column. New Zealand University Press, Wellington, 1970
121. Sullivan PE, Markos PD: Clinical Procedures in Therapeutic Exercise. Appleton & Lange, Norwalk, CT, 1987

14 | Management of Selected Cervical Syndromes

Patricia H. Trott

This chapter builds on the previous chapters of this book, particularly those relating to pain mechanisms and clinical reasoning. Physical therapists are required to evaluate and manage patients with cervical disorders of varying complexity. These range from those with clear neuroanatomic patterns, typified by peripherally evoked nociception, to those that seem bizarre in their presentation and are typical of centrally evoked nociception and affective mechanisms.

Discussion is restricted to the presentation of basic concepts underlying the recognition of certain clinical patterns, and to the selection of passive movement techniques for treating cervical syndromes. This is followed by the presentation of selected cervical conditions frequently seen by physical therapists, and in the overall management of which manipulative therapy has a major role.

ISOLATION OF CERTAIN CERVICAL SYNDROMES

Patients who have a history of *symptoms occurring spontaneously* or following some trivial incident have symptoms, signs, and histories that are easily recognized. These conditions have clear neuroanatomic patterns that are evoked by peripheral mechanisms. They follow a predictable course and their response to manipulative therapy is also predictable. Knowledge of the structures that can cause pain, the response to posture and movement, and the expected signs to be found on physical examination also assist the therapist in recognizing those conditions marked by a spontaneous onset of symptoms. This contrasts with patients who have a *history of injury*, such as a direct blow to the head, a fall, or surgery. Here the symptoms and signs vary, depending on which tissues are injured and the force of the injury. In these cases the response to treatment is less predictable.

The suggestion that all patients fit neatly into specific categories is invalid; indeed, as stated above, patients often present with symptoms and signs of more complex nociceptive patterns. As discussed in depth in Chapter 6, the organization of knowledge into schemata, such as clinical patterns or syndromes, facilitates the recall of that knowledge for use in the clinical setting and the building and retention (memory) of new knowledge with each patient encounter. The separate presentation of some of these conditions in this chapter can help inexperienced therapists to more easily recognize the components of two or more coexisting conditions and to direct their treatment appropriately.

SELECTION OF PASSIVE MOVEMENT TECHNIQUES

The principles of selecting a technique for the diagnosis and treatment of conditions affecting the cervical spine are similar to those outlined for the lumbar spine,[1] but are presented again with specific examples of disorders of the cervical spine.

Diagnosis

The specific diagnosis of a disorder of the cervical spine can be difficult to achieve, since the etiology of such disorders is frequently multifactorial. For example, mechanical, inflammatory, and viral causes may coexist. Also, a pathologic process can produce differing patterns of symptoms and signs. For example, a patient with a diagnosis of "cervical spondylosis" may present with severe low cervical and medial scapular pain that restricts cervical movement in all directions, or with no pain but marked restriction of extension, rotation, and lateral flexion to one side. Pain patterns can range from more easily recognized peripherally evoked nociception to complex patterns including centrally evoked nociception, autonomic, and affective mechanisms (see Ch. 11).

For these reasons, the selection of physical treatment modalities for a disorder of the cervical spine is based on the patient's symptoms and signs and on the history of the disorder rather than on a diagnostic title. Particular attention is paid to the patterns of pain response that can occur during test movements, since these are important in the selection of passive movement techniques. These considerations are discussed in more detail below.

Pain-sensitive Structures and Their Pain Patterns

The reader is referred to Chapter 4, in which available research on cervical pain mechanisms is discussed.

Range/Pain Response to Movement

Test movements of the cervical intervertebral joints and neuromeningeal tissues produce the common patterns described in the following sections.

Stretching or Compressing Pain

Unilateral neck pain may be reproduced by either stretching (e.g., lateral flexion to the contralateral side) or by compressing the faulty tissues (e.g., lateral flexion toward the painful side).

End-of-range or Through-range Pain

Pain may be reproduced at the limit of a particular movement (i.e., when the soft-tissue restraints are stretched) or during the performance of a movement, increasing near the limit of the movement (this is common in joints in which there is a constant ache).

Local and Referred Pain

In patients who have referred pain, the response to test movements influences the selection of passive movement techniques. For example, a patient in whom test movements immediately cause distal symptoms requires treatment with very gentle movement that does not provoke the distal symptoms. Test movements that cause latent referred pain or cause the referred pain to linger also indicate caution in treatment. In cases in which a test movement must be sustained at the end of a range of movement before the referred symptoms are provoked, sustaining the treatment technique will also be necessary.

History

The history of a disorder includes information about its onset and progression. Conditions that have a spontaneous (non-traumatic) onset have a characteristically progressive history; a degenerating disc or postural ligamentous pain, for example, have a typical pattern of progression. Knowing the history that is typical for these conditions helps the therapist to recognize the current *stage of the disorder* and to match this with the symptoms and signs to form a syndrome. Typical histories are presented at the end of this chapter.

A detailed history also gives information about the stability of the disorder. This will guide the extent and strength of the techniques used in identifying and treating it, and may contraindicate certain techniques. This is particularly important in cases of radicular pain with worsening neurologic signs, in which injudicious treatment may further compromise the affected nerve root.

The progression of the disorder allows prediction of the *outcome of treatment*, the number of treatment sessions needed, and the long-term *prognosis*.

The following case history illustrates these aspects of history taking. A 40-year-old truck driver presents with a 10-year history of recurrent episodes of neck stiffness and left-sided low cervical pain. These occur for no apparent reason and last for a day or two. In the previous two years the pain has spread to his left shoulder and on each occasion has required treatment (heat and exercise). One week ago, after driving a long distance, the patient experienced his worst episode of severe neck pain, which spread further into his left arm, and also experienced paresthesia in his left thumb and index finger. His symptoms are not responding to heat and exercise, but he is able to continue his work driving and lifting merchandise.

This history is typical of worsening zygapophyseal joint arthropathy, and the patient now has symptoms of C6 nerve root irritation. His cervical disorder is relatively stable in that he can continue his work without worsening of his symptoms. More specific treatment will be required, and can be performed quite firmly without risk of exacerbating his symptoms. One would expect to make him symptom-free, but would also anticipate further episodes of his condition due to its progressive nature.

Symptoms

The area and the manner in which a patient's symptoms vary in relation to posture and movement assist in the recognition of their source, and, if they match the response to physical examination, can assist in the selection of passive movement techniques. A movement or combination of movements that simulates a position or movement described by the patient as one that causes pain can be used as the treatment technique. The following case history illustrates this.

A woman complains of left sided mid-cervical pain each time she twists to reach for her car seatbelt. In this position her neck is extended, laterally flexed, and rotated to the left. Examination confirms that this combined position reproduces her pain, and testing of intervertebral movement reveals hypomobility of the left C3-4 zygapophyseal joint. An effective treatment technique would consist of placing the patient's neck in this combined position and passively stretching one or more of its components (localizing the movement to the C3-4 joint by use of local thumb pressures).

Two other important aspects of the patient's symptoms are the *severity of the pain* and the *irritability of the disorder*. *Severity* relates to the examiner's interpretation of the severity of the pain based on the patient's description and the functional limitations caused by the pain. The *irritability* or "touchiness" of a disorder is explained in Chapter 6. In relation to treatment, the most significant factor in irritability is the length of time the pain takes to subside after provocation. If in the example given above, the patient experiences a momentary pain each time she reaches for her seatbelt, her condition is non-irritable and the treatment suggested is appropriate. However, if she is left with a residual ache for an hour after reaching once for her seatbelt, her condition is irritable and the initial treatment technique should be performed with the patient's neck in a position of comfort, and should not provoke pain.

Signs

Signs refer to physical examination findings and are discussed in Chapter 7. It is important to reach a mechanical diagnosis of neuromusculoskeletal tissue dysfunction through isolation of the structures at fault, on the basis of knowing the distribution of pain and the response to physical tests. Knowledge of the movements that increase and decrease the pain response is a major determinant of the method to be used for applying passive movement in treatment.

Selection Based on the Effects of the Technique

Passive movement as a treatment technique can be broadly divided into its use as *mobilization* (passive oscillatory movements) or *manipulation* (small-amplitude thrust and stretch performed at speed at the limit of a range of movement). Mobilization is the method of choice for most cervical conditions because it can be used as a treatment for pain or for restoring movement in a hypomobile joint. It can be adapted to suit the severity of the pain, the irritability of the condition, and the stability of the disorder. Also, gentle mobilization may be safely applied in conditions in which a manipulation is contraindicated [e.g., vertebrobasilar insufficiency (VBI)].

Manipulation is the treatment of choice when an intervertebral joint is locked. When the aim is to regain mobility of an irritable joint, a single manipulation may be less aggravating than repeated stretching by mobilization.

Position of the Intervertebral Joint and Direction of the Movement Technique

Treatment by passive movement involves careful positioning of the affected intervertebral segment and selection of the most effective direction of movement. These are based on a knowledge of spinal biomechanics and the desired pain response.

A manipulation is applied in the direction of limitation to stretch the tissues in that particular direction. Using biomechanical principles, the cervical spine is positioned (in lateral flexion and contralateral rotation) to isolate movement to the desired intervertebral segment, and a thrust is applied in the appropriate direction. When using *passive mobilization,* both the position of the intervertebral joint and the direction of movement are varied according to the desired effect of the technique. Some examples are given below.

Avoiding Discomfort or Pain

In cases in which pain is severe or a condition is irritable, the provocation of symptoms should be avoided. The cervical spine is positioned so that the painful intervertebral segment is pain-free, and the movement technique that is employed must also be pain-free.

Causing or Avoiding Referred Pain

Provocation of referred pain is safe when that pain is chronic, non-irritable, and not originating from a nerve root. To alter the condition, provocation of the symptoms in treatment may be necessary, by positioning, by application of the treatment technique that is selected, or both. However, if the pain is of nerve root origin (i.e., is worse distally, and neurologic changes are present), and particularly if the examination of movements reproduces distal pain, treatment techniques that provoke the distal pain should not be used.

Opening One Side of the Intervertebral Space

Techniques that open one side of the intervertebral space (i.e., widen the disc space and the foraminal canal) should be chosen in cases of nerve root irritation/compression and in cases of a worsening unilateral disc or zygapophyseal joint disorder.

Stretching Contracted Tissues

Joints that are both painful and hypomobile can respond differently to passive mobilization. The pain response during the performance of a technique, and its effect over a 24-hour period, will guide the therapist about the direction in which to move the joint and how firmly to stretch the contracted tissues. A favorable response to gentle oscillatory stretching occurs when there is a decrease in the pain experienced during the technique, thus allowing the movement to be performed more strongly. A worsening of the pain response indicates that this direction of movement is aggravating the condition.

Moving Intervertebral Joint(s) or the Intervertebral and Foraminal Canal Structures

If, during the physical examination, movements of both the intervertebral joints and neural structures in the foraminal canals reproduce the patient's arm pain, treatment should be directed to the intervertebral joints in the first instance. The effect on the intervertebral joint signs and neural signs is noted, and if the latter do not improve, movement of the neural tissues should be added.

Performance of the Movement Technique

Selection of a treatment technique does not merely relate to the direction of movement, but also to the manner in which it is applied.

The *amplitude* of a movement can be varied from barely perceptible to full use of the available range. The rhythm can be varied from smooth and evenly applied to staccato. Similarly, the *speed* and *position in range* in which the movement is performed can be altered.

A passive movement technique must be modified according to its desired effect, and this is based on the symptoms experienced by the patient during the technique, the quality of the movement, the presence of spasm, and the end-feel. It is not possible to discuss these details in this chapter, but merely to present the two ends of the symptom spectrum, from a constant ache with pain experienced through the range of movement, to stiffness with mild discomfort felt only at the end of the range of certain movements. A full description may be found in Maitland.[2]

Constant Aching with Pain Through Range

The cervical spine must be placed in a position of maximal comfort (usually one of slight flexion and midposition for the other movements). The treatment technique will be of small amplitude, performed slowly and smoothly (so that there is no discomfort or increase in the degree of aching). The movement technique may be a physiologic or an accessory movement, and should result in an immediate reduction in the degree of aching. In those patients in whom there is no immediate effect, the effect should be noted over a 24-hour period.

Stiffness with Mild Discomfort Felt Only at the End of Range of Certain Movements

The cervical spine is carefully positioned at or near the limit of the hypomobile directions of movement (i.e., in the position that best reproduces the symptoms of stiffness and discomfort). The treatment should put maximal stretch on the hypomobile intervertebral segment. The technique should be firmly applied, of small amplitude, and sustained. Should the level of discomfort increase with the firm stretching, large amplitude movements can be interspersed every 40 to 60 seconds.

CERVICAL SYNDROMES

In this section, some of the common clinical presentations with a history of spontaneous (nontraumatic) onset are discussed, using typical case histories. The clinical reasoning related to management of these conditions by manipulative physical therapy is emphasized. It is beyond the scope of this chapter to describe patient self management in detail, but it must be stressed that the latter is integral to the management of all patients. Cervical vertigo, cervical headache, and thoracic outlet syndrome are not included, since these conditions are discussed in Chapters 8, 13, and 15, respectively.

Zygapophyseal Joint Arthralgia

The zygapophyseal joints are a common source of pain in the cervical spine, particularly in the upper cervical spine, where they can cause local neck pain and pain referred to the head (see Ch. 4). Joints between C3 and C7 can refer pain to the supraspinous fossa and into the arm.[3] The area of pain strongly suggests the intervertebral source of the pain, but this must be confirmed by specific palpation for soft-tissue changes (thickening of the tissues in the interlaminar space and around the zygapophyseal joint) and altered intervertebral movement (most frequently hypomobility). Seldom does pain arise from one joint alone; more commonly it arises from two or three adjacent joints. Joints may become symptomatic bilaterally or only on one side.

Osteoarthrotic changes (joint space narrowing, sclerosis, and osteophytosis) may or may not be evident on plain radiography, but Rees[4] found these changes to be common features in his tomographic studies of 2,000 patients with cervical headache.

In the elderly, low cervical (C4 to C7) spondylitic changes are more common than osteoarthrotic changes of the zygapophyseal joints, but the two kinds of changes often coexist. Specific examination will help to determine whether symptoms are arising from the disc and/or the zygapophyseal joints.

Case Study

A 55-year-old housewife presented with a 3-year history of right sided neck pain of gradual onset. When severe, the pain spread to the supraspinous fossa and upper lateral arm. The patient could not recall any incident having caused the onset of her pain, but it had been worse since she had hit her head 10 days earlier. Radiographs showed moderate spondylosis at C5-6 and mild bilateral osteoarthrosis of the C4-5 and C5-6 zygapophyseal joints.

Symptoms. The patient's mornings were symptom free, but by the end of each afternoon her neck ached, and the ache was worsened by activities involving cervical extension.

Physical Signs. Cervical flexion and left rotation (70°) were slightly restricted but painless on passive overpressure. Extension was limited to half the normal range by right neck pain, and rotation to the right (40°) reproduced pain in the right neck and supraspinous fossa. Intervertebral movement tests revealed hypomobility at the C3 to C6 zygapophyseal joints, which was more marked on the right. The pains in the cervical and supraspinous fossa were reproduced by right unilateral posteroanterior gliding (C3 to C6), whereas posteroanterior gliding on the left side revealed painless hypomobility.

Interpretation. The patient is a middle-aged woman with a stiff, degenerative, low cervical spine. The condition has been made worse by jarring of her neck. The area of pain and the patient's physical signs strongly suggest a zygapophyseal joint disorder. It would be appropriate to treat this with passive movement because both the symptoms and signs have a mechanical presentation. There are no contraindications to this, but at the first application it would be prudent to mobilize the joints short of producing discomfort. The presence for 3 years of symptoms in hypomobile degenerative joints suggests that a number of treatments (for example 5 to 10) may be required to progress both the firmness of stretching and the precision of application to the point of pain-free mobility. A home exercise program will be required to reduce the frequency of recurrence of the patient's symptoms.

Treatment

Day 1 (Treatment 1). With the patient prone and her neck supported comfortably in slight flexion, large amplitude, unilateral posteroanterior (PA) oscillatory pressures were applied over the right C3 to C6 zygapophyseal joints (Fig. 14-1). The oscillations were slow and rhythmic, with care being taken not to cause any discomfort during the technique. Re-examination showed an improvement of 10° in the range of both cervical extension and right rotation. The patient was asked to perform mobility exercises twice daily after heating her neck under a warm shower. She was instructed

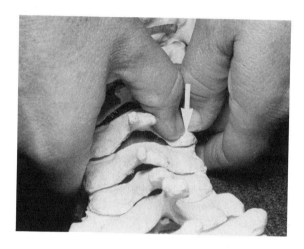

Fig. 14-1.   Unilateral PA gliding of the facets of the right C2-3 zygapophyseal joint.

to extend and to rotate her neck to each side, taking the movements to the onset of slight discomfort only.

Day 3 (Treatment 2).   The patient reported that she had more mobility of her neck and less aching in the late afternoons. Physical examination showed that she had maintained the increased range gained at her first treatment. Unilateral PA pressures were applied further into range so that they stretched the hypomobile right C3 to C6 zygapophyseal joints, causing some discomfort. Two applications of this technique improved the range of right rotation to 60°, but extension remained unaltered. The patient was asked to continue with her mobilizing exercises.

Day 5 (Treatment 3).   The patient reported that her condition was improved. She had a mild ache on right side of her neck at the end of the day, but no referred pain to the supraspinous fossa or arm. Cervical extension remained at three-fourths of the normal range, and right rotation at 60°. Firmly applied unilateral pressures to the right C3 to C6 zygapophyseal joints restored a full pain-free range of right rotation, but extension of the patient's neck remained unchanged. (Full range refers to the full range for a patient's age and somatotype).

Interpretation.   Intervertebral movement tests demonstrated long-standing hypomobility of the C3 to C6 zygapophyseal joints bilaterally, but treatment had so far been directed unilaterally. Right rotation improved, since it was restricted predominantly at the symptomatic right zygapophyseal joints, which after treatment had improved mobility. However, extension involves movement of the zygapophyseal joints symmetrically, and might have been restricted by the stiffness on the patient's left side. Therefore, treatment bilaterally would have been necessary to increase the patient's mobility, even though her symptoms were experienced unilaterally.

Day 5 (Treatment 3) Continued. Firm, sustained central and unilateral PA pressures (applied to each side) effected a marked increase in the range of low cervical extension and of both rotations (now 80°).

Day 7 (Treatment 4). The patient was delighted with her progress. She had experienced only two episodes of right neck aching, after cleaning windows. Her cervical extension and right rotation were full range, causing slight right low cervical discomfort. By directing the right unilateral PA pressure medially (a technique that glides the facets under some compression) on C4 and C5 (Fig. 14-2), sharp local pain was elicited. This technique was used as treatment. Three repetitions of oscillations lasting 30 seconds each were firmly applied to stretch the right zygapophyseal joints. Sharp pain was experienced on each occasion, but there was no aching afterward. Following this, extension and right rotation were painless on passive overpressure. Mobilizing exercises were reduced to once daily to maintain mobility of the patient's neck.

Day 12 (Treatment 5). The patient was asymptomatic and felt that her neck mobility was the best it had been for years. Slight discomfort was provoked by placing her neck in the combined position of extension and right rotation. With her neck in this combined position, firm unilateral PA pressures over the right C5-6 zygapophyseal joint caused sharp pain. Four repetitions of this technique for 30 seconds each restored full range extension and right rotation with no discomfort on passive overpressure.

Treatment was discontinued, with an explanation to the patient that recurrences of her neck pain and stiffness were likely, but would be less

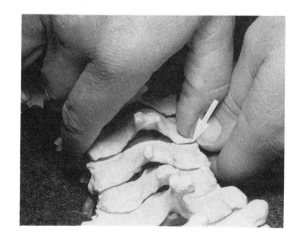

Fig. 14-2. Medially directed unilateral PA gliding of the facets of the right C2-3 zygapophyseal joint.

frequent if she maintained her cervical mobility with once-daily mobilizing exercises.

Acute Locking of Zygapophyseal Joint (Wry Neck)

Acute locking can occur at any intervertebral level, but is most frequent at C2-C3.[5] When locking occurs above this intervertebral level there is usually a history of trauma, whereas locking in the low cervical levels is usually secondary to a disc disorder. Classically, locking follows an unguarded movement of the neck, with instant pain over the articular pillar and an antalgic posture of lateral flexion to the opposite side and slight flexion, which the patient is unable to correct. Locking is more frequent in children and young adults. In many, the joint pain settles within 24 hours without requiring treatment (because the joint was merely sprained or because it unlocked spontaneously), but other patients will require a localized manipulation to unlock the joint. Some authors[5–7] postulate that the locking is due to impaction of synovial villi or meniscoids between the facets of the zygapophyseal joint. In older subjects the locking may result from the mechanical catching of roughened arthritic articular surfaces.[8] In both cases the innervated synovium and capsule would be stretched.[9]

Case Study

A 26-year-old man presented with a history of sharp left-sided neck pain of sudden onset when he turned his head rapidly to the right to catch a ball that morning. He found that he was unable to hold his head erect because of this sharp pain. He had no past history of cervical symptoms.

Symptoms. When the patient held his head flexed laterally to the right and in slight flexion, he had no pain but only a dull ache along the left side of his neck. On attempting to hold his head erect he experienced sharp, deep pain localized over the left C2-3 zygapophyseal joint. There were no symptoms of vertebrobasilar insufficiency.

Physical Signs. The patient's head was held in right lateral flexion and slight flexion. Attempts to correct this position actively or passively caused sharp pain over the left C2-3 zygapophyseal joint. With the patient's head in slight lateral flexion to the right, flexion and right rotation were of full range and painless; upper cervical extension was slightly limited, and left rotation was 40° with both of these movements causing sharp left-sided cervical pain.

With the patient in the supine (non-weight-bearing) position, it was possible to place his head in the midline position. With the head and neck

in the neutral position, sharp pain was elicited on full upper cervical extension and at 50° of left rotation. Testing of left lateral flexion at each intervertebral level confirmed a mechanical block to the movement at C2-3 with
pain and spasm, while the movement was full range at the adjacent levels.

Treatment

Day 1 (Treatment 1). With the patient supine and his neck in a neutral
position for the upper cervical spine, gentle manual traction was applied
as a slow oscillation, sustained for 30 seconds, and then released. This
was repeated four times, causing no discomfort. Because there was no
improvement in the range of motion of his head, a relaxation technique
was employed in an attempt to reduce the spasm and so allow the joint to
unlock spontaneously. The patient's head was rotated 45° to the left, short
of any discomfort, and a technique of reciprocal relaxation for the right
cervical rotators was applied. Passive intervertebral lateral flexion to the
left at C2-3 remained unchanged.

Interpretation. Because the patient's zygapophyseal joint will not unlock easily, it will be necessary to "gap" the facets, using a manipulation
localized to the C2-3 intervertebral level. This is one condition in which it
is not possible to fully perform the premanipulative screening tests for
VBI[10] or for instability of the upper cervical spine[11] (see Ch. 7). In this
particular case there was no history of symptoms suggestive of VBI or
of trauma or disease that might weaken ligamentous tissue. By careful
positioning of the spine, the "thrust" technique should place minimal
stretch on the segments above C2. Informed consent for the use of manipulation must be obtained from the patient.

Day 1 (Treatment 1) Continued. A transverse thrust manipulation was
applied to open the left C2-3 zygapophyseal joint. A description of the
method of this technique can be found in Maitland.[2] Before the manipulation, the end position of the technique was sustained for 10 seconds to
ensure that there would be no provocation of vertigo or nystagmus, and
was then released in order to note whether any latent symptoms occurred.
The manipulation was performed after this.

Following the manipulation, there was a full passive range of left lateral
flexion at the left C2-3 zygapophyseal joint, but on assuming the sitting
position the patient again adopted a wry neck position. Active left lateral
flexion was full but still painful. Following the application of large amplitude unilateral PA oscillatory pressures and ultrasound to the left C2-3
zygapophyseal joint, only slight discomfort was experienced on active left
lateral flexion.

A soft collar was applied to protect the joint from jolting in the patient's car. The patient was advised to rest, with his head comfortably supported on one pillow, for the remainder of the day.

Day 2 (Treatment 2). The patient reported that because his neck ached on the way home, he had taken analgesics and rested. He had subsequently experienced one or two twinges of pain when turning in bed. On the morning of his second treatment his neck had felt "normal." In sitting, full left lateral flexion was painful over the left C2-3 joint. Passive left lateral flexion at this joint was painful when subjected to non-weight-bearing testing but was of full range. Treatment consisted of three repetitions of large amplitude unilateral PA pressures, each applied for 60 seconds over the left C2-3 joint, after which left lateral flexion, performed in sitting, was pain-free to passive overpressure. On the following day the patient telephoned to cancel his appointment because he had regained full pain-free mobility of his neck.

Recurrent Locking of Cervical Zygapophyseal Joints

Some individuals experience recurrent cervical zygapophyseal joint locking. Many are women who exhibit generalized joint hypermobility. The recurrence rate of this condition can be lessened by teaching these individuals exercises to improve both the strength and coordination of their cervical muscles.

Discogenic Pain

The low cervical spine is a common site of spondylosis. From in vitro studies[7,12] it has been noted that horizontal fissuring of the disc from the uncovertebral region begins in the first decade of life and is quite extensive by the age of 20 to 30 years. In many cases this degenerative process remains asymptomatic, but in others symptoms develop either spontaneously or after postures involving sustained extension or flexion. Cases of spondylosis of traumatic origin are excluded from this discussion.

The clinical picture varies considerably. Stiffness of the low cervical spine is common to all cases. This may progress to the stage at which loss of mobility interferes with daily activities; thus, for example, loss of extension and rotation make it difficult to turn around so as to drive a car in reverse. Frequently, stiffness of the cervicothoracic region causes the development of a kyphotic (dowager's hump) deformity. In other cases, aching and pain may develop. The stiff low cervical joints may be the source of pain, which is frequently described as a burning pain across the base of the neck, or the mobile mid-cervical joints may become symptomatic, the typical complaint being a central, deep mid-cervical pain. Pain may also be experienced in the medial scapular area.[13]

It is unusual for patients with spondylosis to complain of nerve root symptoms or to develop neurologic signs. This contrasts with discogenic disorders of the lumbar spine, which often progress to the prolapse of nuclear material, causing nerve root symptoms and signs. In cervical discs the small nucleus pulposus is gradually lost via the posterior and lateral fissures, and at the same time undergoes metaplastic change from a soft gel into fibrocartilage.[7] Any nuclear material remaining in young adults is more likely to herniate posteriorly into the spinal canal than laterally through the uncovertebral joints.[7]

Case Study

A 60-year-old housewife presented with central low cervical pain of gradual onset over the preceding 3 weeks. She associated this with long hours of sustained neck flexion while sewing. Discogenic pain is likely to arise from mechanical stress (e.g., sustained flexion and anterior shear forces) on the annulus, the outer fibers of which are innervated.[14,15] The patient's symptoms began as stiffness on straightening her neck and some short-lived stiffness in the mornings. Movements of her neck would readily ease this. Her symptoms were worsening in that for the previous week she had been able to sew only for increasingly short periods before her symptoms appeared. Three days before presenting she awoke with a very stiff neck and experienced left medial scapular pain each time she flexed her neck. She was unable to recall any neck symptoms in the past, but for 2 or 3 years had awakened with neck stiffness that she considered to have been "normal as one gets older." Radiographs of the cervical and thoracic spine showed mild narrowing of the C4-5 and C5-6 disc spaces.

Symptoms. The patient was unable to flex her neck because of sharp pain experienced medial to the spine of her left scapula. This pain would ease immediately on returning her neck to the upright position. This pain interfered with many of her daily activities, and by noon of each day, a constant, deep central ache (C5 to C7) had developed. Lying supine with her head on a thick pillow eased her pain after half an hour, but the ache would soon return once she was again upright and attempting household activities. In the mornings her neck was stiff and ached for half an hour.

Signs. The patient had a pronounced forward head posture (Fig. 14-3A), attempted correction of which by passive posterior gliding (Fig. 14-3B) reproduced both the low cervical and sharp left medial scapular pain. The following movements also reproduced both areas of symptoms: flexion (half range), extension (one-fourth range), left rotation (45°). The patient was instructed to perform these active movements only to the onset of discomfort.

On palpation, the spinous process of C4 was depressed while that of C5 was prominent. The deep interspinous soft tissues between C4-5 and C5-6 were thickened, and this thickening was most pronounced on the

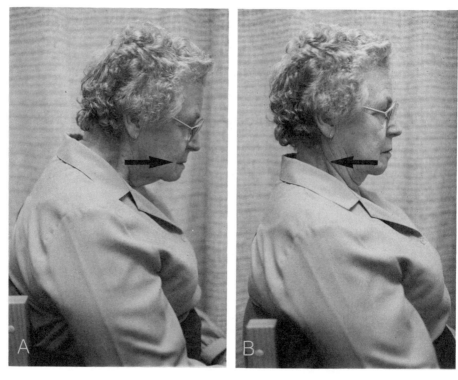

Fig. 14-3. (A) Lateral view of forward head posture. (B) Correction of forward head posture by posterior gliding.

left between C4 and C5. The C4 vertebra was very mobile to central PA pressures, while C5, was by contrast markedly hypomobile. Deep pain was elicited at both levels. The C4 to C7 zygapophyseal joints were of normal mobility and only mildly painful with unilateral PA pressure and testing of segmental physiologic movements. Tests for the upper and mid-thoracic spine demonstrated painless hypomobility.

Because of the irritability of the patient's condition, muscle length and strength tests were deferred until the condition was no longer irritable.

Interpretation. Discogenic disorders often commence insidiously, in this case with morning stiffness. A forward head posture coupled with long periods of sustained flexion puts an anterior shearing force on the low cervical discs and, in time, symptoms may develop. The area of pain, pattern of movement restriction, and palpation findings in this case were typical of a discogenic disorder. The lack of unilateral neck pain and normal mobility of the zygapophyseal joints for the patient's age and somatotype failed to implicate these joints as the source of her pain. Her disorder was worsening and irritable.

While the symptomatic joints in a case such as this should settle in a week or two with treatment, the long-term relief of symptoms requires attention to correcting both the muscle imbalance and the forward head posture.

Treatment

Day 1 (Treatment 1). Following the examination, the patient experienced a constant deep central ache in the low cervical area. Because this was relieved by gentle manual traction, traction was chosen as the treatment technique. Traction was applied with the patient supine and with her head and neck supported comfortably on two pillows so that the head-on-neck position was neutral between flexion and extension, and the neck-on-thorax position was in approximately 35° of flexion, which was the neutral position for the C4-5 intervertebral joint. Four pounds of traction was chosen because with that strength, movement could be palpated in the soft tissues in the interspinous space between C4 and C5, and because this effected a reduction in the patient's neck ache. Traction was applied for 7 minutes, and because of the irritability of the patient's disorder, her movement signs were not reassessed afterward.

The patient was given a soft collar as a temporary measure to support her neck and to prevent painful flexion. She was asked to wear the collar while upright but not when resting in bed.

Day 2 (Treatment 2). When seen the next day, the patient reported that her neck was more comfortable and that she had slept well. Her cervical movements were unaltered. Traction was repeated at 4 pounds for 15 minutes, after which all of the patient's cervical movements improved in range before medial scapular pain was produced. She was asked to continue wearing the collar.

Day 3 (Treatment 3). The patient had experienced no left medial scapular pain, and her neck felt less stiff on the morning of her third day of treatment. Flexion, extension, and posterior gliding of her low cervical spine were now at three-fourths of range, and left rotation was at 70° before sharp medial scapular pain was produced. Movement further into range was possible with central PA pressures over C4 and C5 before eliciting deep pain.

For treatment, central PA pressures (Fig. 14-4) were applied slowly and rhythmically to C4 and C5 for 60 seconds, keeping short of producing any discomfort. This resulted in a definite improvement in the range of all movements. Because a second application of this technique caused a deep ache to develop, the technique was stopped and traction was applied using the same dosage as on the previous day. Reassessment showed a full range of all movement except posterior gliding, which remained at three-fourths range and still produced sharp medial scapular pain. The patient was ad-

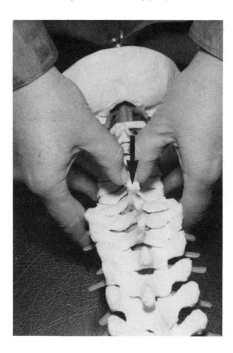

Fig. 14-4. Central PA oscillatory pressures on spinous process of C5 vertebra.

vised to wear her collar only if her neck or medial scapular pain returned, and she was taught correction of her forward head posture, taking the movement only to the onset of discomfort.

Day 4 (Treatment 4). The patient had been symptom-free until late afternoon, when her central low cervical ache developed. This was helped by the collar. Stiffness was now present for 5 minutes only in the mornings, and was eased by a warm shower. Flexion and left rotation were full and painless to passive overpressure, extension was almost full range but caused pain centrally over C7, and the extreme range of posterior glide still caused slight left medial scapular pain. If PA pressures to C5 were directed toward the right (Fig. 14-5), deep sharp pain was elicited. Treatment consisted of three repetitions of central PA pressures applied for 30 seconds to C5, including some directed toward the right. This technique was performed as small oscillations at the end of the range of movement, so as to obtain greater mobility. The treatment caused local pain that settled as soon as the stretching stopped. After each application, extension and posterior gliding improved, becoming full and painless to overpressure.

Interpretation. With a long-standing forward head posture, there is often an associated poking chin with adaptive shortening of the suboccipital muscles and weakness of the short flexor muscle group. Now that disco-

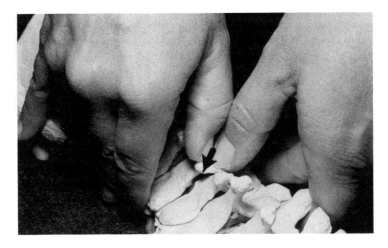

Fig. 14-5.   Central PA oscillatory pressures directed toward the right.

genic disorder is no longer irritable, the neck muscles should be examined for tightness and weakness.

Day 4 (Treatment 4) Continued. With this particular patient, the short extensors were not tight, but there was marked weakness of the short flexor muscles. The strength and endurance of these flexors should be improved first by a gravity-assisted exercise. Figure 14-6 illustrates correction of the forward head posture, to which is added scapular depression and adduction and resisted upper cervical flexion. The chin is tucked down and held against the resistance of the patient's hand. The patient was asked to perform 10 isometric contractions three times per day, holding each contraction for 5 seconds.

Day 12 (Treatment 5). The patient reported only two occasions when her neck had ached. Each occasion had followed sewing for 1 hour, and she had been able to stop the aching by repeated posterior gliding of her low cervical spine. On examination, her cervical movements were full and painless to passive overpressure, with the exception of sustained overpressure to posterior gliding, which caused a deep ache over C7. Posteroanterior pressures to C5, when directed to the right, were stiffer than when directed to the left.

Treatment consisted of four repetitions of PA pressure applied to C5 centrally and directed to the right. The oscillatory pressures were applied firmly and sustained for 60 seconds to stretch the restricted range of C5 on its adjacent vertebrae. At the end of the third and fourth application a deep ache developed, but was eased by larger amplitude PA pressures. Following the mobilization, sustained overpressure to posterior gliding was pain free. Because the short flexor muscle strength had improved, the

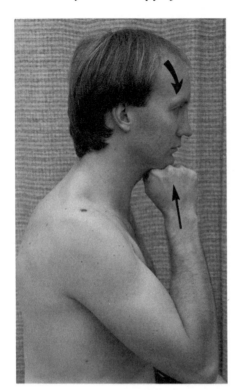

Fig. 14-6. Gravity-assisted isometric exercise for the cervical short flexor muscles. The chin is tucked in against the resistance of the hand.

isometric exercises were progressed from a hold of 5 seconds to one of 10 seconds.

Advice was given to the patient regarding self management of her cervical disc problem. This included regular posture correction, instruction to break up long periods of sustained cervical flexion by regularly performing full range low cervical extension and posterior gliding and to avoid lifting or pushing when she was tired or unwell (i.e., at times when the muscular protection of her neck is less efficient).

Day 33 (Treatment 6). When seen 3 weeks after her fifth treatment, the patient was symptom and sign free except for some residual hypomobility and soreness with PA pressures on C5. Her short flexor muscles were now sufficiently strong to cope with a progression to gravity resisted exercises. Figure 14-7 illustrates the ability to maintain the chin tucked in (upper cervical flexion) while just taking the weight of the head off the pillow. Together with scapular depression and adduction, the position is held for an increasing number of seconds, and can be combined with slight rotation to each side.

The C5 vertebra was firmly mobilized (as on Day 12). The persistence of continuing hypomobility of C5 was explained to the patient, and the need for regular posture correction and exercise was emphasized.

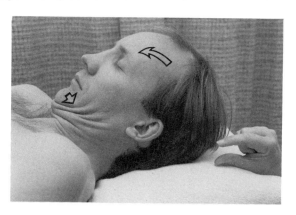

Fig. 14-7. Gravity-resisted isometric exercise for the cervical short flexor muscles. With the weight of the head just clear of the pillow, the upper cervical spine is held in flexion.

Discogenic Wry Neck

The exact pathoanatomic mechanism for the production of medial scapular pain and the associated antalgic posture of contralateral lateral flexion and flexion has not been reported, although the innervation of the outer annulus of the cervical discs has been described in recent studies,[14,15] and Cloward demonstrated that pain can be referred from cervical discs to the medial scapular area.[13]

A wry neck position, or torticollis, secondary to a discogenic condition differs in several respects from that secondary to a locked cervical zygapophyseal joint.

There is no history of a quick or unguarded movement resulting in a sudden onset of pain and locking; frequently, the patient awakens with the pain, having been pain free the night before.

The distribution of the symptoms differs from the case of a locked cervical zygapophyseal joint; most commonly, sharp pain is experienced medial to one scapula with certain cervical movements and postures, but there is no pain in the neck. However, having to hold the wry position against gravity may result in some generalized aching in the cervical musculature.

The physical signs are also different. There is often a marked kyphotic deformity, and in the non-weight-bearing position, a greater range of pain-free movement is possible. In particular, ipsilateral lateral flexion is not mechanically locked, but is limited by sharp referred pain (no local pain). Testing of passive accessory intervertebral movements demonstrates painful hypomobility with the application of central PA pressures, whereas unilateral PA oscillatory mobilization of the zygapophyseal joints is full range and painless.

Differentiation of the two distinct types of wry neck is important because the appropriate treatment for each differs. For a locked zygapophyseal joint, unlocking the joint (often by a manipulation) is essential, whereas manipulation is likely to irritate the discogenic type of wry neck.

Cervical Radicular Pain

A previously injured nerve root can give rise to pain if it is subjected to mechanical stimuli. The low cervical and upper thoracic nerve roots may be subject to injury because of the angulated course of the rootlets. Within the dura the rootlets run downward, but on piercing it they turn abruptly upward, at an angle of between 30° and 45°,[16] to reach their relevant foramen. The angulation of these rootlets is increased during cervical extension,[5] and hence they are prone to injury during hyperextension injuries and if the neck is held in sustained extension (as in painting a ceiling).

The onset of nerve root involvement may be insidious or may follow unrecognized stress or trauma, such as sleeping in an awkward position, unusually prolonged cervical extension or flexion, or traction on an arm. Nerve root symptoms are unusual in young subjects unless there is a history of trauma, in which case the likely causes are posterolateral disc protrusion or zygapophyseal joint effusion.[17] In older individuals with established degenerative changes (regardless of whether they are symptomatic or not), the nerve root may be compromised from foraminal encroachment by osteophyte formation at the margins of the facets of the zygapophyseal joint or disc–vertebral-body margin. Nerve root compression may also be due to fibrotic thickening of the dural sleeve.[18]

Case Study

Six months ago, a 50-year-old farmer experienced right sided low cervical pain and stiffness after shoveling earth for 4 hours. The pain settled after a few days, but the patient subsequently noticed that any physical activity was followed by neck stiffness on the following morning.

Four days ago, the patient painted a ceiling and the next morning awakened with severe right shoulder and arm pain. During the day, this worsened and spread into his forearm. He felt that his condition was worsening in that his fingers felt numb. Routine radiographs showed advanced spondylotic changes at C5-6 and C6-7, but no osteophytic encroachment of the neural foramina.

Symptoms. The patient complained of constant, severe pain that was worse in the right forearm, and from which he was unable to find relief except by medication that gave some short-term relief. Numbness of the right index and middle fingers was also present.

Physical Signs. The patient's head and neck were held rigidly in slight flexion, and he cradled his right arm with his left and supported it across his chest. Only two cervical movements were examined because of the severity of his pain and the irritability of the condition. Both extension (5°) and right rotation (30°) increased the patient's forearm pain. A neurologic examination revealed that his right triceps power was only of half strength, his right triceps reflex was absent, and there was numbness of the pads of his right index and middle fingers. The first component of the upper limb tension test (ULTT) (shoulder girdle depression) increased the intensity of his forearm pain (see Ch. 11). Passive intervertebral movement tests and scanning tests for other sources of arm symptoms were not performed.

Interpretation. The early history of this case is typical of a chronic condition (there is insufficient information to incriminate a disc or a zygapophyseal joint disorder as the cause). Then, following sustained cervical extension, symptoms developed in the arm. The presence of neurologic changes supports a diagnosis of right C7 nerve root compression.

Traction is the treatment of choice for severe nerve root pain of acute onset. It may take several days before the symptoms improve, although a slow, steady improvement in the physical signs is expected.

Treatment

Day 1 (Treatment 1). Traction was given with the patient supine. Positioning for maximum comfort is essential. Two pillows were required to place the low cervical spine in sufficient flexion and another pillow was placed under the patient's right arm (to prevent the weight of the arm from retracting or depressing the shoulder girdle).

Seven pounds of traction was needed for the therapist to palpate movement occurring in the deep soft tissues at C6-7. The patient was asked to assess the intensity of his arm symptoms, after which the 7 pounds of traction was applied and the intensity of the patient's symptoms reassessed. Because the pain then worsened, the strength of the traction was halved and sustained for 10 minutes. Throughout the procedure, the patient's arm symptoms remained unchanged. After the traction was stopped the patient continued to rest for half an hour, after which the traction was reapplied for another 10 minutes at the same strength. At the completion of another rest period, the patient reported that the intensity of his forearm pain had decreased. His physical signs were not reassessed. The patient was advised to rest in bed as much as possible, in a position of maximal comfort.

Days 2 and 3 (Treatments 2 and 3). The patient reported no symptomatic relief, and his cervical and neural signs were unchanged. Cervical traction was repeated, with two applications of 15 and 20 minutes at the third treatment, interspersed with a rest period of 30 minutes. Neural conduction was unaltered, although the patient reported improvement in his forearm pain and finger sensation.

Day 4 (Treatment 4). The patient reported that he could sometimes completely ease his forearm pain by tucking his right thumb into his belt. Examination revealed that in this position his shoulder girdle was elevated, a position that reduces tension on the C7 nerve root. With the patient's right thumb tucked into his belt, his cervical extension and right rotation could be taken an extra 15° before producing forearm pain. His nerve conduction signs were unchanged.

Interpretation. The signs in this case show that there is painful restriction of the normal distal movement of the C7 nerve root and that this is also limiting of the range of cervical extension and right rotation. Rather than continue cervical traction, a more rapid symptomatic improvement is likely to occur from mobilization of the articular tissue (C6-7 intervertebral level) or the neural tissue, using a component of the ULTT. In view of the patient's previously worsening neurologic status, it was decided to treat the articular component of his condition.

Day 4 (Treatment 4) continued. With the patient lying prone, passive accessory movements isolated the maximal hypomobility and local discomfort to the right C6-7 zygapophyseal joint. This was then mobilized, using a combination of small and large amplitude movements and taking care not to refer symptoms to the arm. Following this, the patient was able to hang his right arm by his side for 2 minutes before experiencing forearm pain. His cervical extension and rotation each improved by 15°. A second application of passive mobilization was thought unwise, owing to the patient's unstable neurologic status, but cervical traction, as for Treatment 3, was given. On completion of the traction there was definite improvement in the patient's triceps strength and reflex, and in sensation in his finger pads.

Day 6 (Treatment 5). The patient was delighted with his progress. He experienced only occasional and less intense right forearm pain, and his finger sensation was normal. His triceps was five-sixths of normal strength, and his triceps reflex was slightly depressed. It was necessary to combine low cervical extension with right rotation in order to reproduce his neurogenic forearm pain. Shoulder girdle depression was pain-free, but the addition of 40° of passive abduction brought on sharp forearm pain.

Interpretation. With such improvement in neural conduction, it is safe to more firmly mobilize the low cervical spine. Because neural tension signs more effectively reproduce the forearm pain, it may be necessary to add careful neural mobilization.

Day 6 (Treatment 5) continued. Following three applications of firm passive mobilization of the C6-7 and adjacent levels, the patient's forearm pain could not be reproduced even by right rotation sustaining the combined position of extension and right rotation. After the first application of mobilization, the patient's neural mobility increased slightly (right shoulder abduction to 50°), after which there was no further change. Before changing to neural mobilization as a treatment technique, the patient's neurologic conduction was assessed and found to be unchanged. With the right shoulder girdle depressed, large amplitude abduction, up to the onset of forearm pain, was performed. Only slight resistance to this movement was encountered. The technique was repeated, after which forearm pain was elicited at 65° abduction.

Day 13 (Treatment 6). The patient was asymptomatic and had full recovery of C7 nerve root conduction. With the shoulder girdle depressed, abduction to 90° was pain-free, but the addition of 30° of glenohumeral lateral rotation caused sharp forearm pain. On the left side, by comparison, the addition of lateral rotation and elbow extension components of the ULTT could be taken to full range and were painless. To lessen the likelihood of recurrence of the patient's symptoms, it was decided to stretch the right arm into lateral rotation (three firm stretches). The patient was asked to return in a fortnight, since his neural tissue still lacked full mobility.

Day 27 (Treatment 7). The patient remained asymptomatic. Cervical and neural conduction signs were checked and found to be normal. The ULTT revealed a painless limitation of elbow extension of 20°. Three firm stretches of elbow extension restored a full range of motion and treatment was discontinued.

SUMMARY

The purpose of this chapter has been to highlight the application of manual therapy (passive mobilization and manipulation) in some cervical syndromes. Manual therapy is an effective and safe method of treatment if it is based on careful, thorough examination and regular assessment. In practice, it is essential that manipulative therapy be integrated with techniques for poor posture and inadequate muscle protection.

REFERENCES

1. Trott PH, Grant ER, Maitland GD: Manipulative therapy for the lumbar spine. In Twomey LT, Taylor J (eds): Physical Therapy of the Low Back. Churchill Livingstone, New York, 1994
2. Maitland GD: Vetebral Manipulation. 5th Ed. Butterworth, London, 1986
3. Aprill C, Dwyer A, Bogduk N: Cervical zygapophyseal joint pain patterns. II: A clinical evaluation. Spine 15:458, 1990

 4. Rees S: Relaxation therapy in migraine and chronic tension headaches. Med J Aust 2(2):70, 1975
 5. Grieve GP: Common Vertebral Joint Problems. 2nd Ed. Churchill Livingstone, Edinburgh, 1988
 6. Bourdillon JF: Spinal Manipulation. 3rd Ed. Heinemann, London, 1982
 7. Twomey LT, Taylor JR: Joints of the middle and lower cervical spine. Age changes and pathology. p. 215. In Jones HM, Jones MA, Milde MR (eds): Proceedings of the Sixth Biennial Conference, Manipulative Therapists Association of Australia, Adelaide, 1989
 8. Stoddard A: Manual of Osteopathic Practice. 2nd Ed. Hutchinson, London, 1983
 9. Giles LG, Taylor JR: Human zygapophyseal joint capsule and synovial fold innervation. Br J Rheumatol 26:93, 1987
10. Australian Physiotherapy Association: Protocol for pre-manipulative testing of the cervical spine. Aust J Physiother 34:97, 1988
11. Aspinall W: Clinical testing for the craniovertebral hypermobility syndrome. Journal of Orthopaedic and Sports Physical Therapy 12:47, 1990
12. Taylor JR, Twomey LT: Acute injuries to cervical joints. An autopsy study of neck sprain. Spine 18:1115, 1993
13. Cloward RB: Cervical discography: a contribution to the aetiology and mechanism of neck, shoulder and arm pain. Ann Surg 105:1052, 1959
14. Bogduk N, Windsor M, Inglis A: The innervation of the cervical intervertebral discs. Spine 13:2, 1989
15. Mendel T, Wink CS, Zimny ML: Neural elements in human cervical intervertebral discs. Spine 17:132, 1992
16. Nathan H, Feuerstein M: Angulated course of spinal nerve roots. J Neurosurg 32:349, 1970
17. Simeone FA, Rothman RH: Cervical disc disease. p. 287. In Rothman RH, Simeone FA (eds): The Spine. Vol. 1. WB Saunders, Philadelphia, 1975
18. Frykolm R: Cervical nerve root compression resulting from disc degeneration and root sleeve fibrosis. Acta Chir Scand, suppl. 160, 1951

15 | Neural Injury in the Thoracic Spine: A Conceptual Basis for Manual Therapy

David S. Butler
Helen Slater

Of the three traditional divisions of the spine, the thoracic spine is surely the least studied and understood. Physical therapy remains focused on cervical and lumbar disorders despite some unique aspects of the thoracic spine, especially its neurology, that warrant greater attention.

The importance of the thoracic spine is emphasized by the fact that all central nervous system information to and from the lower limbs, pelvis, and viscera must pass through this spinal area; that substantial areas of innervation of the trunk and viscera arise from it; and that with the exception of the upper three lumbar segments, it houses the sympathetic nervous system as the latter passes to the entire body. Therefore, while there are undoubted thoracic neurogenic sources for symptoms in the thoracic area, this area also houses neural tissue that may be responsible for symptoms in other areas of the body. In addition, the thoracic spine and rib cage are possible sites of referral of symptoms from viscerogenic structures such as the lungs and heart. All clinicians must be aware that visceral pathology may masquerade as being of musculoskeletal origin, and that musculoskeletal disorders may appear to be viscerogenic.[1-5]

Physiologic and mechanical continuity of the nervous system dictates that

313

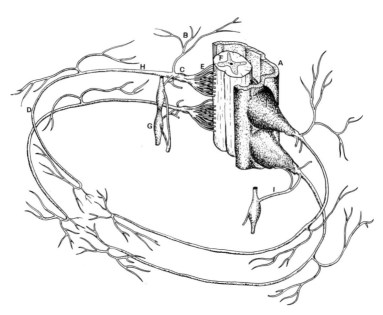

Fig. 15-1. Thoracic neural tissues, diagrammatic view. **(A)** Dura mater; **(B)** dorsal ramus; **(C)** dorsal root ganglion; **(D)** intercostal nerve; **(E)** nerve rootlets; **(F)** spinal cord; **(G)** sympathetic trunk; **(H)** ventral ramus; **(I)** white rami communicantes.

movements of the upper and lower quadrants will inevitably move and put tension on thoracic neural tissues.[6–8] This means that pathologic changes affecting neural tissues or interfacing tissues in the cervical or lumbar regions may have consequences for thoracic neural tissues, and conversely that pathology of the thoracic region may affect disorders of the cervical and lumbar spine. Appreciating this neural continuity offers physical therapists new directions for assessing and treating thoracic neuropathies.

This chapter focuses on the mechanisms of thoracic pain, and proposes some management strategies specific to disorders relating to thoracic neuropathies. The thoracic neural structures considered in this chapter are peripheral nerves, nerve roots, sympathetic trunks and ganglia, and the spinal cord and meninges (Fig. 15-1). Information about thoracic neuropathies is scanty. This chapter utilizes what is known about the thoracic spine, extrapolates from knowledge of the lumbar and cervical spine, and uses the authors' clinical experience.

Definitions

Neurodynamics refers to the study of the mechanical and related physiological properties of neural tissues.

Neurogenic symptoms refers to symptoms originating in any of the neural conducting or connective tissues.

Neuropathic pain is a term used to describe pain that results from pathologic processes affecting neural tissue.

Nociceptive pain (or nerve-end pain) refers to pain produced when the peripheral terminals of nociceptive neurons are stimulated.

Sympathetically maintained pain is defined by Campbell et al.[9] as "pain that is dependent on the sympathetic innervation of the area afflicted with pain."

PAIN MECHANISMS AND NEURAL INJURY

In any pain state, peripheral, central, autonomic, and affective (emotional) mechanisms will be involved.[10–12] Pain mechanisms need consideration just as pain sources do. For example, the pathologic changes that occur in an intercostal nerve entrapment may provide a source of pain. However, because ongoing pain may alter the sensitivity of neurons in the dorsal horn of the spinal cord,[13] central mechanisms may become a feature of such a pain pattern. The interplay of each of these mechanisms will dictate the type of clinical presentation of pain and also influence the management approach taken by the physical therapist.

The notion of neural injury includes damage to the neural conducting and connective tissues themselves as well as persistent alterations in the firing of neurons that may occur as later sequelae to injury. Pain can be conveniently divided into physiologic pain and pathologic pain.[13] Physiologic pain is the result of painful input where no tissue damage occurs. This kind of pain is nociceptor mediated, and its pathway therefore begins at the peripheral terminals of nociceptors. Such pain is usually transient and well localized, but if the inflammatory reaction in the innervated tissues continues, the nociceptors may become sensitized so that they may fire more readily. Physiologic pain serves a protective function.[13] The sequelae of these peripheral neuronal alterations may include changes in the response properties of dorsal horn neurons that make them respond painfully to normally innocuous input such as light touch. Such pathologic pain may occur as a result of persistent target tissue or neural damage, and may be characterized by being prolonged and exaggerated to an extent that is out of proportion to the stimulus. Pathologic pain appears to have no useful biologic function, instead merely serving to perpetrate the pain cycle. Further reading on this subject is available and recommended.[10–12]

Mechanisms of Sympathetically Maintained Pain

It has already been mentioned that the thoracic spine is unique because it houses most of the sympathetic outflow of the body. The sympathetic nervous system (SNS) has a special role in the generation and maintenance of certain pain states.[14] Not all symptoms can be related to alterations in the sympathetic link of the nervous system, although the frequent benefits of chemical and surgical sympathectomy support a sympathetically mediated contribution to many pain states.

The mechanisms by which the SNS causes pain and other sympathetic epiphenoma have evoked much debate (Wright, personal communication, 1993). However, it is generally acknowledged that increased sympathetic tone, or a more-or-less normal sympathetic outflow acting on noradrenaline-sensitive systems that have an increased sensitivity, or a combination of these mechanisms is involved. The SNS may cause a chemical sensitization of peripheral sensory neurons that renders them responsive to normally innocuous stimuli. This can perpetrate the cycle of peripheral-central sensitization with a direct feedback loop to sympathetic neurons in the spinal cord. Ultimately, this closed loop can drive the pain cycle (Fig. 15-2). Abnormal sympathetic responses may also occur if signaled to do so by higher centers or by internuncial neurons, and if the sympathetic neural apparatus is in some way damaged or sensitized.

Nowhere in the literature is there any mention that altered dynamics of the SNS may contribute to SMP states. We feel that there is considerable clinical, neuroanatomic, and pathologic evidence for a hypothesis that loss of the normal movement and tension requirements of the SNS may be another mechanism of SMP.[15] In particular, in areas of the nervous system in which the SNS stands apart from the rest of the system, [i.e., the sympathetic trunks (ST), ganglia, and rami], neural tissue may be more vulnerable to mechanical interference from pathologic changes in interfacing tissues. Tests of the mechanics of other areas of the nervous system have become well established clinical tests. For example, a limited and painful straight leg raise may be indica-

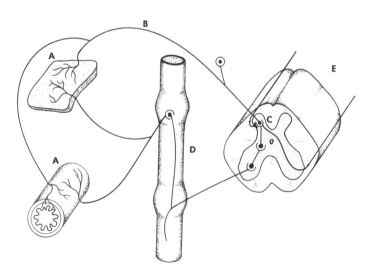

Fig. 15-2. Tissues involved in sympathetically maintained pain. **(A)** target tissues (viscus and skin); **(B)** afferent neuron; **(C)** dorsal horn; **(D)** sympathetic trunk; **(E)** spinal cord.

tive of mechanical compromise of the normal movement and tension requirements of the sciatic nerve and its branches.

Nathan,[16] in a comprehensive cadaveric study, has documented the existence of costovertebral joint osteophytes that distort or entrap the adjacent ST. Mechanical compromise may also exist in the form of unphysiologic postures that insidiously distort, stretch, or irritate the ST. Additionally, lung disorders such as bronchiectasis, tuberculosis, and tumors have been linked with ipsilateral facial flushing due to mechanical irritation of the ST.[17] Appenzeller[17] has reported patches of excessive sweating confined to the shoulder, arm, or chest of patients with severe scoliosis. It was apparently unclear whether these changes were due to spinal cord injury or injury to sympathetic preganglionic neurons; however, it is feasible that mechanical compromise of the ST may have contributed to altered physiology of some of the sympathetic efferents. Since the ST contains a high proportion of preganglionic neurons that diverge when synapsing on postganglionic neurons, any mechanical compromise of the ST has the potential to affect a variety of target tissues over a considerable anatomic area. This helps make clinical sense of the non-dermatomal multitissue nature of some SMP states.

TYPES OF NEURAL INJURY

Neurogenic injury can be considered direct, indirect, or both. Direct injury may involve overstretch or laceration, but more commonly, neural tissue may be indirectly involved in changes in non-neural tissue, such as alterations in the shape of a tunnel, rubbing on the callus of a healing fracture, distortion by postural changes, or blood organizing around the neural tissues. Because of the physiologic and mechanical continuum of the nervous system, a neuropathy in any site is likely to evoke subclinical and symptomatic responses in other areas of the nervous system, such as peripheral nerve, spinal cord, autonomic tracts, and supraspinal centers.

Neural injury can be difficult to measure. Frank injuries, such as cord and nerve root compression or arachnoiditis, may show up with the appropriate imaging technique or be obvious from clear neurologic signs. However, physical therapists are presented with an enormous challenge in addressing neuropathies at the more minor end of the clinical spectrum, where few if any medical investigations are positive. Pain in such cases can be as challenging to treat as that at the more overt end of the spectrum, such as that in reflex sympathetic dystrophy. Examples of minor thoracic neuropathies include nerve irritation, ectopic neural pacemakers in nerve trunks, subtle alterations in dorsal horn processing, abnormal dural adherence to the spinal canal, and osteophytes distorting the sympathetic trunk. Many of these injuries may occur insidiously, their only evidence being pain or neurogenically maintained inflammation in target tissues.

Until such time as physical therapists join up with pain scientists to document a comprehensive account of thoracic pain syndromes, symptom-dominant approaches must be used in managing such syndromes. However, this approach does not have to be reliant on dogma and doctrine, because clinical reasoning skills and an increasing knowledge of pain-related sciences offer management that can be situation specific rather than recipe driven. The recent advent of a more refined neurodynamic examination also offers therapists a more precise access to these minor neuropathies.

THORACIC SPINAL CORD AND MENINGES

In the thoracic spine, trauma and changes in posture may affect the cord and meninges. Although symptomatic disc trauma appears less common in the thoracic than in the lumbar or cervical spine, it may involve varying degrees of cord compression and myelopathy rather than spinal nerve involvement.[5,18]

Spinal Cord

Cord neuropathy raises the two issues of direct injury and incoming peripheral nociceptive input that may cause or maintain altered spinal cord processing of impulses. In some pain states, both events may occur. Although it is well recognized that the cervical cord is the region of the cord most commonly injured or involved in myelopathies, the thoracic cord has features that also make it vulnerable. While the cervical and lumbar spinal canals are spacious, the thoracic spinal canal is much narrower, especially between the T4 and T9 vertebral levels. In addition, the thoracic cord and meninges have a poorer vascularization than the cervical and lumbar cord and meninges, making the mid-thoracic area a "critical vascular zone."[19] Events within the spinal canal, such as arise from thoracic disc herniation, surgery, and postural alterations including scoliosis, may put the cord at risk. Thoracic discs herniations are common, but the great majority are small, and most occur at lower thoracic levels. The rare thoracic myelopathy from disc trauma has been summarized by Skubic and Kostuik.[5]

The thoracic cord and meninges do not have to adapt to the same degree of movement as do the cervical and lumbar neural tissues. During thoracic flexion and extension the length of the thoracic section of the spinal canal changes minimally,[6,7,20] and indeed, the neural tissues contained in it will be more affected by cervical flexion and extension. However, thoracic lateral flexion, and particularly rotation, will impose forces on the cord that are sufficient to alter its diameter.[6]

As a result of physical injury, or even in its absence, persistent barrages of ectopic impulses along nonmyelinated primary afferent neurons may lead to the sensitization of and later to morphologic changes in dorsal horn cells.[21,22] Afferents from the viscera as well as thoracic peripheral nerves may contribute to altered impulse processing within the dorsal horn in some pain states. Ultimately, normally innocuous stimuli such as touch or colonic distension may register as painful sensations. These events may particularly occur in patients in whom descending pain-control mechanisms from the midbrain and brain stem are compromised by injury, or are altered, such as could occur in a state of chronic depression. These central sources of variation in pain have been extensively reviewed by Fields[10] and by Wall and Melzack.[12]

Meninges

The thoracic dura mater is innervated by branches of the sinuvertebral nerves[23] and is therefore a potential source of symptoms. The thoracic meninges are not as richly innervated as the cervical and lumbar meninges, nor are they subjected to the same degree of movement as the meninges in other regions of the spine.[7]

However, the lack of epidural space in this area may potentiate irritative or compressive symptoms. The lumbar and cervical meninges have been identified as sources of pain,[24–26] and although the thoracic meninges have at this stage escaped attention, it is logical that mechanical or chemical changes in these tissues are likely to evoke pain.

Of the meninges, the dura mater in particular takes most of the brunt of mechanical stress. This tissue is well designed to handle mechanical forces, with strong, layered collagen fibers and connections to the spinal canal by dural ligaments and septa. The dural ligaments run from the anterior dura to the posterior longitudinal ligaments and discs. These dural ligaments are innervated in the lumbar spine[27] and therefore probably in the thoracic spine. The thoracic dura mater and ligaments may be injured by overstretch or from accidental or intentional durotomy. Exudate from disc trauma, epidural hematoma, and loss of the normal movement space from spinal stenosis may also injure the dura.

Much weaker than the dura mater are the arachnoid mater and the pia mater. Cerebrospinal fluid (CSF) flows in the subarachnoid space between these two meninges, both of which are innervated.[28] Pial tissue around the anterior spinal artery possesses nerve endings functioning as stretch receptors.[29] While the meninges may sustain mechanically induced injury, changes in the CSF content (blood or inflammatory mediators) can also result in meningeal irritation and the production of pain.

PERIPHERAL NERVE AND THORACIC NERVE ROOTS

In the thoracic spine, the peripheral nerves that warrant attention are the truncal nerves (intercostal nerves and dorsal rami of the spinal nerves) and a number of cervicogenic nerves that innervate tissues of the thoracic spine, especially the long thoracic, dorsal scapular, subscapular, and suprascapular nerves.

Truncal Nerves

Intercostal nerves supply the joints of the vertebral bodies, the ribs, the parietal pleura, and the abdominal and intercostal musculature. These nerves may be injured by blunt trauma that lacerates or overstretches them, particularly in young individuals with springy ribs.[30] Such direct trauma is rare, and the intercostal nerves are more likely to be sensitized and/or damaged by adjacent callus formation,[31] paraspinal or mediastinal tumors, and thoracic surgery, particularly thoracotomy.[32] Abnormally mobile ribs, especially the tenth rib,[33] may move and put tension on the associated intercostal nerve. A thoracic scoliosis would put tension on neural tissue, including intercostal nerves on the convex side, and would compress neural tissue on the concave side.[6]

Mechanically induced neuropathies of the dorsal rami of the spinal nerves are probably more common than reported. The dorsal rami innervate the erector spinae muscles and then penetrate any overlying muscles and fascia. Posturally related muscle tension and spasm are probably the greatest causes of these neuropathies.[33] Clinically, the lateral cutaneous branch of a dorsal ramus, rather than the medial cutaneous branch, seems more vulnerable to mechanical stress owing to the sudden change in direction required by the former at the fascial opening.

The Cervicogenic Nerves

Any of the cervicogenic nerves listed previously may be injured and cause symptoms and disordered function of the target muscles. Despite their being primarily motor nerves, pain may arise from these nerves connective-tissue sheaths, or may be modulated by chemicals liberated at the terminals of the neurons. The long thoracic nerve has reportedly been injured by compression bandages, backpacks, activities such as strenuous axework or carrying heavy objects on the shoulders, and axillary lymph node surgery.[33–35] The suprascapular nerve appears vulnerable at the scapular notch, where it turns medially at an angle of approximately 90° to innervate the infraspinatous muscle. Activities involving cross-body shoulder adduction and shoulder girdle depression will stress the nerve.[33,35,36] Reports of injury to the dorsal scapular, thoracodorsal, and subscapular nerves are rare, possibly because minor injury to these nerves can be easily masked by local soft-tissue signs such as muscle tightness or trigger points. These nerves and their roots have a greater potential for injury at the cervical spine, particularly in the intervertebral foramina and in their passage through the scalene muscles.

Thoracic Nerve Roots

Grieve[37] noted the rarity of reports of thoracic nerve root compression and suggested that the reason for it might be the difficulty of demonstrating a deficit in the region supplied by a single root. Nevertheless, given that degenerative changes in thoracic joints are common, thoracic root injury surely exists. Nerve root compression may be clinically detectable when associated vertebral segments are palpated or positioned, or when the mechanics of the nervous system are tested, as in the slump test which will be described. Because the spinal cord is shorter than the spinal canal, nerve roots, and particularly those that are located more caudally, descend in the canal before ascending to emerge through their respective foramina. Any further angulation may predispose the roots to injury.[38]

Injury to intercostal nerves and roots may mimic a variety of syndromes, such as angina pectoris in the case of T5 or T6 nerves,[39] and intra-abdominal syndromes, as in the case of injury to lower thoracic nerves.[40,41] Strategies that involve scanning of other systems (e.g., digestive, cardiovascular), and physical examination including structural differentiation (see below), should assist in the differential diagnosis of such injury.

SYMPATHETIC NERVOUS SYSTEM

Many clinicians are aware that impaired intervertebral thoracic joint mechanics appear to be linked with pain and sympathetic epiphenomena. Restoration of movement of the hypomobile segment is often associated with the amelioration of symptoms.[42-44] Maitland[42] has referred to this symptom complex as the "T4 syndrome." Less frequently considered is the possibility that in addition to loss of normal mechanics of the neighboring thoracic joints, abnormal sympathetic neurodynamics may be present from compromise to the sympathetic trunk, particularly in the area of the costovertebral joints[16] and vertebral body.[45] This may well explain some of the more bizarre patient presentations in which apparently viscerogenic symptoms resolve in response to thoracic treatments. Clearly there are somatovisceral and viscerosomatic reflexes that can influence certain pain states, and these may well be activated by techniques of manual therapy.

The STs are continuous structures that consist predominantly of preganglionic neurons that have emerged from the lateral gray matter of the spinal cord and joined the trunk via the white rami communicantes. Preganglionic sympathetic neurons destined for the head arise from spinal segments T1 to T5, those for the upper limb from T1 to T9, and those for the lower limb from T9 to L3.[46] In the thorax, the sympathetic trunks lie on or just lateral to the costovertebral joints. Considering the neuroanatomy of the STs and hypothesizing about their neurodynamics, in conjunction with clinical observations in symptomatic individuals, the sympathetic chains appear to undergo mechanical deformation during trunk and body movement.

This concept gains support when the position of the ST is superimposed on the bones of the thorax (Figs. 15-3 and 15-4). In Figure 15-3 it is clear that the effect of lateral flexion of the thoracic spine will be a tightening of the contralateral sympathetic trunk. An analysis of Figure 15-4, shows that cervical extension will put tension on the cervical part of the ST and that thoracic flexion

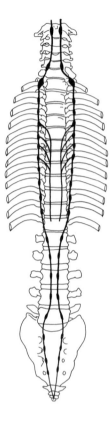

Fig. 15-3. The sympathetic trunk; anterior view with ribs resected. (From Butler,[58] with permission.)

will put tension on the thoracic part of the chain. High-velocity injuries such as motor vehicle accidents will have mechanical implications for the ST. Macnab,[47] in whiplash experiments involving monkeys, showed that the extension phase of the incident would tear the cervical sympathetic trunk with a probable focus of trauma at the low cervical and cervicothoracic junction, where the ST takes a dramatic change in direction from anterior in the cervical spine to lateral and posterior in the thoracic spine. The cervicothoracic junction is also the area in which the stellate ganglia lie. Most of the sympathetic supply to the head, neck, and arms has to pass through these ganglia. Those individuals who sit with a forward head posture and in thoracic kyphosis may be putting insidious stresses on their sympathetic trunks.

A subtle and for physical therapists a more common minor neuropathy of the ST appears to exist in patients in whom the sole symptom is pain that is slow to resolve or is out of proportion to the initial pain-producing stimulus, or in patients in whom the injured target tissues take longer to heal than expected for the nature of the presumed pathology. Careful strategies of enquiry and a physical examination (described below) that includes seeking subtle clues of sympathetic symptoms is often fruitful. Some of the chronic injuries from occupational and sporting overuse may fall into this category. Some of these

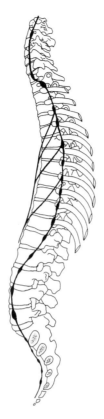

Fig. 15-4. The sympathetic trunk; lateral view. (Adapted from Butler,[58] with permission.)

hypotheses are currently being tested in research at the University of South Australia and the University of Queensland.

PHYSICAL THERAPY EXAMINATION

The aim of the physical therapy examination is to determine whether any mechanical compromise exists, and to identify any associated abnormal sensitivity of thoracic neural structures and any relevant changes in target tissues. Subjective and physical examination and analysis will be necessary to help identify any abnormality in neural tissues. The nervous system is examined for signs and symptoms indicating that its mechanics (i.e., its ability to move in relation to surrounding structures and to handle loading without abnormal responses) are normal. This should be routine during the physical examination, and if the examination gives rise to hypotheses that suggest neuropathy, then a more refined and detailed examination of the nervous system will be required. Such an examination will be part of the general procedure for thoracic examination as outlined by Magarey (see Ch. 7) and others,[37,42,48,49] or can be integrated into the examination protocols of most approaches to manual therapy.

It is important to emphasize here that, as with other hypothesis categories in clinical reasoning (Ch. 6), the mechanisms of symptoms are constantly reviewed and updated as the examination proceeds, to reflect the contribution to the symptoms of each of the mechanisms of pain. For example, a patient who presents with local rib-area pain of recent onset following a rib fracture 6 weeks earlier, may have an irritated intercostal nerve. This could be an example of acute, predominantly peripherally evoked nociception and neurogenic pain. There is minimal contribution from central mechanisms, no overt signs of an abnormal sympathetic response, and perhaps a minor affective contribution. However, if the same patient were to again present after 6 months, with continuing pain, and an abnormal sensitivity to light touch over the ribs, but a good thoracic range of movement, the suggestion would be of a dominance of central mechanisms. In this presentation there may also be a strengthening affective component as the patient becomes more anxious about the pain.

Physical therapists may determine the presence of neuropathies in various ways. These include:

History taking. Symptom patterns will emerge to strengthen or weaken hypotheses about sources and mechanisms involved in a neuropathy (see chs. 6 and 11).

Examination of the status of the target tissues in the innervation fields. This will involve sensory and motor tests of nerve conduction.

An examination of thoracic neurodynamics. This entails testing the mechanical abilities of the various neural components to ascertain whether the tissues can stretch and glide in relation to interfacing structures without producing symptoms. Some of these assessment techniques will also serve to restore normal thoracic neurodynamics.

EXAMINATION OF CONDUCTION

Meninges and Cord

According to the observations of Cyriax,[50] the thoracic dura mater can refer pain to the head and neck. There is no evidence for this, although referral of meningeal pain will be extrasegmental owing to the multilevel, somatic, and sympathetic innervation provided by the sinuvertebral nerves. Perhaps the symptoms experienced need not be pain. The sensation of stiffness has been attributed to the dura mater.[25]

Lesions of the thoracic cord may mimic root pain and paresthesias. Rarely, paraplegia, disturbances of the bladder, bowel, and sexual function, and gait ataxia may occur, as well as sensory loss below the lesion site.[5,51] Spinal cord pain, either from direct injury or indirectly mediated and occurring without neurologic signs, will be non-dermatomal, poorly localized anywhere in the trunk and legs, and spontaneous, and not necessarily influenced by mechanical events. This pattern of pain is discussed in greater detail in Chapter 11 and elsewhere.[10-12] Cord signs such as hyperreflexia are not a necessary accompaniment of spinal cord pain. The physical tests for thoracic cord myelopathy are the Babinski test and tests for hypertonus (reflexes, clonus) and lower limb coordination. These are described in many texts.[42,52]

Peripheral Nerve/Nerve Root

Since there are no plexus formations in the thoracic spine, the dermatome for an intercostal nerve is the same as for a nerve root. Sensory loss due from a lesion to an intercostal nerve is more likely to be in the distal innervation field, whereas nerve root compromise is more likely to involve the proximal field. Lesions involving the first thoracic root may cause sensory disturbances to the medial arm. In addition, sympathetic outflow to the cervical sympathetic chain may be interrupted, causing disturbances in visual accommodation, facial flushing, and alterations in sweating, or a complete Horner's syndrome.

Intercostal muscle weakness will be hard to exhibit, and is probably best examined by palpating the muscle in the intercostal space and asking the patient to cough. Minimal weakness of the abdominal musculature will be difficult to demonstrate unless there is paralysis of a number of nerves or the patient is very slim. The thoracic primary rami may be affected by alterations of interfacing fascial tunnels or effects on the rami as they pass through muscles such as the multifidus, erector spinae, latissimus dorsi, and lower trapezius. Altered function of the erector spinae due to neuropathy of the thoracic primary rami will be difficult to demonstrate. The more likely incriminating evidence will be a hyper- or hyposensitive cutaneous innervation field. This condition has been referred to as nostalgia paresthetica.[53]

The cervicogenic nerves innervating muscles in the thoracic region are primarily motor nerves. Minor weakness will be hard to detect, and the only manifestation of neuropathy may be pain along the course of the nerve or dull, ill-defined pain in surrounding muscles, owing to compromised function. Isolated mononeuropathies are rare. Among these cervicogenic nerves, the long thoracic nerve has had the most attention. It descends along the lateral thoracic wall, supplying the serratus anterior muscle. Injury to the nerve may lead to a winging scapula. Weakness of the latissimus dorsi (thoracodorsal nerve) can be masked by compensation on the part of the pectoralis major and teres major. Atrophy in the supraspinatus and infraspinatus muscles, supplied by the suprascapular nerve, can be observed because of occasional weakness in the early stages of shoulder abduction and in external rotation of the shoulder, respectively.

Sympathetic Nervous System

The physical therapist needs to be aware that features such as pain and altered sweating or swelling in any part of the body may be thoracogenic because the entire sympathetic outflow derives from this area. Segmental deficits in sweating occur with lesions of the sympathetic chain or white rami communicantes. These may be detectable on the chest wall. The deficits will be more global with cord injury.[54] Features that strengthen a hypothesized sympathetic mechanism for symptoms include hyper- or hypohidrosis, changes in skin color and temperature, trophic changes (e.g., dry skin, brittle nails), easily provoked skin redness on palpation, sensations of swelling, and visceral sensations such as bloating. It should be emphasized that these symptoms and signs are not necessary accompaniments of a sympathetic stress syndrome. Pain or stiffness may be the only symptoms.

EXAMINATION OF THORACIC NEURODYNAMICS

The thoracic components of the nervous system are examined for signs and symptoms indicating that its mechanics (i.e., its ability to move in relation to surrounding structures and to handle loading without abnormal responses) are normal. Inevitably, the continuum of the nervous system dictates that examination of one part, such as a peripheral nerve, will involve loading other components, such as a nerve root or meninges. Tension testing will therefore be performed while keeping hypotheses related to sources and mechanisms of symptoms firmly in mind and subject to continual revision by the clinician.

Passive Neck Flexion

Passive neck flexion (PNF) stresses neural and non-neural tissue in the neck, and moves and tensions neural tissues in the thorax and lumbar spine.[55,56] The test therefore loads thoracic neuromeningeal structures and moves them in relation to the surrounding spinal canal. Passive neck flexion is often positive in evoking lumbar symptoms,[57] and it will be noted that it often reproduces thoracic symptoms.

Upper Limb Tension Tests

The upper limb tension tests (ULTTs) described in Chapter 11 and elsewhere[58–60] can also be done for cases of thoracic neuropathy, and this is particularly true for symptoms originating in the upper thoracic spine. Restrictions in the ranges of movement or abnormal symptom reproduction during testing may well indicate a high thoracic neuropathy perhaps involving the sympathetic nervous system. A ULTT with a bias to the ulnar nerve[54] (see Ch. 11) is more likely to evoke upper thoracic symptoms than tests with a bias to the radial and median nerves. Many clinicians have noted that thoracic mobilization yields improved ranges of movement and of symptom responses to the ULTTs. These responses may well be related to mechanical and physiologic changes in thoracic neural tissues, including the sympathetic system, and in the mechanics of non-neural tissues.

Straight Leg Raise

Although an integral part of the lumbar spine examination, the straight leg raise test (SLR) should also be considered a routine neurodynamic test for the thoracic spine. The SLR can be performed in combination with PNF and also with a ULTT to prestress the nervous system. If a neurogenic component of thoracic symptoms is suspected, the thoracic spine may be positioned in a symptom-provoking position such as lateral flexion, after which the SLR can be added. Alterations in thoracic pain as a result of these structurally differentiating maneuvers strengthens the hypothesis of a neurogenic component to the symptoms. This will be considered further in the section below on tension test analysis. In some cases in which the nervous system is extremely mechanosensitive (perhaps after whiplash trauma), the prone knee bend test will provoke thoracic pain.

The Slump Test

The slump test, originally described by Maitland,[42] is particularly useful as an examination and treatment tool for the thoracic spine. It is likely to be more sensitive (although not exclusively) than the SLR and PNF because more tension can be placed on the nervous system, and the test may be performed with the thoracic spine in a variety of positions. However, the slump test is an inappropriate examination for acutely injured and irritated spines. The test is usually performed with the patient in the sitting position; however, the most commonly useful variation of the test for the cervical and thoracic spine involves performing it in a long-sitting position (slump LS). The suggested base sequence for examination of a non-irritable condition is: Long-sitting with the knees extended, plus lumbar and thoracic flexion, plus cervical flexion (Fig. 15–5 A to C). This may be considered a test for all thoracic neural structures contained in and around the spinal canal. There are two useful variations to this suggested sequence. First, movements such as thoracic lateral flexion/rotation and cervical flexion/lateral flexion or rotation can be added to this base test (Fig. 15-5D). Second, the neurodynamic sequencing can be altered. For example, cervical flexion may be added first, followed by trunk flexion. Clinically and experimentally,[61] it appears that the neural tissue in the component that is added first (e.g., neck flexion) will be most challenged by the test.

It has been postulated that the slump test can be refined so as to put more tension onto the sympathetic trunk,[15,58] with this variation referred to as the "sympathetic slump" (Fig. 15-6). This is effected by lengthening the trunk in relation to its interfacing bony structures. Thoracic lateral flexion can increase the load on the contralateral ST, as can thoracic rotation. Further tension can

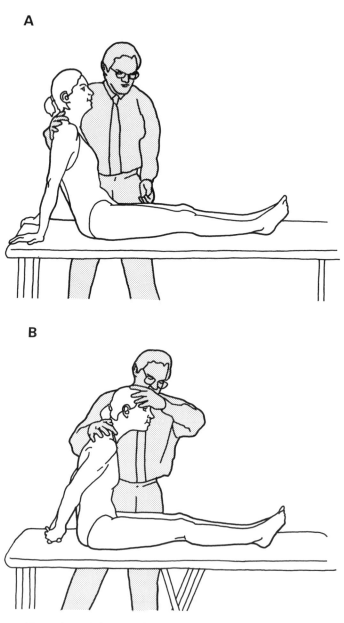

Fig. 15-5.   (**A**) Slump longsitting starting position; (**B**) addition of thoracic and lumbar flexion.

C

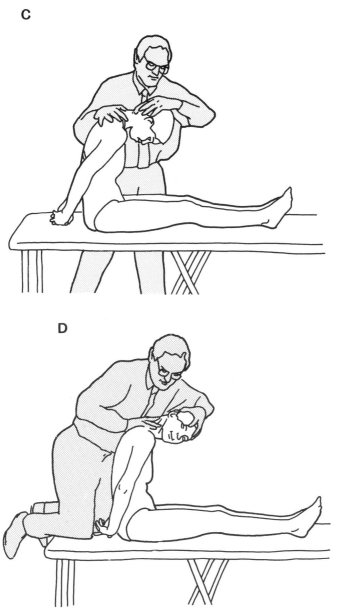

D

Fig. 15-5. (C) addition of neck flexion; (D) vary neck position. (From Butler,[58] with permission.)

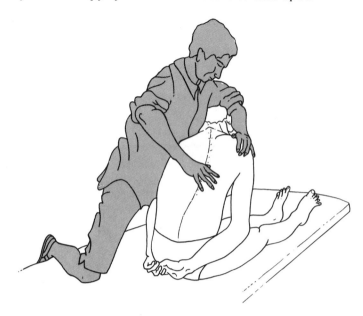

Fig. 15-6. The "sympathetic slump."

be applied by contralateral lateral flexion of the cervical spine. Tension that is more localized to the cervical sympathetic trunk can be effected by extending the neck with the thorax kept in flexion and lateral flexion. The ST can also be moved and tensioned by loading neural tissue to which it is attached. An example of this is the addition of a SLR[6] (Fig. 15-7). In patients with acutely injured and irritated neural and non-neural tissues, these tests should be performed with the greatest care, and may often be inappropriate. Gentle SLR or PNF may be more relevant and safer, but these too should be performed with great care.

Individual Nerve Tests

By reviewing the peripheral neuroanatomy and analyzing positions that provoke and ease pain, it is possible to mechanically load most peripheral nerves. The slump LS test combined with left thoracic lateral flexion and a deep breath from the patient has been shown clinically to be an adequate test for stressing the right intercostal nerves. The neurodynamics of the long thoracic nerve are tested by combining thoracic lateral flexion with cervical flexion and lateral flexion away from the test side, combined with a deep inspiration. The dorsal scapular nerve will be tested by employing the same standard test undertaken to establish the length of the levator scapulae. Horizontal flexion of the shoulder with lateral flexion of the neck away from the test side and shoulder girdle depression puts tension on the suprascapular nerve.[36]

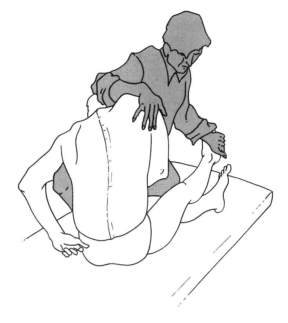

Fig. 15-7. Addition of a straight leg raise to a "sympathetic slump" position.

ANALYSIS OF THORACIC TENSION TESTS

Some of the essential considerations in an analysis of thoracic tension tests are covered in the following sections. More detailed information is available.[58,62]

Multistructural Considerations

It will be unlikely, and perhaps impossible, to have a patient present to a physical therapist with neural tissue as the only tissue exhibiting pathologic changes. Changes in joint, muscle, and fascia will need assessment and perhaps treatment. For example, pathologic changes involving an intercostal muscle may be responsible for an intercostal neuropathy, or an arthritic costovertebral joint may have deleterious effects on the adjacent sympathetic trunk.

Structural Differentiation

If a patient can be put in a pain-provoking position such as thoracic flexion, and this position can be held and knee extension that is found to decrease or increase the pain can be added, it may be inferred that an abnormality of neurodynamics exists. However, this is only one piece of data contributing to the substantiation of a hypothesis about the nature of tissues involved in a disorder. Other data, including the area of symptoms, history, and pattern of symptom fluctuation will be required. Another example of structural differentiation involves a PNF test that results in a tugging sensation in the left mid-thorax. This is an asymmetric and abnormal response to PNF, and so heightens the suspicion of altered neurodynamics. Closer analysis, to determine the site(s) of neuropathy in the thorax, will require interpretation of the area of symptoms, history of the injury, nature of the tissues surrounding the nervous system and, if appropriate, any available objective tests, such as imaging techniques.

Clarification of Responses

During physical examination, the precise reproduction of symptoms may not be possible. Physical therapists are urged to include a categorization of test responses (i.e., physiologic, clinical physiologic, and neurogenic responses) as discussed in more detail in Chapter 11. When a patient's symptoms are severe, it may sometimes be undesirable to reproduce them. Limiting movements to produce a clinical physiologic response may be sufficient.

A physiologic response (usually pain or discomfort) is the response that occurs at the physiologic limit of any movement. In the case of a SLR, physiologic sources of pain could be neural or musculoskeletal. Structural differentiation can be used to infer the presence or absence of a neuropathy and to categorize the response as neurogenic.

The clinical physiologic response to a test is an important one. Consider, for example, a patient who presents with left-sided intermittent anterior chest pain and is referred to a physical therapist by a medical specialist to determine whether there is a neuro-orthopedic contribution to the symptoms. Physical testing reveals no movement abnormalities. However, when the slump LS position is applied with right thoracic lateral flexion, the patient complains of a pulling in the left mid-posterior thorax. No symptoms are reproduced with the slump LS position and flexion to the left. Although the anterior chest pain has not been reproduced, the test has evoked a symptom that may be relevant, and which is not normally expected and is evoked only when testing one side. This can be considered a clinical physiologic response. By treating and altering this response and ascertaining if the pattern of anterior chest pain changes, a hypothesis may be supported or challenged.

PHYSICAL THERAPY MANAGEMENT

Treatment guidelines specific to the ULTTs are outlined in Chapter 11, and additional management details are available elsewhere.[58,63] Some management guidelines in relation to selected disorders are given below.

Clinical reasoning strategies must be utilized in interpreting symptoms, selecting treatment, and assessing the effect of treatment. This is particularly so with the thoracic spine because assumptions have to be made about pathologic changes, and also and more generally because of the enormous variation in the presentation of pain. The management strategy can only be an intelligent hypothesis, and its effectiveness or failure can only be clinically demonstrated by reassessment.

The neural tissues can be mobilized. This is an inevitable consequence of any manual treatment, but the techniques for accomplishing it can be refined to direct treatment more specifically at neural tissues. Simply put, the aim is to restore the normal elasticity and range of movement of the nervous system wherever possible. The intimate link between neural and non-neural tissues means that a powerful way of mobilizing the nervous system and improving ranges and responses to tension tests is to mobilize any extraneural sources of compromise. Most commonly, a multitissue (neural and musculoskeletal) and multilevel (peripheral and vertebral) approach to mobilization will be required.

SELECTED DISORDERS—TREATMENT POINTS

Thoracic Nerve Root/Intercostal Nerve Entrapment

In addition to examination of the neural structures, changes in the movement and sensitivity of the surrounding ribs, costovertebral joints, costotransverse joints, and intervertebral joints need assessment and perhaps treatment by mobilization and manipulation. Some suitable techniques for this have been described.[48] These may be sufficient to free constrained neural tissue. However, there are also techniques specifically designed to mobilize the neural tissue in more chronic symptom states and states in which abnormal neural mechanics are clearly the major component in the pain pattern. The slump LS position is useful here. Perhaps even more effective is mobilization of the ribs with the thorax in a tension position (Fig. 15-8). Forced inspiration can be used as an adjunct to treatment. The patient could even perform this technique at home, accomplishing mobilization by using deep breathing in a tension position.

Sympathetic Nervous System Contribution to a Headache

With all head and neck pain, the sympathetic nervous system and its bony environs, particularly in the upper thoracic spine, should be assessed and treated if necessary. If a potential source of sympathetic maintenance of headache lies in the trunk, rami, and ganglia, some of the examination techniques described previously will be useful. Intervertebral joint mobilization can be performed using a wedge. In the thoracic spine, the wedge can be placed under a level requiring mobilization, after which an anteroposterior pressure is applied through the ribs via the sternum. For higher thoracic levels up to the cervicothoracic junction, wedge mobilization can be done carefully by retracting the head with careful guidance through the jaw. Wedge techniques often expose the large range of available intervertebral movement, and are useful mobilizing

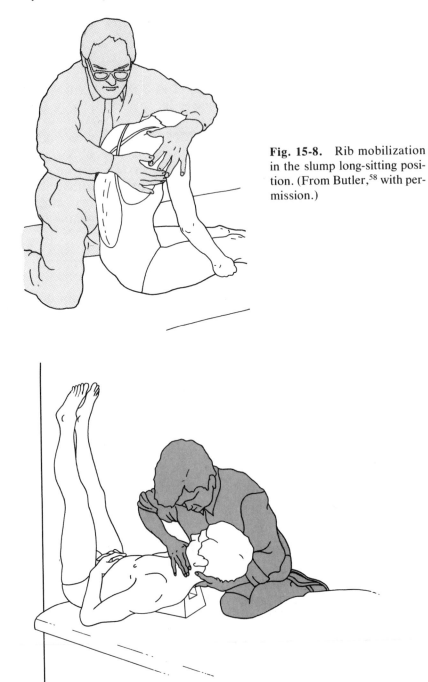

Fig. 15-8. Rib mobilization in the slump long-sitting position. (From Butler,[58] with permission.)

Fig. 15-9. Antero-posterior pressures on the upper thoracic spine, in the bilateral straight leg raise with guidance through the jaw.

techniques in themselves. Tension can be incorporated into the treatment by adding bilateral SLR (Fig. 15-9) or by altering the patient's neck position.

Meningeal Tethering Following Thoracic Fracture

The thoracic spinal canal is much smaller than the cervical and lumbar canals, and any compromise of the thoracic canal space may lead to altered neurodynamics. In the absence of frank cord signs and in the presence of reasonable fracture stability, there should be no obstacle to keeping the meninges, cord, and nerve roots mobile. The advantage of this treatment approach is that the thoracic spine will not initially be moved because the treatment will employ variations of the SLR and PNF. Symptom provocation is not necessary. Techniques suggested for this example include treating "from above" the area of neural compromise, using PNF or passive cervical lateral flexion. Treatment "from below" the area of neural compromise can be performed via knee extension techniques while the hip is held in flexion. Logically, early movement should minimize the occurrence of meningeal and root scarring. In later stages (perhaps some months after initial treatment), the slump LS-based techniques described above can be utilized.

SUMMARY

Neural injuries in the thoracic spine are probably underestimated, often being masked by concurrent injury to non-neural tissues. This may have consequences for management. The lack of research on the neuroanatomy of the thoracic spine and its role in pain states requires that physical therapists take an approach of a clinical reasoning to patient presentations. By using this approach and including the growing knowledge of pain mechanisms, physical therapists are challenged to continue to explore new perspectives in the management of thoracic pain. However, there can be no substitute for clinical research linked with neuroscience research to establish a basis for the concepts on which this chapter is built.

REFERENCES

1. Ashby EC: Abdominal pain of spinal origin. Value of intercostal block. Ann R Coll Surg 59:241, 1979
2. Banyai AL: Anterior chest pain. Chest 70:69, 1976
3. Marinacci AA, Courville CB: Radicular syndromes simulating intraabdominal surgical conditions. Am Surg 28:59, 1962
4. Greive GP: The masqueraders. In Boyling J, Palastanga N (eds): Grieve's Modern Manual Therapy of the Vertebral Column. 2nd Ed. Churchill Livingstone, Edinburgh, (In press)

5. Skubic JW, Kostuik JP: Thoracic pain syndromes and thoracic disc herniation. In Frymoyer JW (ed): The Adult Spine: Principles and Practice. Raven Press, New York, 1991
6. Breig A: Biomechanics of the Central Nervous System. Almqvist and Wiksell, Stockholm, 1960
7. Breig A: Adverse Mechanical Tension in the Central Nervous System. Almqvist and Wiksell, Stockholm, 1978
8. Reid JD: Effects of flexion-extension movements of the head and spine upon the spinal cord and nerve roots. J Neurol Neurosurg Psychiatry 23:214, 1960
9. Campbell JN, Meyer RA, Davis KD, Raja SN: Sympathetically maintained pain: a unifying hypothesis. In Willis WD (ed): Hyperalgesia and Allodynia. Raven Press, New York, 1992
10. Fields H: Pain. McGraw Hill, New York, 1987
11. Wells JCD, Woolf CJ: Pain. Mechanisms and Management. Churchill Livingstone, Edinburgh, 1991
12. Wall PD, Melzack R: The Textbook of Pain. 3rd Ed. Churchill Livingstone, Edinburgh, 1994
13. Woolf CJ: Generation of acute pain: Central mechanisms. Br Med Bull 47:523, 1991
14. Janig W: The sympathetic nervous system in pain: physiology and pathophysiology. In Stanton-Hicks M (ed): Pain and the Sympathetic Nervous System. Kluwers, Boston, 1990
15. Slater H: Adverse neural tension in the sympathetic trunk and sympathetically maintained pain syndromes. Proceedings of the Seventh Biennial Conference of the Manipulative Physiotherapists Association of Australia, Sydney, 1991
16. Nathan H: Osteophytes of the spine compressing the sympathetic trunk and splanchnic nerves in the thorax. Spine 12:527, 1986
17. Appenzeller O: The Autonomic Nervous System. An Introduction to Basic Clinical Concepts. Elsevier, Amsterdam, 1990
18. Stewart JD: Focal Peripheral Neuropathies. Elsevier, New York, 1987
19. Dommisse GF: The blood supply of the spinal cord. A critical vascular zone in spinal surgery. J Bone Joint Surg 56B:225, 1970
20. Lous R: Vertebromedullar and vertebroradicular dynamics. Anat Clin 3:1, 1981
21. Wall PD: Neuropathic pain and injured nerve. Central mechanisms. Br Med Bull 47:631, 1991
22. Susimoto T, Bennet GJ, Kajander KJ: Transynaptic degeneration in the superficial dorsal horn after sciatic nerve injury. Effects of chronic constriction injury, transection and strychnine. Pain 42:205, 1990
23. Groen GJ, Balget B, Drukker J: The innervation of the spinal dura mater: anatomy and clinical considerations. Acta Neurochir 92:39, 1988
24. Smyth MJ, Wright V: Sciatica and the intervertebral disc: an experimental study. J Bone Joint Surg 40A:1401, 1958
25. El Mahdi MA, Latif FYA, Janko M: The spinal nerve root innervation and a new concept of the clinicopathological interrelations in back pain and sciatica. Neurochirurgia 24:137, 1981
26. Kuslich SD, Ulstrom CL, Michael CJ: The tissue origin of low back pain and sciatica: a report of pain response to tissue stimulation during operations on the lumbar spine using local anesthesia. Orthop Clin North Am 22:181, 1991
27. Parke WW, Watanabe R: Adhesions of the ventral dura mater. Spine 15:300, 1990
28. Janig W, Koltzenburg M: Receptive properties of pial afferents. Pain 45:300, 1990
29. Parke WW, Whalen JL: The pial ligaments of the anterior spinal artery and their stretch receptors. Spine 18:1542, 1993

30. Dunkin LJ: Intercostal nerve damage following closed chest injury. Br J Anaesthesiol 42:463, 1970

31. Bathakur AK, Harden A: Entrapment neuropathies of the intercostal nerve. JAMA 53:593, 1961

32. Moore DC: Anatomy of the intercostal nerve: its importance during thoracic surgery. Am J Surg 144:371, 1982

33. Mumenthaler M, Schliack H: Peripheral Nerve Lesions. Thieme, New York, 1990

34. Sunderland S: Nerves and Nerve Injuries, 2nd Ed. Churchill Livingstone, Edinburgh, 1978

35. Narakas A: Compression syndromes about the shoulder, including the brachial plexus. In Szabo RM (ed): Nerve Compression Syndromes. Slack, Thorofare, NJ, 1989

36. Kopell HP, Thompson WAL: Peripheral Entrapment Neuropathies. William and Wilkins, Baltimore, 1964

37. Grieve GP: Common Vertebral Joint Problems. 2nd Ed. Churchill Livingstone, Edinburgh, 1988

38. Nathan H, Feuerstein M: Angulated course of spinal nerve roots. J Neurosurg 32: 349, 1970

39. Hamberg J, Lindahl O: Angina pectoris symptoms caused by thoracic spine disorders: clinical examination and treatment. Acta Med Scand, suppl. 644:84, 1981

40. Krag E: Other causes of dyspepsia—especially abdominal pain of spinal origin. Scand J Gastroenterol, suppl. 79:32, 1982

41. Bechgaard P: Segmental thoracic pain in patients admitted to a medical department and a coronary unit. Acta Med Scand, suppl. 644:87, 1981

42. Maitland GD: Vertebral Manipulation. 5th Ed. Butterworths, London, 1986

43. McGuckin N: The T4 syndrome. In Grieve GP (ed): Modern Manual Therapy of the Vertebral Column. Churchill Livingstone, Edinburgh, 1986

44. Fraser DM: T3 syndrome. In Paterson JK, Burns L (eds): Back Pain. An International Perspective. Kluwer, Dordrecht, 1990

45. Giles LGF: Paraspinal autonomic ganglion distortion due to vertebral body osteophytosis: a cause of vertebrogenic autonomic syndromes. J Manip Physiol Ther 15: 551, 1992

46. Williams PL, Warwick R: Gray's Anatomy. 36th Ed. Churchill Livingstone, Edinburgh, 1980

47. MacNab I: The whiplash syndrome. Orthop Clin North Am 2:389, 1971

48. McNair JKS, Maitland GD: Manipulative therapy techniques in the management of some thoracic syndromes. In Grant R (ed): Physical Therapy of the Cervical and Thoracic Spine. Clinics in Physical Therapy. Churchill Livingstone, New York, 1988

49. Blair JM: Examination of the thoracic spine. In Grieve GP (ed): Modern Manual Therapy of the Vertebral Column. Churchill Livingstone, Edinburgh, 1986

50. Cyriax J: Textbook of Orthopaedic Medicine. 8th Ed. Vol. 1. Ballierre Tindall, London, 1982

51. Brazis PW, Masdeu JC, Biller J: Localization in Clinical Neurology. 2nd Ed. Little Brown and Company, Boston, 1990

52. Dale AJD et al (eds.) Mayo Clinic and Mayo Foundation. Clinical Examinations in Neurology. 6th Ed. Mosby, St Louis, 1991

53. Pleet AB, Massey EW: Notalgia paresthetica. Neurology 28:1310, 1978

54. Fealey RD: The thermoregulatory sweat test. In Low PA (ed): Clinical Autonomic Disorders. Little Brown and Company, Boston, 1993

55. Breig A, Marions O: Biomechanics of the lumbosacral nerve roots. Acta Radiol 4: 602, 1963
56. Tencer AF, Allen BL, Ferguson RL: A biomechanical study of thoracic spine fractures with bone in the canal. Part III. Spine 10:741, 1985
57. Troup JDG: Biomechanics of the lumbar spinal canal. Clinical Biomechanics 1:31, 1986
58. Butler DS: Mobilization of the Nervous System. Churchill Livingstone, Melbourne, 1991
59. Elvey RL: Treatment of arm pain associated with abnormal brachial plexus tension. Aust J Physiother 32:225, 1986
60. Kenneally M, Rubenach H, Elvey R: The Upper Limb Tension Test: The SLR of the arm. In Grant R (ed): Physical Therapy of the Cervical and Thoracic Spine. Churchill Livingstone, New York, 1988
61. Shacklock MO, Butler DS, Slater H: The dynamic central nervous system—structure and clinical neurobiomechanics. In Boyling J, Palastanga N (eds): Grieve's Modern Manual Therapy of the Vertebral Column. 2nd Ed. Churchill Livingstone, Edinburgh, 1994
62. Slater H, Shacklock MO, Butler DS: The dynamic central nervous system—examination and assessment using tension tests. In Boyling J, Palastanga N (eds): Grieve's Modern Manual Therapy of the Vertebral Column. 2nd ed. Churchill Livingstone, Edinburgh, 1994
63. Butler DS, Shacklock MO, Slater H: Treatment of altered nervous system mechanics. In Boyling J, Palastanga N (eds): Grieve's Modern Manual Therapy of the Vertebral Column. 2nd Ed. Churchill Livingstone, Edinburgh, 1994

16 | A Movement System Balance Approach to Management of Musculoskeletal Pain

Steven G. White
Shirley A. Sahrmann

It is not unusual to be able to recognize from a distance someone known to us even without being able to see their facial features. Many individuals have characteristics about their gait, posture, and movement patterns that are peculiar to them. The grace and elegance of the movements made by many an elite dancer or performer may be contrasted with the unrefined motion of those less expert.

A multitude of different patterns of movement are potentially available to us. Questions arise about whether or not one movement pattern is "better" than another, and whether there is a relationship between how we move and how long our movement system (MS) lasts.

In the movement system balance (MSB) theory Sahrmann proposes that there is an ideal mode of movement-system function, and that any deviation from that ideal is less efficient and more stressful to the components of the system.

The consequences of gross forms of overuse of structures (e.g., stress fractures) and faulty biomechanics (e.g., overpronation of the foot leading to knee disorders) are well recognized and have been appropriately managed for some time. The MSB theory suggests that many more of the syndromes that are seen clinically are the result of cumulative microtrauma and are not simply cases of "age related degeneration" or the result of a single, relatively trivial incident, as is so frequently described.

This chapter outlines the principles of the MSB theory described by Sahrmann, and relates these to the management of pain originating from the cervical spine.

THE CONCEPT OF MOVEMENT SYSTEM BALANCE

The underlying premise of the MSB theory is that of mechanical efficiency. The human neuromusculoskeletal system is required to function day in, day out, week after week, month after month, in some individuals for up to 100 years. A machine required to operate for a similar period and subjected to as wide a variety of stresses and strains would have to be both superbly designed and maintained. For a number of reasons, our bodies are often not able to cope with the requirements put on them, and consequently break down.

The MSB theory suggests that if movements were performed precisely and did not become altered, the elements of the human musculoskeletal system would adapt and be able to withstand the rigors of everyday life.

Several factors are necessary to ensure efficient and ideal operation of the movement system. These include

1.   The maintenance of precise movement of rotating parts. This is characterized by movement of the instantaneous axis of rotation (IAR) of a joint along a path that falls within normal bounds for that particular joint.
2.   Correct muscle length
3.   Correct motor control
4.   Correct relative stiffness of both contractile and non-contractile tissue
5.   Correct kinetics

Each of these will be discussed in this chapter.

Cumulative Microtrauma

Noyes[1] put an increasing load on the anterior cruciate ligament of the knee and plotted the force–elongation curve that represented the progressive failure of the ligament. The results demonstrated that microtrauma starts with stresses that are within normal physiologic loads.

In joints that have an altered IAR, these loads are enhanced, and the repetition of movements involving such a joint can accelerate the effects of microtrauma. Depending on the magnitude of the shift in IAR and the load that is being placed on the joint in terms of the frequency and vigor of a movement, either failure or adaptation of the structures under stress will result.

Sahrmann suggests that the majority of musculoskeletal pain syndromes (MPS) seen clinically are the result of an altered IAR and cumulative microtrauma. We recognize the most obvious examples of this in disorders such as stress fractures and tendonitis, but may not be paying sufficient attention to the contribution of these factors to many other clinical problems.

Treatment of the patient's pain usually involves methods designed to reduce inflammation and pain and to stimulate repair. Such treatment will be inadequate if the cause of the pain is not addressed. A recurrence of the disorder causing the pain, the development of some related problem, or the need to curtail aspects of activities of daily living (ADL), work, or recreational activity is very likely if MSB is not achieved.

Instantaneous Axes of Rotation

In a study of patients with neck pain, Amevo, Aprill, and Bogduk[2] showed that 77 percent exhibited abnormal IARs. They commented that muscle spasm has the capacity to decrease range of movement and to alter IARs. Their findings are discussed in greater detail in Chapter 2.

Frankel and associates[3] demonstrated displacement of the IAR in all of 30 knees with internal derangements. They also showed that in knees with abnormal IARs, the tibial and femoral joint surfaces did not glide tangentially during knee flexion and extension (as they do in the normal knee), but were instead either compressed or distracted. Thus, stresses were imposed on articular cartilage and/or soft tissue surrounding the joint. These authors and others have demonstrated significant relationships between displaced IARs and pathologic changes. The MSB theory proposes that any deviation of the IAR from the norm constitutes a state of movement imbalance. In such a situation the joint is not operating as efficiently as it could, and with movement of the joint, inappropriate stress will be placed on some component of the joint or associated tissue.

Factors Determining the Position of the IAR

A number of factors together determine the position of the IAR during the movement of any given joint. These are discussed in the following sections.

Shape of the Joint Surfaces

The shape of the surfaces of a joint is a structural element and a factor that physical therapy does not change. Pathologic processes that lead to changes in the joint surface configuration (e.g., osteophytic lipping) will alter the IAR. Oliver[4] demonstrated alterations in the IAR in the lumbar spine in the presence of osteophyte formation in the zygapophyseal joints.

Interestingly, bony change does occur, especially in immature bone, as a result of loads that are transmitted through that bone. This property is the basis for the conservative treatment of congenital dislocation of the hip, for example, in which sustained mechanical stress is used to keep the head of the femur against the pelvis so as to ensure proper formation of the acetabulum.

Sahrmann suggests that in accord with Wolf's Law, incorrect postural alignment and/or faulty force transmission through the musculoskeletal system leads to maladaptation of components of that system. Correction of kinetics at an early stage would contribute to the normal development of bones and joints.

Length and Mobility of Soft Tissue Crossing the Joint

Injury to a ligament, tendon, or skin may lead to changes in its length or mobility. Adhesions may form that bind the ligament or tendon to surrounding structures. The relative inextensibility of scar tissue restricts the elongation of the skin in particular. These factors may influence movement in an underlying joint in such a way as to cause a deviation from the normal movement pattern for that joint.

The importance of nerve mobility is well recognized. Tests such as the straight leg raise (SLR) test, the slump test,[5] and the upper limb tension test (ULTT) first described by Elvey[6] and considered in detail in Ch. 11) are based on the mobility that is normally present in neural tissue and between nerves and their neighboring tissues. Any restriction of this mobility may limit the normal excursion of underlying joints. In addition, there are likely to be changes in recruitment patterns in muscles that cross the same joints, as part of the mechanism that protects nerves from abnormal stresses. These factors may alter the way in which movement can be performed at the involved joints, and may thus alter the IAR.

Muscle tissue is often the site of adaptation of the body to stress. The ability of muscle to adapt its resting length in particular can have dramatic effects on the movement patterns of the joints affected by muscles. This is discussed below.

Relative Participation of Muscles Around the Joint.

The relative participation of muscles around a joint will be discussed under the heading "Motor Control."

Muscle Length

Identification of shortened muscles has been a part of physical therapy examination for many years. The MSB theory recognizes the importance of the effect of shortened muscles on movement, but puts more emphasis on the identification of lengthened muscles.

Normally, a muscle fiber will generate its maximum tension at its normal resting length (which is between 2.0 and 2.25 μm). If the fiber is held temporarily in a lengthened position, there is less overlap of its actin and myosin filaments, and therefore fewer cross-bridges can form between them. This reduces the tension that can be generated at that length.[7] In a shortened position, the amount of overlap between actin and myosin is so great that it too interferes with cross-bridge formation, once again reducing the amount of tension developed.

Several authors[8–10] have shown that muscles maintained in either a shortened or a lengthened position adapt to that position. A muscle maintained in a lengthened position will show an increase in its number of sarcomeres and a reduction in individual sarcomere length. In this process, the muscle adapts to the lengthened position and becomes able to develop its maximum tension at this "new" length.

Similarly, a muscle held in a shortened position loses sarcomeres and the remaining ones are lengthened. The adapted muscle is now capable of generating maximum tension at this new length.

This relationship has important ramifications for the movement system. Muscles that are lengthened will not be able to generate normal tension if they are put into a shortened position. Thus for example, a poor sitting posture, with abducted (protracted) scapulii, puts the middle and lower parts of the trapezius muscle into a posturally lengthened position. The muscle can adapt by adding sarcomeres, and can thus generate its maximum tension at its new resting length, but with the scapula abducted.

If the scapula is now placed in an adducted position, the trapezius muscle will be shortened and its filaments overlapped, and it will be unable to generate its usual tension. If the arm is now loaded, the scapula will move into abduction until the filaments of the trapezius can generate sufficient tension. This abducted position may well be undesirable for the glenohumeral joint, and could lead to inappropriate stress on structures around this joint.

The MSB theory suggests that there is an ideal resting length for each muscle, and that this (and variances from this ideal), will be reflected by the posture of the joints over which each crosses. For example, clinical testing indicates that swimmers often have weaker, lengthened external rotators of the glenohumeral joint as compared to the internal rotators. The arms are observed to be in an internally rotated position. This position is the result of the opposing amounts of tension that these antagonists can generate at their altered resting lengths.

Motor Control

Efficient, effective movement about a joint requires precise participation by a number of muscles. Some of these control only that joint itself, while others control other joints as well. The timing of the participation of each muscle and the amount of tension it generates are critical in ensuring precise movement.

Celli[11] described three types of muscle groups about the shoulder: "moving" muscles, "stability" muscles, and "non-involved" muscles. The deltoid and upper trapezius, for example, exhibited increasing EMG activity during shoulder abduction, while supraspinatus, infraspinatus, and teres major muscles showed constant EMG activity as they stabilized the head of the humerus in the glenoid cavity. By contrast, the subscapularis, biceps, and pectoralis major were electrically silent.

Without the stabilizing effect of the supraspinatus and infraspinatus muscles, the deltoid, through its line of action, would move the humerus cranially and cause compression of the structures in the subacromial space. Plotting the IAR for this motion would clearly demonstrate a deviation from within "normal" bounds.

Muscles may become dominant or "dominated" for a number of reasons. These include

1. Paralysis
2. Alteration in a muscle's length–tension relationship such that it is unable to develop the required tension in the position maintained by the joint or body posture. This may necessitate the use of a movement synergist to help control the action normally governed primarily by that muscle.
3. Pain that may either inhibit or exaggerate muscle participation (as in muscle spasm)
4. Practiced or repetitive actions in which muscles are continually used in specific patterns. This may lead to a muscle becoming stronger and more easily recruited than its movement synergists.

Richardson[12] theorized that some muscles have a predisposition to becoming dominant because of their biomechanical and physiologic features. She described the neuromuscular plasticity of muscles in terms of the ability of muscle fibers to change their characteristics in response to neural impulses reaching a particular muscle from motor neurons.

Relative Stiffness

The MSB theory suggests that the body takes the line of least resistance during movement. A simple analogy suffices to illustrate this point. Consider a length of wire and a piece of rubber tubing joined together (Fig. 16–1). This simple system may be held at one end and pressure exerted at the other end. The movement that occurs will be in the less stiff of the two components, the rubber tubing. This occurs whichever end is held or compressed, and occurs even though the wire and the rubber are individually both quite flexible.

The clinical application of this analogy may be illustrated by the following example. A patient develops restriction of movement at the atlantoaxial joint. What may be found on examination is the development of increased movement at a lower cervical level, commonly C5–C6, and the development of symptoms arising from this relatively hypermobile segment. Similarly, a patient with a

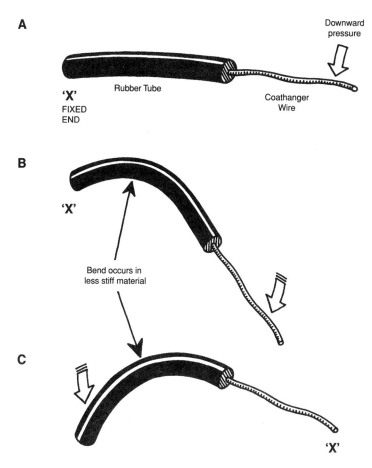

A

Downward
pressure

'X'   Rubber Tube
FIXED
END

Coathanger
Wire

B

'X'

Bend occurs in
less stiff material

C

'X'

Fig. 16-1. Relative flexibility. (**A**) A piece of rubber attached to a length of wire. Both are flexible, but the rubber bends more easily than the wire. (**B**) Fixation (X) at the rubber tubing end. Pressure applied to the wire. (**C**) Fixation at the wire end. Pressure applied to the rubber. Regardless of which end is fixed, the rubber will always bend, since it is less stiff than the wire.

"frozen" shoulder attempting glenohumeral elevation will move predominantly at the scapulothoracic complex. The relative stiffness of the structures involved determines where the movement occurs.

Restricted range of movement is not the only factor determining the movement pattern under conditions of relative stiffness. If the scapulothoracic joint of the patient described above is "looser" or less "stiff" than the glenohumeral joint, then unless the scapula is actively stabilized, movement will occur at the scapulothoracic joint because it moves more easily than the glenohumeral joint.

With repetition of these compensatory movements over time, there will be adaptation of soft tissue around the joint. Further, the new movement pattern becomes "learned." Muscles that normally stabilize the scapula now allow it to move. These muscles may become weakened through disuse, and lengthened as they are stretched to allow the scapulothoracic movement now necessary because of the movement restriction at the glenohumeral joint.

The importance of the principle of relative stiffness is that in addressing faulty movement patterns, attention must be paid to the hypermobile segment of a movement system. How this might be undertaken will be presented in the section on Treatment Principles.

Kinetics

Orthotics have been used for many years to alter foot posture and function in order to relieve symptoms from shin, knee, hip, and back disorders, as well as foot problems. Biomechanically, the foot clearly affects joints further up the kinetic chain. Therefore, correction of foot biomechanics is necessary to reduce the likelihood of recurrence of a problem in the more proximal segments of this movement system.

The MSB theory also stresses the importance of the physical therapist's reversing the direction of observation along the kinetic chain. In addition to calling for consideration of the foot and knee when there is hip pain, for example, the MSB theory stresses the importance of examining joints proximal to the site of the disorder or symptomology to determine the efficiency and correctness of their function. This process may identify faults that are predisposing if not prime factors in the cause of the patient's symptoms.

Using the glenohumeral/scapulothoracic example previously described, the alteration in the biomechanics of the upper quarter brought on by the relative stiffness of the glenohumeral joint may lead to stress being applied to other sites, with pathologic changes developing at those sites.

ASSESSMENT

The first section of this chapter briefly outlined the concepts of the MSB theory. This section describes the examination physical therapists should conduct to determine movement system imbalance.

Posture

The MSB theory proposes that the relative resting length of antagonistic muscles determines the posture of joints. Consequently, it is important to assess postures that are relevant to the patient's problem. For the cervical and thoracic spine this will include examination in the standard and sitting positions and also with the patient in a crawling position on the hands and knees. Standing posture is important because the position of the pelvis and lumbar spine significantly influences that of the cervical and thoracic spine, and vice versa. Sitting posture is especially important when the patient's symptoms are related to the sitting position, as in the case of a typist who has neck pain. The hands-and-knees posture permits assessment of the dominance of the levator scapulae and trapezius muscles over the longus cervicis, as well as providing information about the stability of the scapulothoracic joint.

Once posture has been carefully assessed, some assumptions can be made about the length and length–tension properties of key muscles. Thus, for example, a patient with a forward head posture may well have a lengthened longus cervicis because of the increased cervical lordosis created by this posture. Likewise, there may be shortening of the sternocleidomastoid (SCM), scalene, trapezius, and/or levator scapulae muscles, since these muscles are all in a shortened position when there is an increased lordosis.

If the longus cervicis is lengthened, it will be weak upon testing if the patient is placed supine with the upper cervical spine flexed. The longus cervicus, along with the rectus capitus anterior major (RCAM) muscle, is important in providing stability to the cervical spine.[13] Together the two muscles decrease the lordosis of the cervical spine and provide a stable base for muscles such as the SCM and the supra- and infrahyoid muscles to be able to flex the neck on the thoracic spine. Without this stability, the role of the SCM changes from flexing the neck on the thoracic spine, and flexing the head on the neck, to extending the head on the neck and increasing the cervical lordosis. Because the trapezius and levator scapulae both extend the neck and increase the cervical lordosis, they too need the antagonistic pull of the longus cervicis to counterbalance their action.

At this point, hypotheses are being made about muscle length. Observing posture only in one position, however, can be deceptive. Thus, for example, a patient with an increased cervical lordosis from a forward head posture could be assumed to have shortening of the upper fibers of trapezius muscle. Yet this would be unlikely if the patient's occupation required regular cervical flexion, such as in the case of a jeweller.

Nevertheless, the information gained from an initial observation of posture is still useful since the posture must be altered if it reinforces a significant factor in a patient's movement imbalances.

Flexibility, relative stiffness and movement patterns

Testing of the length of key muscles and other structures crossing joints follows from the postural assessment. Hyperflexibility is as important to identify as hypoflexibility. There is a tendency for postural muscles to become lengthened to an extent that results in their inability to generate sufficient tension when placed in a shortened position.

With regard to hypoflexibility, the emphasis is less on the muscle shortness and more on the way in which a patient compensates for a lack of movement caused by that shortness. Knee extension while sitting may be used by way of example. In this situation a patient with short or "stiff" hamstring muscles may be unable to straighten the knee, or may be able to straighten the knee only by rotating the pelvis posteriorly and thus shifting the origin of the hamstrings caudally.

If the patient has to flex the lumbar spine to achieve knee extension, then the muscles that stabilize the lumbar spine will become stretched, or may even be inhibited, and thus suffer the consequences of disuse if activities such as driving or prolonged sitting in a bed or bath are performed frequently. On examination, the underlying lumbar joints are often found to become hypermobile in flexion (and commonly in rotation in flexion) because they are frequently moved in this way. This sets up a vicious cycle in which the lumbar intervertebral joints become less "stiff" than the hamstrings. Consequently, whenever there is a choice between flexion of the lumbar spine and lengthening of the hamstrings, the movement will occur in the lumbar spine, where there is less "stiffness."

Palpation of the cervical spine during movement of the shoulder can be very revealing. During elevation of the arm through abduction, one might expect the cervical spine to remain stable throughout its length, so as to provide a base from which the upper trapezius and levator scapulae muscles can work. When the upper trapezius contracts to upwardly rotate the scapula, movement may be induced in the upper and mid-cervical spine if there is relatively more flexibility in the spine than in the scapulothoracic complex in elevation and upward rotation.

The levator scapulae muscle must lengthen to allow upward rotation of the scapula. If it is shortened or unable to relax in a manner appropriate to allow eccentric lengthening, then either scapular motion will be noted to halt or movement will be seen to be induced in the cervical spine. The latter fault is particularly likely if the cervical spine is not stabilized appropriately by the longus cervicis. (As described previously, the longus cervicis is the antagonist to the increase in cervical lordosis induced by the levator scapulae).

Identification of this fault may be achieved in the following way. As the patient actively elevates the arm, first through abduction and then through flexion, the cervical spinous processes or zygapophyseal joints should be palpated. This palpation should then be repeated while resistance is applied to the abduction and flexion movements. Applying such resistance aids in revealing more subtle faults. Palpation should be continued as the patient returns the arm to the side, since this allows an analysis of the quality of eccentric muscle control.

The movement of a joint may change significantly if there is reduced neural mobility in a nerve crossing that joint. For example, with glenohumeral abduction/external rotation, the scapula may well have to elevate to reduce tension on components of the brachial plexus.[14] Upper limb tension tests[6,14] will indicate whether there is an adverse neural tension component to the patient's movement pattern. These tests may also reveal the strategies that patients use in trying to avoid stressing painful tissue.

In this situation the continued excessive scapular elevation to relieve adverse neural tension can become an habitual pattern. As a result, a fixed pattern of excessive activity in the scapular elevators occurs whenever glenohumeral abduction/external rotation is attempted. Faulty recruitment patterns can develop not only from attempts to avoid pain, but also because of environmental conditions. For example, an individual working at a high desk will have to maintain the scapulae in an elevated position. As a result, the upper trapezius, rhomboid, and levator scapulae muscles can become recruited in many more activities than is ideal. With time, the structures around the scapulae (including components of the brachial plexus) adapt to this cephalad positioning of the scapulae and become another factor that contributes to the movement pattern.

Patients move in certain ways for a variety of reasons, including:

A shortened tissue that may not allow movement in a particular direction.
A weakened muscle that may provide insufficient power to undertake the movement.
"Take-over" of the movement by a dominant muscle.
Repeated actions at work or in recreational pursuits that may result in the learning of certain movement patterns.
The avoidance of pain.

The relevant reason why a patient moves in a certain way must be correctly identified so that the patient can be taught how to restore normal movement.

Strength

In the MSB approach, the relative strength and endurance of muscles is more important than the overall strength that any muscle or group of muscles can develop. Testing of both antagonists and synergists of specific muscles should be undertaken. In the presence of a comparatively weak muscle, one often notes clinically that a muscle with a similar action (a movement synergist) is used to compensate for the weakness. This is particularly likely to occur if that synergist is relatively strong. The use of this stronger muscle reinforces its dominance and, in accord with the old maxim, allows "the strong to get stronger and the weak to get weaker."

Once a muscle becomes dominant it influences the way in which the joint or joints underlying it will move. This will often be away from the ideal and toward a less efficient and more stressful movement pattern. An assessment of MSB must therefore analyze the relative strength of both stabilizing and movement synergists.

Relative strength can be determined by observing an imbalanced movement. Palpating muscles with the patient maintaining a specific position can give further information. The individual muscle testing positions described by Kendall and McCreary[15] are recommended. These authors also described many of the common strategies for substitution that occur if a muscle is particularly weak or dominant.

In the cervical spine, the strength of the longus cervicis muscle relative to the SCM, the scalenes, the upper trapezius, and the levator scapulae is of great importance. As previously described, these muscles tend to increase the cervical lordosis as compared to the action of the longus cervicis, which is to flatten the lordosis.[12]

The longus cervicis and the RCAM muscles may be tested in their shortened positions with the patient supine and by placing the cervical spine passively into flexion with the chin tucked in. With active maintenance of this position the chin will begin to protrude (i.e., extension of the head on the neck will occur) and/or the cervical lordosis will increase if these muscles are weak or are not being adequately recruited. Normally the patient should be able to maintain the correct position (without chin protrusion or any increase in cervical lordosis) even with the therapist applying moderate resistance to the patient's forehead. During the performance of the test the therapist should palpate the superficial muscles for more information with which to determine those that are predominating.

Strength and endurance should also be assessed in positions of significance to the patient. For example, a swimmer needs appropriate strength of the scapular stabilizers at the moment the hand catches the water and throughout the "pull" phase of a swim stroke. If these muscles were tested in their shortened position only, a stabilization fault elsewhere in the range of movement might not be detected.

When testing the ability of a swimmer to pull the arm through the swimming stroke, it is necessary to concentrate on the swimmer's ability to prevent movement of the scapula regardless of the position in which the therapist places the scapula. For example, the therapist may elevate or depress the scapula and note the ability of the scapular stabilizers to hold that position. This gives a good guide to their relative strength. If the intent is to test for endurance, then it is desirable to test the swimmer immediately after or during a training session rather than repeating the clinical tests to the point of fatigue. Quite apart from the time factor it entails, testing to fatigue in the clinical setting may give an inaccurate picture, since it does not reproduce an actual activity.

The MSB concept emphasizes the desirability of developing movement, especially powerful and rapid movement of the limbs, from a stable base. This base is the scapulothoracic joint, the cervical and thoracic spine in the case of the upper limb. In the case of the lower limb it is the lumbar spine and pelvis.

Isokinetic testing provides a relatively high degree of objectivity in the assessment of strength, endurance, power, and velocity throughout the range of movement (ROM) of a structure.[16] However, this form of testing has the disadvantages of being unable to test individual muscles and of being insufficiently adaptable to simulate functional testing positions (e.g., the closed kinetic chain).[17] Also of concern is the lack of specificity of isokinetic testing. The action of a strong muscle may mask the lack of contribution of a weakened synergistic muscle.

ASSESSMENT PROTOCOL

The following assessment is used to identify movement imbalances and the factors contributing to them.

Patient Standing

1. Posture. Note the position of the scapula on the chest wall (abducted/adducted, elevation/depression, upward/downward rotation, winging/tipping) and the humerus with relation to the scapula. Note also the position of the head on the neck and neck on the thoracic spine, and the contours of the thoracic spine.
2. Movement of the scapula during glenohumeral abduction and flexion. Note the timing of scapulohumeral rhythm, and scapulothoracic motion, and whether there is sufficient scapular upward rotation, abduction, and elevation.

Patient Sitting

1. Posture
2. Physiologic movements of the cervical spine, specifically rotation and flexion. Note the ROM and any deviation from the normal path of movement (rotation off a fixed vertical axis). Observe whether cervical ROM or movement patterns change as the therapist passively elevates, depresses, upwardly rotates, or downwardly rotates the patient's scapula. Note also the weight and/or resistance to correction of scapular position. This assists in determining the length and effect of stretch of the SCM, upper trapezius, and levator scapulae. Similarly, cervical rotation in flexion, extension, and side flexion should be carefully observed.
3. Palpate the spinous processes or zygapophyseal joints from C1 to C7 as the patient elevates the arm through abduction and then returns the arm to the side. Similarly, palpate the spine while the patient elevates the arm through flexion. This should also be done with the patient holding a weight in the hand to increase the load.
4. Assess the strength of serratus anterior, upper trapezius, and levator scapulae muscles.

Patient on Hands and Knees

1. Posture
   (a) Position of the scapula. Winging may suggest weakness or perhaps insufficient activity of the serratus anterior muscle. If there is pronounced winging this suggests that the muscle is lengthened. Elevation of the scapula from the superior border to the acromion may suggest dominance by the upper trapezius. Elevation of the superior border of the scapula with depression of the acromion (downward rotation) suggests shortness of the levator scapulae. This position could indicate shortening of the elevators or lengthening of the depressors.

Upward/downward rotation and the muscle lengths associated with abduction or adduction of the scapula should be deduced in the same way.

(b) Position of the head on the neck and the neck on the thoracic spine. Extension of the head on the neck with an increased cervical lordosis suggests dominance by the upper trapezius and levator scapulae muscles over the longus cervicis and RCAM muscles.

To further test the relative strength of these two muscle groups the patient should be encouraged to adopt and maintain a dorsal glide position of the head on the neck (flatten the cervical curve). Moderate resistance should then be added to the occiput.

Observe and palpate to determine which muscles the patient uses to maintain this position.

Patient Lying Prone

1. Test the ability of the middle and lower trapezius to maintain the scapula in upward rotation and with the medial end of its spine approximately 5 cm from the thoracic spinous processes, while holding the weight of the arm. The glenohumeral joint should be positioned at 90° of abduction and 90° of external rotation, and the elbow should be extended. Look for drift from this starting position in order to determine which muscles are attempting to stabilize the scapula.

2. With the patient's elbow flexed to 90°, observe the patient internally, and then externally rotate the glenohumeral joint in 90° abduction, with the humerus supported along its full length. Note whether the patient prefers to move at the scapulothoracic joint or more correctly at the glenohumeral joint. Note whether the patient moves correctly when instructed to do so. If the patient is unable to do so, assess the factors contributing to the faulty control. Which muscles are dominant and thus causing the faulty movement direction? Correspondingly, identify the muscles whose activity is insufficient to counteract the activity of dominant muscles.

Patient Supine

1. Test the relative strength of the longus cervicis and RCAM versus the SCM and the scalenii muscles.

2. Perform the ULTTs[6,14] if the findings from the history or physical examination suggest that neural tension may be a factor in the patient's movement imbalance.

3. Assess the length of the pectoralis major and minor and latissimus dorsi muscles.[15] Observe carefully for any movement strategies by the patient to substitute other muscles for the muscle being tested.

4. Assess the length and strength of the infraspinatus and teres minor (lateral rotators) and teres major and subscapularis muscles (medial rotators). Testing of passive accessory and passive physiological intervertebral movements of the relevant spinal joints should be included in the examination.

The protocol described above is a starting point for the assessment of imbalances in muscle function and active movement.

TREATMENT PRINCIPLES

Once the assessment has been completed, the factors most relevant to the patient's problem must be identified.

Many of the faults identified in the assessment may not be major contributors to the patient's pain. Because the approach to treatment will be one that requires tissue adaptation (lengthening, strengthening, shortening, and retraining) for any effective change in posture and movement patterns, the factors most crucial for change should be identified. Identifying those faults that are producing pain and that can change most easily is important. Prioritizing in this way avoids what may seem an overwhelming task for both patient and therapist. The explanation to the patient must include

The concepts of balance and cumulative microtrauma
The need to change bad habits
The time required for change
The "new" pains that may be experienced as a consequence of that change
The importance of active participation in the therapeutic program

Priorities

Management from the viewpoint of MSB theory means that some factors must be addressed before others. These priorities, as based on the concepts discussed in this chapter, are listed below.

1. Explain to the patient the posture and movement faults that are perpetuating the condition, including a description of those tissues that have become lengthened from poor posture. If the patient does not correct these faulty habits, progress will be difficult to achieve.

2. The patient must be able to correct the faulty postures and movement patterns. Teaching the patient how to correct poor posture and faulty movement patterns is most important, just as McConnell[18] has promoted in the management of patellofemoral joint pain. The patient should be aware that effecting the necessary changes takes time and effort, as does the learning of any new skill.

3. Teach the patient to shorten lengthened tissue by active contraction with the muscle in a posturally shortened position.[12] Emphasis on good posture and correct movement patterns will go a long way to achieving this goal. Posture

is determined by the resting length of muscles and the tension that these muscles generate automatically at this resting length. Actively contracting a muscle to correct and maintain a desired posture requires the concentration of the patient and with respect to endurance, puts a demand on this muscle that may not yet have been developed. Splinting, taping, and/or orthotics are often necessary to prevent continued lengthening of tissue during the many lapses in active effort by the patient.

4. Strength or flexibility should not be over-emphasized. Patients generally prefer performing an exercise to correcting a posture or movement pattern. Patients often believe that the harder they work at an exercise the better the result. This attitude contributes to greater emphasis on strengthening and less attention to correcting faulty postures and movements.

5. Clearly weakened muscles should be strengthened. The initial emphasis on strengthening should be on those muscles that stabilize relatively hyper-mobile joints. In the early stages of treatment, weakened muscles should not be stressed, and adding resistance may be counterproductive. Resistance above 40 percent of maximum voluntary contraction (MVC) is likely to recruit inappropriate activity from synergistic muscles.[12] Once the patient has mastered precise muscle control, resistance can be added progressively. Functional training is also necessary, through exercises that relate closely to the sport or other activity during which the problem became apparent, or in which the patient participates. Richardson details further progressions that incorporate closed-kinetic-chain exercises and other useful strategies to aid rehabilitation.[12,17]

6. Be precise. With any exercise that entails movement, it is important to maintain the normal axis of rotation and appropriate muscle participation in performing the movement. Biofeedback units, mirrors, and muscle stimulators may be useful in eliciting appropriate muscle activity. The emphasis is on recruiting a specific muscle and not one of its movement synergists.

7. Shortened tissue must also be addressed, but should not be overemphasised. Most often the MSB approach suggests that stretching be done actively, using antagonists of a shortened muscle. Whenever possible, the exercise should promote stability proximally. For example, the scapular elevators may be stretched by flexing the neck both toward the chest and laterally just sufficiently to feel the onset of resistance in the scapular elevators. This should be followed by asking the patient actively to depress and abduct the ipsilateral scapula by using the lower trapezius and serratus anterior muscles to stretch the upper trapezius muscle.

Therapists should use their knowledge of functional anatomy for specificity in prescribing exercise. For example, cervical lateral flexion to the left, plus right rotation and flexion, will stretch the right upper trapezius more than will left lateral flexion combined with left rotation in flexion, which will stretch the right levator scapulae muscle.

There is no need to force a muscle to the end of its range of movement to lengthen it. Indeed, this may be painful and may lead to reflex contraction of the muscle. Working the antagonist may contribute to reflex inhibition of the stretched muscle. End-of-range activity may also lead to movement occurring elsewhere because of increased flexibility and/or poor stabilization of the secondary site.

8. Patients will need to be reviewed so that their exercises are corrected and graduated as necessary. As the patient develops control of new movement or posture, modification of the exercises will be required until these become functional (i.e., performed in a manner as near to everyday situations as possible). This will require varying the speed, position, direction, load, and timing of movements.[12]

9. Reduce pain or swelling that alters a normal movement pattern or significantly limits movement. Pain and swelling may inhibit some muscles and may result in others working constantly to splint the symptomatic area. Correcting movement patterns will prevent further aggravation, which in itself may reduce or eliminate the pain and swelling. This can occur because cumulative microtrauma is often the reason for movement imbalance, stiffness, and other problems in the first place. It may, however, be necessary to also utilize other physiotherapeutic approaches in order to reduce pain and swelling.

Preferably, the patient should be the one to control pain and manage other problems. Successful self management convinces the patient of the value of the movement-correction program and the importance of long-term participation in it.

10. When there are signs of adverse neural tension[14] it is often necessary to address this first. Successful retraining of movement patterns is less likely to occur in the presence of these neural signs.

11. Manual therapy complements the MSB approach to patient management. In particular, the need to mobilize hypomobile joints that are contributing to hypermobility elsewhere, or to a faulty movement pattern. For example, a "frozen shoulder" may perpetuate scapular instability, with the patient moving at the scapulothoracic joint in order to compensate for loss of mobility at the glenohumeral joint. Specific joint mobilization is often necessary in cases of spinal hypo or hypermobility, since patients do not have the ability to actively stabilize one cervical level while moving at another in an attempt to undertake self-mobilization.

SUMMARY

The MSB approach to managing musculoskeletal pain syndromes challenges the physical therapist to reconsider some of the traditional methods of assessment, and to question the interpretation of the findings of such assessment as well as the rationale behind treatment based on those findings.

The concept of an "ideal" mode of operation for the neuromusculoskeletal system is postulated. An IAR falling within the normal centrode of motion for a joint is suggested as a definition of the ideal for that joint. This challenges researchers to define normal centrodes of motion for each joint, and physical therapists to address the factors that push the IAR outside these norms.

Emphasis is put on the management of lengthened skeletal muscle. The MSB approach demands consideration of the effects of the different relative stiffnesses of tissues on the determination of where movement will occur during activity.

The principles of the MSB theory and the rationale behind this theory have been presented. We have also sought within this chapter to provide an outline for integrating these principles with others that are widely used by physical therapists in the management of cervical and thoracic pain syndromes.

REFERENCES

1. Noyes FR: Functional properties of knee ligaments and alterations induced by immobilization. Clin Orthop 123:210, 1977
2. Amevo B, Aprill A, Bogduk N: Abnormal instantaneous axes of rotation in patients with neck pain. Spine 17:748, 1992
3. Frenkel VH, Burstein AH, Brooks DB: Biomechanics of internal derangement of the knee. Pathomechanics as determined by analysis of the instant centres of motion. J Bone Joint Surg 53A:945, 1971
4. Oliver M: Extension and hyperextension of the lumbar spine—an anatomical and biomechanical study. Unpublished M. App. Sc. thesis. Curtin University of Technology, Perth, Australia, 1990
5. Maitland GD: The slump test: examination and treatment. Aust. J Physiother 31: 215, 1985
6. Elvey RL: Treatment of arm pain associated with abnormal brachial plexus tension. Aust J Physiother 32:224, 1986.
7. Gordon AM, Huxley AF, Julian FJ: The variation in isometric tension with sacromere length in vertebrate muscle fibres. J Physiol 184:170, 1966
8. Williams PE, Goldspink G: Changes in sarcomere length and physiological properties in immobilised muscle. J Anat 127:459, 1978
9. Tabary JC, Tabary C, Taradiew C, et al: Physiological and structural changes in the cat soleus muscle due to immobilization at differ lengths by plaster casts. J Physiol 224:231, 1972
10. Tardieu C, Tabary JC, Tardieu G, et al: Adaptation of sarcomere numbers to the length imposed on muscle. p. 99. In Guba F, Marechal G, Takacs O (eds): Mechanism of Muscle Adaptation to Functional Requirements. Pergamon Press, Elmsford, NY, 1981
11. Celli L, Balli A, de Luise G, Rovesta C: Some new aspects of functional anatomy of the shoulder. Ital J Orthop Traumatol 11:83, 1985
12. Richardson C: Muscle imbalance: principles of treatment and assessment. Proceedings of the New Zealand Society of Physiotherapists Challenges Conference, Christchurch, August 1992.
13. Kapandji IA: The Physiology of the Joints. 2nd Ed. Vol. 3. The Trunk and Vertebral Column. Churchill Livingstone, New York, 1974
14. Butler DS: Mobilization of the Nervous System. Churchill Livingstone, Melbourne, 1992.

15. Kendall FP, McCreary E: Muscles testing and Function 3rd Ed. Williams & Wilkins, Baltimore, 1983.
16. Guffey J, Burton B: A critical look at muscle testing. Clin Management 11:15, 1991
17. Palmitier RA, An KN, Scott SG, Chao EYS: Kinetic chain exercise in knee rehabilitation. Sports Med 11:402, 1991
18. McConnell J: The management of chondromalacia patellae. A long term solution. Aust J Physiother 32 1986

17 | Mechanical Diagnosis and Therapy for the Cervical and Thoracic Spine

Rodney N. Grant
Robin A. McKenzie

Neck pain, and pain referred from the neck to the upper back, shoulders and arms, is so widespread throughout both eastern and western societies that it could almost be said to be universal. In addition, mechanical disorders affecting cervical segments may cause pain in the head in the form of occipital, frontal and temporal headaches. Few of us escape such symptoms during our lifetime. Fortunately, rather more frequently and more rapidly than occurs in the lumbar region, most of us recover spontaneously.

However, a sufficient number of people suffering from neck and referred pain are so affected by either the persistence or by the severity of the symptoms, or as in the case in the lumbar spine, by the recurrent nature of the problem, that they seek assistance. Therapists and clinicians worldwide respond to this request for assistance, and in doing so are helping to create patient dependence. The patient rightly or wrongly attributes his recovery to the treatment he is receiving at the time the symptoms resolve, and returns for more of the same at the first sign of recurrence. Such is the nature of our treatments that they are seen by the patient as the source of healing. Perhaps this is what is wrong with our present therapies.[1]

ORIGINAL PRINCIPLES

A chance clinical observation in 1956, when a patient whose back and referred leg pain were dramatically reduced after lying in a certain position, stimulated a study of the symptomatic response to movement and position in patients with disorders of the low back, neck, and thoracic spine.

Following this, predictable patterns of symptomatic response to certain movements and positions became apparent. Subsequent clinical analysis over a period of 30 years enabled Robin McKenzie to identify three mechanical syndromes, describe the centralization phenomenon, expound the philosophy that self-treatment provides a tool for prophylaxis, and develop a rational and progressive system of conservative patient care that quickly identifies those patients who require spinal manipulative therapy.[1,2] These developments have become widely known as the McKenzie system. Recent investigations have provided some support for these new concepts,[3-12] but few clinical trials of them have met stringent scientific requirements.

Of the numerous pathologic conditions of the spine, nonspecific ailments marked by pain in the lumbar, dorsal, and cervical regions, with or without radiation of pain, comprise the vast majority of problems found among workers.[13] It is estimated that over 90 percent of mechanical disorders of the spine fall into this category,[13] and despite modern imaging procedures, their specific diagnosis remains elusive. Mechanical diagnosis enables the categorization of these patients according to clinically identifiable syndromes. Furthermore, identification of these mechanical syndromes does not depend upon naming the structure involved, nor upon a specific diagnosis.

For the clinician involved in the diagnosis and treatment of nonspecific pain, it soon becomes apparent that many patients who experience such pain have similar signs and symptoms. Yet treatment that is effective for one patient may not be effective for another with an apparently identical disorder. Thus, one patient will be helped by cervical flexion mobilization, while another with the same apparent set of symptoms will be worsened.

For those clinicians wishing to improve assessment procedures and methods of treatment, the Quebec Task Force (QTF) on Activity Related Spinal Disorders[13] recommends the adoption of a system of classification of patients by pain patterns. An understanding of the mechanisms of pain production and recognition of patterns of symptomatic response to movement or position enables the clinician to classify patients in the nonspecific spectrum into subgroups based on the mechanics of their condition, and to determine the direction and force of the mechanical therapy required.[1,2,14]

A group of patients exist, usually with chronic disorders, in whom specific mechanical classification is difficult. Delay in providing appropriate treatment may complicate the patient's mechanical disorder and produce confounding psychological distress. It is not appropriate to apply specific mechanical therapy to this group, about whom, provided serious pathology has been eliminated, it may be said have true nonspecific pain. These patients may require general physical reactivation and possibly individual psychological assistance.

However, the static and dynamic mechanical evaluation procedures developed by McKenzie enable classification of the majority of patients, in whom the symptomatic response to mechanical therapy may be predicted and an early prognosis made.[15–17] Recognition of atypical symptomatic responses to movement or position allows the clinician to identify those patients who will fail to respond to mechanical therapy,[1,2] possibly because of mechanically irreversible or more sinister pathology.[18] Further, atypical responses can assist in identifying patients who may require surgical management.[17]

THE MECHANISMS OF PAIN PRODUCTION

Chemical or mechanical stimulation of nociceptive receptors causes pain, signaling the presence of stimuli that are potentially harmful.[19] Chemical stimulation of nociceptive receptors produces pain that is constant and unvarying in location, provided the concentration of irritant chemicals is sufficient for this. Chemical pain occurs in the presence of infective, inflammatory, and other disease processes[18,19] and during the healing phase following trauma.[20] It is not possible to lastingly reduce pain of chemical origin through movement or positioning, and McKenzie has used this principle to identify patients with pathologies unsuited to mechanical therapies.

Mechanical deformation of any innervated tissue that is sufficient to stimulate nociceptive receptors induces pain of mechanical origin. Such mechanical pain will be produced or abolished, increased or decreased, and/or change location in direct relation to the degree of the applied force. Commonly, mechanical pain is intermittent, appearing and disappearing as the patient moves or adopts certain positions. Constant mechanical pain may occur if sufficient mechanical deformation is present within the tissue irrespective of the position the patient adopts. If mechanical deformation increases, decreases, or changes location in response to movement or position, the pain will also increase, decrease, and/ or change location. If mechanical deformation is permanently changed through movement or positioning, the pain will remain increased, decreased, and/or changed in location after the movement has been performed or the position adopted.

Historical and observed symptom behavior in response to movement or position enables the clinician to classify the patient into one of three clearly defined mechanical subgroups.[1,2]

THREE MECHANICAL SUBGROUPS IN THE NONSPECIFIC SPECTRUM

The Postural Syndrome

Few patients have pain of postural origin alone. However, all patients with mechanical neck or back pain will have a postural component to their problem. That component must be eliminated before the underlying mechanical cause can be accurately identified.

Patients with pain of postural origin describe pain felt locally and separately or simultaneously in the cervical, thoracic, or lumbar areas. They are, however, able to move fully and freely in all directions. Pain does not limit their movement. Historically these patients have intermittent pain, felt only when they are stationary and when static loading has been prolonged. These patients will be symptom free when moving. Routine examination of these patients is unrewarding, for they move without discomfort or limitation in any direction and will frequently comment, "I don't seem to have it right now!" Reproduction of their pain is possible only by statically loading the affected area for a period of time in the posture described as being painful. This commonly occurs in the sitting and standing postures, but infrequently in lying. The pain is abolished immediately on change of position or on movement. These patients are usually under 30 years of age, have sedentary occupations, and undertake little or no exercise. Some may be described as being hypermobile.

One must ask: What causes pain to behave in this manner? What pathologic process could cause pain only with prolonged end-range static loading and in the absence of limitation of movement?

The Conceptual Model

In the search for answers to these questions, a conceptual model is presented that provides the basis for the clinical reasoning used in treating nonspecific mechanical disorders of the back and neck. The answers may seem simple in retrospect. Spinal pain arising from the postural syndrome is provoked by mechanical deformation that occurs when normal periarticular soft tissues are subject to prolonged static loading at end range.[21] No pathologic condition need exist. Pain of similar origin can be induced in the index finger by bending it backward excessively or for prolonged periods (Fig. 17-1).

The Dysfunction Syndrome

Patients classified as having the dysfunction syndrome usually describe a history of a traumatic event or a previous episode of acute neck pain. Intermittent pain persists within or adjacent to the spine, with the single exception of

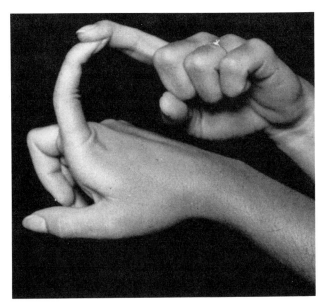

Fig. 17-1. The bent finger syndrome. Pain is produced when normal periarticular soft tissues are subject to prolonged static loading at end range. (From McKenzie,[1] with permission.)

cases in which referred or radiating symptoms are experienced. Pain develops insidiously in the absence of a precipitating incident. In addition to their pain, however, these patients have limitations of movement, unlike those patients with the postural syndrome. Historically, their pain is felt consistently when performing certain movements or adopting certain positions. Thus, movements or positions that are painful to them today were so yesterday and will be so tomorrow. These patients describe pain that is felt immediately when movement reaches the end of their limited range. The pain stops immediately when the end-range position is released. The pain is thus not felt in mid range or during motion. The intensity of the pain of which patients with the dysfunction syndrome complain is the same each day provided their activity levels are consistent. These patients are usually over 30 years of age, except where trauma or derangement can be identified as the original cause of their problem. They commonly exhibit poor posture and frequently undertake little or no exercise.

Examination will always reveal a restriction of motion, and the pain of which the patient complains will be felt only at the end of the available range of movement. Repetition of end-range movement will produce the same pain, which does not either progressively worsen or improve, nor change location, nor will their limited range of movement increase.

What is the cause of this pain? What pathologic processes produce pain only when movement reaches the extreme point in a limited range?

The Conceptual Model

A conceptual model also allows understanding of the dysfunction syndrome. The pain described by patients with the dysfunction syndrome is produced when, upon attempting full movement, they mechanically deform adaptively shortened, scarred, or contracted soft tissues. Such inelastic soft tissue, when adjacent to spinal motion segments, restricts movement.

Adaptively shortened, scarred, or contracted soft tissue may arise from two common causes. First, poor postural habits maintained during the first few decades of life lead to adaptive shortening and a gradual reduction of mobility with aging. This is especially so when the individual rarely moves through a full range of movement. Restriction of movement usually affects those sagittal movements essential for the maintenance of the very erect posture.

Second, contracture of scar tissue develops during the repair following trauma or intervertebral joint derangement. Thus, an inextensible scar can form within or adjacent to otherwise healthy surrounding elastic structures, restricting mobility.

Pain from dysfunction is always felt intermittently, and is not referred except in patients with nerve root adherence.[1,2] Pain resulting from the stretching of contracted tissue appears only when the shortened structure is subjected to tension, and ceases immediately when the tension is released. Pain is therefore felt only at end-range and not during the motion itself. Episodic exacerbation of symptoms does not occur in the dysfunction syndrome unless exercise levels have been excessive, causing further damage to the already contracted tissue. This type of exacerbation usually subsides within a few days.

With rare exceptions it is not possible to identify the structure causing the pain of dysfunction. Any of the soft tissues adjacent to the vertebral column may be damaged and may subsequently contract. Thus, the pain of dysfunction may result from adaptive shortening or from contracture resulting from the repair process following injury of any periarticular tissue, including the zygapophyseal joint capsule, intervertebral disc annulus, or superficial or deep muscles or their attachments. Pain may also result from adherence of the nerve root or dura following intervertebral disc herniation or prolapse, or from fibrosis following surgery.

The Derangement Syndrome

A third subgroup can be identified from among patients with nonspecific disorders of the neck and back. These subjects most commonly develop pain suddenly as a result of performing certain movements or activities, or from adopting certain positions. Less commonly, patients with the derangement syndrome develop pain for no apparent reason. These patients are usually aged between 20 and 55 years, and invariably have poor sitting posture. They comprise the majority of people seeking treatment for neck or back pain.[1,2]

Frequently these patients describe having had similar symptoms previously but, unlike patients with the dysfunction syndrome, patients with the derangement syndrome may be completely symptom free for months, during which time they can move without limitation.

During episodes of pain, these patients may experience severe symptoms that can be felt within or adjacent to the spine, or that may radiate and be referred distally in the form of pain, paraesthesiae, or numbness.[1,22] Most episodes remit spontaneously within 3 to 5 days. However, many patients experience symptoms persisting for 16 to 20 weeks or longer.[22] In severe cases, the deformities of torticollis or kyphosis may be evident.[22]

Pain arising in patients with the derangement syndrome may be constant, but may increase or decrease in response to movement or change of position. In these cases the patient will be unable to find any pain-free position.

The pain of derangement is otherwise intermittent, and may appear only as a result of the performance of certain movements or on the adoption of certain positions. Patients with the derangement syndrome may describe certain movements or positions as being painful on some occasions but pain-free on others. Their pain may be local or referred. They may describe their pain as being able to change location; for example, it may move from the right side of the neck to the left. It may also vary in area, intensity, and frequency. A change in the location of pain as a result of the performance of certain repeated movements occurs only in the derangement syndrome, and depending on whether the pain moves centrally or peripherally is described as *centralization* or *peripheralization*, respectively.[1,2]

Many patients with the derangement syndrome describe a change in their condition as a result of the passage of time. Symptoms may resolve spontaneously or worsen progressively. What may start as a minor problem, such as local neck pain or stiffness, may progress to a severe problem with referred pain, deformity, and neurologic deficit.[23]

Examination reveals symptoms that can be produced or abolished, increased or decreased, or centralized or peripheralized in response to repeated movements or sustained positions. Pain will be felt during movement itself, and obstruction to movement (movement loss) will increase or decrease commensurately with symptoms. A rapid and lasting alteration of symptoms and range of movement following the adoption of certain positions or the performance of certain repeated movements is possible only in patients with the derangement syndrome.

The Centralization Phenomenon

First identified by McKenzie in 1956, *centralization* is that phenomenon whereby as a result of the performance of certain repeated movements or the adoption of certain positions, radiating symptoms originating from the spine

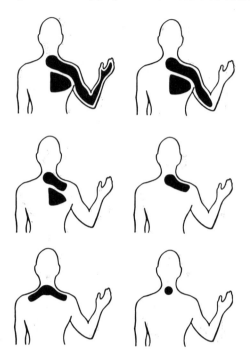

Fig. 17-2. Centralization of pain. (From McKenzie,[1] with permission.)

and referred distally are caused to move proximally toward the midline of the spine[1,2] (Fig. 17-2).

Conversely, other movements, usually in the opposite direction to those that cause centralization, may cause pain to radiate distally. This has been termed *peripheralization*. If repeated or sustained, such movements may produce a neurologic deficit.[1,2]

Movements or positions that cause centralization, when used therapeutically, may cause rapid improvement in patients with the derangement syndrome. In some cases complete resolution of symptoms can be achieved within a few hours. The recovery process depends on avoidance of those movements or positions that cause peripheralization. Of note is that movements that cause peripheralization are typically the same as those reported to have caused the onset of the original pain.[24]

Analysis of the centralization phenomenon during clinical examination will enable the clinician to identify the patient with a rapidly reversible mechanical disorder, reliably determine the appropriate direction of force for treating the disorder, and predict the treatment outcome.[5,6,24]

How do centralization and peripheralization occur? What causes asymptomatic people to be suddenly transformed into severely disabled beings as a result of apparently simple, everyday movements or activities? What pathologic processes are responsible for the progression to referred or radiating pain, deformity, and neurologic deficit from localized spinal pain?

The Conceptual Model

McKenzie suggests that the only mechanical disorder that may be capable of producing pain that changes location in direct response to movement or change of position is excessive displacement of components of the fluid nucleus or fibrous annulus complex of the intervertebral disc. The cervical intervertebral disc annulus is innervated,[25,26] and the cervical disc alone has been reported to be a potent[25,27] and common[28] source of pain of spinal origin. However, the mechanism of internal derangement of the intervertebral disc is not fully understood, and its relationship to the production of pain is unproven.

Excessive displacement of the fluid nucleus/annulus complex from the area of greatest to the area of least load may result from the adoption of prolonged static positions[22] or the performance of certain repetitive movements.[10] Such derangement may be productive of pain, since the innervated annulus is subject to mechanical deformation from the altered disc mechanics. McKenzie has proposed[1,2] the probability of an embryonic stage in the process of intradiscal tissue displacement, during which migration of nuclear material is minimal and when such displacements are reversible given the appropriate mechanical environment.

Stimulation of the central or lateral aspects of the cervical intervertebral discs produces central or unilateral referred pain, respectively,[27] and the location of displacement within the disc may determine the location of pain of which the patient with the derangement syndrome complains. Conceptually, a progressive increase in the displacement of intradiscal material posterocentrally may cause an increase of pain centrally or symmetrically. A change in the location of displacement from posterocentrally to posterolaterally may change the location of pain from central to unilateral, and the pain may radiate or be referred distally.[1,2] Posterocentral or posterolateral displacement causing disc bulging may involve the spinal cord or nerve root complex, respectively, causing radiating pain and paresthesia or numbness.[25]

Excessive displacement may impede translation or rotation of the vertebral bodies and lead to the obstruction of certain movements. If the volume of displacement is sufficient, the normal resting position of adjacent vertebrae may be disturbed and deformity may result. Excessive displacement may also affect the ability of the joint surfaces to move in their normal pathways, and deviation to the right or left of the sagittal plane may result on attempting flexion or extension. Sudden loss of spinal mobility and the appearance of deformity in the case of acute neck pain may be likened to the locking that can occur in the knee joint, in which internal derangement of the meniscus is common. Described simply, the pain of derangement results from anatomic disruption and displacement within the intervertebral segment.

Mechanical treatment of the derangement syndrome depends on the integrity of the annulus fibrosis, which if competent may favor a reduction of displaced tissue following the application of appropriate forces. In some patients, particularly those with constant brachialgia, no movement or position can be found that will reduce, centralize, or abolish their pain. Frequently, all movements worsen a patient's symptoms. In such cases it is probable that the hydrostatic mechanism of the disc is impaired, the annulus fibrosis incompetent, and the reversal of displacement is therefore impossible. In these cases mechanical therapy has no place.

This conceptual model has yet to be validated scientifically. One should be cautious when extrapolating from those lumbar investigations supportive of this model[29-40] to the cervical spine, since there are considerable morphologic differences between the two regions[41] (see also Ch. 1). One should be equally cautious when attempting to generalize from cadaveric studies[10,41] to subjects with nonspecific painful disorders of the neck or back.

Unfortunately, the conceptual model presented as a rationale for the treatment of those patients with the derangement syndrome has polarized many clinicians and researchers interested in nonspecific painful disorders of the neck or back. A better explanation may exist for the clinical observations that have been described, and the current model may eventually be altered, but until that new explanation is forthcoming, the existing model is a reasonable model on which to base mechanical therapy.[1]

TISSUE REPAIR AND REMODELING: THE PLACE OF TREATMENT

The intent of any treatment program is to assist and enhance the process of recovery. Measures must also be taken to ensure that no disruption of repair either retards or delays recovery. It is our strong clinical impression, particularly with respect to nonspecific disorders of the cervical spine, that many patients recover despite treatment rather than because of it. Clinicians involved in the treatment of disorders of the spine should be fully aware of the natural history of these disorders,[23] the body's own recuperative powers,[20,42] and the true effects of their treatments on these processes.

To illustrate this subject further, it may help to recite a case history first described by Sir Astley Cooper in 1831 ("A treatise on dislocations and fractures of the joints." Sir Astley Cooper, Bart., F.R.S., Sergeant Surgeon to the King, 1831). A thatcher in the early eighteenth century fell from a steeply pitched roof, dislocating his right hip. Reduction of the dislocation was attempted by the local doctor, but the femoral head remained in the obturator foramen (Fig. 17-3). After many months the thatcher returned to work, climbing ladders and squatting to weave straw despite his injury. The pain and movement in his hip improved over the ensuing months and he lived a normal life before succuming several years later to "the plague." Subsequent autopsy by Sir Astley Cooper exposed the results of his reductive attempt years earlier. As a result, we have the unique opportunity of seeing the marvelous capacity of the body for repair. It is suggested that movement provided the stimulus for the

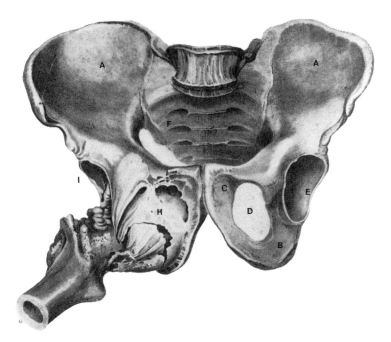

Fig. 17-3. ''Shews a dislocation into the foramen ovale which had never been reduced, and beautifully exhibits the resources of nature, in forming a new socket for the head of the bone, and allowing the restoration of a considerable degree of motion. **(A)** Right and left ilium. **(B)** Ischium. **(C)** Pubes. **(D)** Foramen ovale. **(E)** The left acetabulum. **(F)** Sacrum. **(G)** Os femoris. **(H)** The new acetabulum, formed in the foramen ovale, in which the head of the thigh bone was contained, and in which it was so completely enclosed, that it became impossible to remove it, unless a portion of the new socket was broken away. It was lined by a ligamentous substance, on which the head of the bone moved to a considerable extent. **(I)** The original acetabulum, situated above the level, and to the outer side of the new cavity.'' (From Sir Astley Cooper, Bart., F.R.S., Sergeant Surgeon to the King. A treatise on dislocations and fractures of the joints. 1831.)

complete remodeling of soft tissue and bone that resulted in the formation of a new acetabulum (Fig. 17-4).

From the work of Merrilees and Flint[43] we understand how the mechanical environment may determine the quality of connective tissue repair and remodelling. The physiologic constitution of connective tissue, especially the type and concentration of glycosaminoglycan (GAG) and the diameter and arrangement of collagen fibers, is partly determined by the mechanical environment existing at the time of collagen and GAG synthesis. Effective treatment methods must ensure that an appropriate mechanical environment is present during or shortly after the healing process is complete, in order to maximize the natural healing and remodelling capabilities of connective tissue. During the process of repair following injury to connective tissue, optimal synthesis of extracellular material

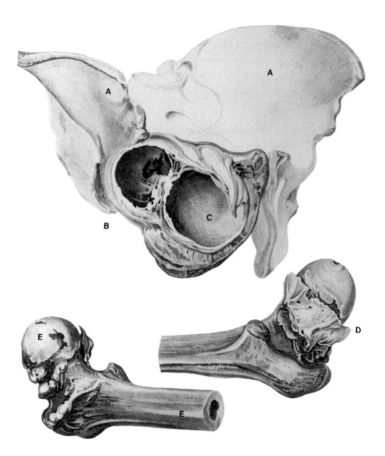

Fig. 17-4. "Exhibits another view of the same preparation, shewing the relative situation and appearance of the new and original acetabulum. **(A)** Ilia. **(B)** The original acetabulum, little more than half its natural size, the edge of the new acetabulum occupying its lower and anterior part. **(C)** The new acetabulum formed in the foramen ovale, a deep ossific edge surrounding it; its internal surface is extremely smooth. The ligament of the foramen ovale has disappeared, and ossific matter has been deposited in its stead. **(D)** The thigh bone removed, and the portion of the new acetabulum is shewn, which was obliged to be broken off to separate the thigh-bone from its new socket. **(E)** Head and neck of the thigh-bone; the former a little changed by absorption, and the latter by ossific deposit." (From Sir Astley Cooper, Bart., F.R.S., Sergeant Surgeon to the King. A treatise on dislocations and fractures of the joints. 1831.)

(particularly GAG and collagen) is stimulated if the tissue is progressively subject to those forces it would normally be required to withstand. Thus, cartilage must resist compressive forces, tendon must resist tensile forces, and fibrocartilage must resist both compressive and tensile forces. Once tissue repair is complete, remodelling of contracture can also only be achieved by progressively stressing the newly layered collagen.

The remodelling process is an important consideration during the treatment of any mechanical disorder in which contracture contributes to the persistence of symptoms. This is especially relevant in subacute and chronic conditions. The therapeutic forces required to enhance the repair or remodelling processes can only be applied by movement and loading, but must neither disrupt healing nor cause injury.

Prolonged rest in the treatment of mechanical disorders can no longer be justified.[44-46] The deleterious effects of rest may enhance degenerative change,[47] induce secondary complications, and foster chronicity. Physical therapists have at their disposal a range of mechanical forces with which to treat and manage mechanical disorders of the neck and back. Using appropriate mechanical force, therapists can progressively apply stress to healing tissue, remodel shortened fibrous tissue, and reduce internal derangement. Disrupting and damaging external forces must be eliminated or at worst reduced. Too frequently, however, progressive therapeutic force is not applied in a structured and logical manner.

THE SELF TREATMENT PHILOSOPHY

Clinical observations by McKenzie of the ability to bring about rapid and effective changes in pain intensity and location in patients suffering from mechanical back and neck pain without the use of manipulative techniques have provided new concepts in patient management. Self-treatment provides the vehicle for patient independence and long-term benefit.

McKenzie has described the chance observations in 1956 that led to these developments.[1] A patient with a 3-week history of back and leg pain unresponsive to treatment lay prone on a treatment table, fixed in an extended position. After 5 minutes in the hyperextended position his symptoms had diminished dramatically. On standing he remained better, all pain having disappeared from his leg. Furthermore, the pain in his back had moved from the right side to the center. The procedure was repeated the following day as the only method of treatment, and in this period he became completely symptom free. On another occasion, a former patient who had received treatment for recurring episodic back pain stated that she no longer required assistance when her symptoms recurred. On such occasions she would perform the exercises shown to her previously, and was able to effectively treat herself. If she performed the exercises at the first signs of recurrence, she was able to abort the impending episode.

Evolving from these and other clinical observations was the realization that patients, without assistance, could significantly affect the course of their own disorder, and if instructed properly could rapidly reverse situations that were productive of pain.[48] The special skills of the physical therapist, although valuable, were therefore seen not to be essential for treating the vast majority of patients with mechanical disorders of the neck or back. Simple maneuvers, performed by the patient, were sufficient.

In a randomized prospective study on the treatment of whiplash, McKinney[7] showed that at the 2-year follow-up, there was a statistically significant benefit for patients treated by advice and a self-treatment protocol incorporating those procedures developed by McKenzie,[49] over those treated by physical therapy or rest.

"If there is the slightest chance that a patient can be educated in the methods that enable him to reduce his own pain and disability using his own understanding and resources, he should receive that education. Every patient is entitled to the information and every therapist should be obliged to provide it."[1]

THE PLACE OF EXERCISE IN TREATMENT

> Many hospitals run a 'back class' at which spinal exercises are carried out under physiotherapists' supervision. Many hospitals order extension exercises only; others insist on flexion exercises; the chaos is complete.[50]

The static and dynamic mechanical evaluation procedures proposed by McKenzie enable clinicians to determine whether the symptoms of which a patient complains arise from the postural, dysfunction, or derangement syndromes. The indications for and the direction in which to apply therapeutic motion are determined by the patient's symptomatic response to the mechanical evaluation.[1] It is no longer acceptable to apply the same specific exercise to all persons with neck or back pain.

The Postural Syndrome

The only treatment required for pain of postural origin is correction of the offending posture. The patient must be provided with a sound explanation for such simple management. As postural pain is produced by prolonged end-range stress on normal tissue, passive therapeutic modalities, exercise, mobilization, or manipulation, are inappropriate to its treatment. Bed rest or medication will not provide a solution for pain of postural origin. Only the patient, by correcting his/her posture, can successfully remove the causative postural stresses and resolve the pain of the postural syndrome.

Postural pain is the simplest of the three causes of persisting pain in patients with chronic neck or back pain. Education about the cause of the pain (the "bent finger" analogy) and the adoption of corrective postures are the only treatment strategies required in the management of such problems.

The Dysfunction Syndrome

Pain arising from contracted soft tissues may create in the mind of patients and clinicians alike the notion that injury persists and that the patient must avoid painful motion in order to permit the injured tissue to heal. Passive therapies are frequently dispensed, providing, if anything, short-term symptomatic relief. The consequences of rest and inappropriate therapy during the healing process may be far-reaching, as immobility results in adaptive tissue shortening, which in turn may subsequently accelerate degenerative change at adjacent levels. Advice to withdraw from activity may create or amplify disability and may induce secondary complications, while doing little to aid recovery.

The aim of treatment for patients with the dysfunction syndrome is to stretch and remodel the shortened repair or contracted soft tissue. Therapeutic motion is needed to progressively stretch adaptively shortened tissue without damaging it, and the direction of the motion must be that which *produces* the pain of which the patient complains. To be effective, therapeutic motion must reach the end of the available range of motion, for it is only at the end of range that shortened tissue is stretched. Repetition of the stretching exercise should be performed from 5 to 15 times per session if remodelling is to be achieved. Sessions should be spread at approximately 2 hour intervals throughout the day.[1] Because such stretching causes more frequent pain, patients being treated in this way must be provided with appropriate explanations of why painful exercise is beneficial and essential for their recovery.

The patient must understand that only appropriate exercise, performed frequently, permits the remodelling of shortened tissue. As remodelling progresses, mobility improves and pain diminishes. Pain from such stretching should last no more than 10 to 20 minutes. Pain lasting into the following day may indicate overstretching and possibly microtrauma. Pain arising from exercise should never increase progressively or peripheralize, both of which indicate derangement or tissue disruption. The force of the therapeutic motion need only be sufficient to produce mild pain indicating that tension is being applied to the shortened tissue. In most cases patients are able to apply appropriate force to themselves without assistance. Postural correction to eliminate coexisting postural pains should be routine, as should prophylactic advice.

The patient must be reassured that the tissue causing pain is no longer injured and that the healing process is complete. A time frame must be provided so that there are no unrealistic expectations from treatment for this slowly reversible condition. Six to 20 weeks are normally required for the remodelling process to restore function in patients with the dysfunction syndrome. All circumstances must be favorable for treatment and the patient strictly directed[1] and compliant for a successful outcome to result.

Patients must be helped to understand that neither health-care providers nor pills nor bed rest will provide a solution to problems caused by shortened or contracted tissues. Only by performing exercises that stretch the shortened tissue can remodelling occur, and only the patient can apply this process with sufficient frequency and adequate control.

The Derangement Syndrome

The initial aim of treatment for patients with the derangement syndrome is to reduce the derangement. Reduction of derangement is accomplished when therapeutic motion is applied in the direction that reduces, centralizes, or abolishes the patient's pain. This motion must be applied to end-range, for it is only at the end of the available range of motion of the affected part that force sufficient to reduce derangement is achieved. In most cases, patients are able to apply adequate force without assistance.

In the treatment of cervical or thoracic derangement, repetition of the reductive exercises must be performed often enough to maintain maximal reduction. On average, ten exercises repeated at 2-hour intervals is sufficient to maintain reduction, provided all circumstances are favorable for this. Other movements or positions should be avoided while they cause the pain of derangement to return. Thereafter, function should be recovered by restoring normal spinal mobility. Finally, the therapist should ensure that the patient has an adequate understanding of the disorder and knowledge of the appropriate prophylactic measures.

The stages of treatment for a patient with the derangement syndrome are therefore[1,2,50]:

Reduction of derangement by applying appropriate movements.
Maintenance of reduction by correcting posture and avoiding inappropriate movements.
Recovery of function before adaptive changes develop.
Education of the patient in self treatment and prophylaxis.

THE ROLE OF MANIPULATION IN TREATMENT

We should keep an open mind about the possibility that spinal manipulation may benefit at least a subgroup of patients, but it remains unclear how this therapy should fit into medical decision making.[51]

The dynamic mechanical evaluation and centralization of pain determines the preferred direction for therapeutic motion and identifies the few patients who require spinal manipulation.

Manipulative therapy in the form of mobilization is only occasionally required in treatment of the dysfunction syndrome. The force of the mobilization should be applied in the same direction as the movement that produces the pain of dysfunction. Mobilization, when applied, must reach end-range and must always be accompanied by an appropriate self-treatment remodelling program. Manipulative thrust techniques have no place in the treatment of patients with the dysfunction syndrome, since they may cause microtrauma, thus perpetuating the dysfunction cycle.[1]

By contrast, therapist assistance in the form of overpressure, mobilization, or manipulation is more frequently required in treating patients with the derangement syndrome in order to apply sufficient reductive pressures. The direction of applied force is always the same as the movement that reduces or centralizes the patient's pain.[1]

REGIONAL DIFFERENCES AND IMPLICATIONS FOR TREATMENT

Regional differences in the anatomy of the cervical and thoracic spine require different movements to remodel dysfunction or reduce derangement in these two regions. Therapeutic motion in the sagittal plane should be fully explored before resorting to movements in the frontal plane. The academic debate about the direction of coupled movement required for therapeutic purposes ceases to be important when the clinician determines the direction of therapeutic motion by symptomatic response and the centralization phenomenon. This applies equally when deciding the direction of therapeutic exercise or the type of manipulation to apply.

CONCLUSION

The McKenzie concepts about the diagnosis and treatment of nonspecific disorders of the cervical and thoracic spine have been outlined. This approach leaves no place for passive palliative treatment methods that provide short-term pain relief and may create patient dependence. The capacity of the human body for its own repair must be harnessed by professions that seek to provide solutions to those who suffer from disorders of the spine. Those simple therapeutic procedures that the patient can perform should be explored before the application of mobilizing or manipulative techniques. In this way it may be possible for the patient to maintain independence from the therapist and for the therapist to provide long-term benefit to the patient.

REFERENCES

1. McKenzie RA: The Cervical and Thoracic Spine: Mechanical Diagnosis and Therapy. Spinal Publications, Waikanae, New Zealand, 1990
2. McKenzie RA: The Lumbar Spine. Mechanical Diagnosis and Therapy. Spinal Publications, Waikanae, New Zealand, 1981
3. DiMaggio A, Mooney V: Conservative care for low back pain: what works? J Musculoskel Med 4:27, 1987
4. DiMaggio A, Mooney V: The McKenzie Program: exercise effective against back pain. J Musculoskel Med 4:63, 1987
5. Donelson R, Silva G, Murphy K: Centralisation phenomenon. Its usefulness in evaluating and treating referred pain. Spine 15:211, 1990
6. Donelson R, Grant W, Kamps C, Medcalf R: Pain response to sagittal end-range

spinal motion: a prospective, randomised multi-centred trial. Spine, suppl. 16:S206, 1990
7. McKinney LA: Early mobilisation and outcome in acute sprains of the neck. Br Med J 299:1006, 1989
8. Nwuga G, Nwuga V: Relative therapeutic efficacy of the Williams and McKenzie protocols in back pain management. Physiother Pract 1:99, 1985
9. Ponte DJ, Jensen GJ, Kent BE: A preliminary report on the use of the McKenzie protocol versus Williams protocol in the treatment of low back pain. JOSPT 6:130, 1986
10. Shepperd J: Patterns of internal disc dynamics, cadaveric motion studies. Proceedings of The International Society for the Study of the Lumbar Spine, Boston, 1990
11. Stankovic R, Johnell O: Conservative treatment of acute low-back pain. A prospective randomised trial: McKenzie method of treatment versus patient education in "Mini Back School." Spine 15:120, 1990
12. Williams MM, Hawley JA, Van Wijmen PM, McKenzie RA: A comparison of the effects of two sitting postures on back and referred pain. Spine 16:1185, 1991
13. Spitzer WO (ed): Scientific approach to the assessment and management of activity-related spinal disorders. A monograph for clinicians. Report of the Quebec Task Force on Spinal Disorders. Spine, suppl. 12:S10, 1987
14. McKenzie RA: A perspective on manipulative therapy. Physiotherapy 75:440, 1989
15. Kopp JR, Turocy RH, Levrini MG, Lichtman DM: Predictive value of the physical examination for patients with acute diagnosis low back pain. Surgical Forum 33:532, 1982
16. Alexander AH, Jones AM, Rosenbaum DH: Nonoperative management of herniated nucleus pulposis. Patient selection by the extension sign—long term followup. Proceedings of The North American Spine Society, Monterey, 1990
17. Kopp JR, Alexander AH, Turocy RH, Levrini MG, Lichtman DM: The use of lumbar extension in the evaluation and treatment of patients with acute herniated nucleus pulposis: a preliminary report. Clin Orthop 202:211, 1986
18. Portnoy RK: Cancer pain: pathophysiology and syndromes. Lancet 339:1026, 1992
19. Wyke B: The neurology of low back pain. p. 265. In Jayson M (ed): The Lumbar Spine and Back pain. 2nd Ed. Pitman Medical, Kent, 1980
20. Evans P: The healing process at a cellular level. Physiotherapy 66:256, 1980
21. Harms-Ringdahl K: On assessment of shoulder exercises and load elicited pain in the cervical spine. Scand J Rehabil Med [Suppl] 14, 1986
22. Kramer J: Intervertebral disk diseases. Causes, diagnosis, treatment and prophylaxis. 2nd Ed. George Thieme Verlag, New York, 1990
23. Hult L: The Munkfors investigation. Acta Orthop Scand, suppl 16:1, 1959
24. Donelson RG, McKenzie RA: Mechanical assessment and treatment of spinal pain. p. 1627. In Frymoyer JW (ed): The Adult Spine: Principles and Practice. Raven Press, New York, 1991
25. Bogduk N: Innervation and pain patterns of the cervical spine. p. 1. In Grant R (ed): Physical Therapy of the Cervical and Thoracic Spine. Churchill Livingstone, New York, 1988
26. Mendel T, Wink CS, Zimmy ML: Neural elements in human cervical intervertebral discs. Spine 17:132, 1992
27. Cloward R: Cervical discography. Ann Surg 150:1052, 1959
28. Aprill CE, Bogduk N: The prevalence of cervical zygapophyseal joint pain. A first approximation. Spine 17:744, 1992
29. Mixter WJ, Barr JS: Rupture of the intervertebral disc with involvement of the spinal canal. N Engl J Med 211:210, 1934

30. Whitecloud TS, Seago RA: Cervical discogenic syndrome. Spine 12:313, 1987
31. Murphey F: Sources and patterns of pain in disc disease. Clin Neurosurg 15:343, 1968
32. Vanharanta H, Sachs BL, Spivey MA, et al: The relationship of pain provocation to lumbar disc deterioration as seen by CT/discography. Spine 12:295, 1987
33. Kuslich SD, Ulstrom CL: The tissue origin of low back pain and sciatica. Orthop Clin North Am 22:181, 1991
34. Hirsch C, Ingelmark BE, Miller M: The anatomical basis for low back pain. Acta Orthop Scand 33:1, 1963
35. Kornberg M: Discography and magnetic resonance imaging in the diagnosis of lumbar disc disruption. Spine 14:1368, 1989
36. Mooney V: Where is the pain coming from? Spine 12:754, 1987
37. Naylor A: The biochemical changes in the human intervertebral disc in degeneraiton and nuclear prolapse. Orthop Clin North Am 2:343, 1971
38. Krag MH, Seroussi RE, Wilder DG, Pope MH: Internal displacement distribution from *in vitro* loading of human thoracic and lumbar spinal motion segments: experimetnal results and theoretical predictions. Spine 12:1001, 1987
39. Vernon-Roberts B, Pirie CJ: Degenerative changes in the intervertebral discs of the lumbar spine and thier sequelae. Rheumatol Rehabil 16:13, 1977
40. Schnebel BE, Watkins RG, Dillin W: The role of spinal flexion and extension in changing nerve root compression in disc herniation. Spine 14:835, 1989
41. Twomey LT, Taylor JR: Joints of the middle and lower cervical spine: age changes and pathology. Proceedings of the Sixth Biennial Conference of the Manipulative Therapists Association of Australia. Adelaide, 1989
42. Hardy MA: The biology of scar formation. Phys Ther 69:1014, 1989
43. Merrilees MJ, Flint MH: Ultrastructural study of tension and pressure zones in a rabbit flexor tendon. Am J Anat 157:116, 1980.
44. Deyo RA, Diehl AK, Rosenthal PH: How many days of bed rest for acute low back pain? A randomised clinical trial. N Engl J Med 315:1064, 1986
45. Nachemson A: A critical look at conservative treatment of low back pain: p. 453. In Jayson M (ed): The Lumbar Spine and Back Pain. 2nd Ed. Pitman Medical, Kent, 1990
46. Salter R: Motion, not immobility, advocated for healing synovial joints. JAMA 246: 2005, 1979
47. Videman T: Connective tissue and immobilisation. Key factors in musculoskeletal degeneration? Clin Orthop 221:26, 1987
48. McKenzie RA: Mechanical diagnosis and therapy for low back pain: toward a better understanding. p. 157. In Twomey LT, Taylor JR (eds): Physical Therapy of the Low Back. Churchill Livingstone, New York, 1987
49. McKenzie RA: Treat Your Own Neck. Spinal Publicatons, Waikanae, New Zealand, 1983
50. Cyriax J: Textbook of Orthopaedic Medicine. 6th Ed. Williams & Wilkins, London, 1975
51. Deyo RA: Letter to the editor. N Engl J Med 326:12, 1992

18 | Neck and Upper Extremity Pain in the Workplace

Barbara McPhee
David R. Worth

Musculoskeletal complaints are ubiquitous; almost everyone experiences symptoms of these conditions at some time in their lives, with the likelihood of occurrence increasing with age. The population at large perceives these conditions as a normal part of life, and this had led to a tendency to consider them as inevitable rather than potentially preventable.

Musculoskeletal disorders arising in the workplace are proving to be a particularly perplexing problem because they are poorly understood and research into their nature, causes, and prevention is difficult and inadequate. Although designed to do otherwise, workers' compensation and health care systems, interacting with personal and social factors, may encourage some workers, to continue to receive disability payments and discourage an early return to work. As a result, it is increasingly recognized in many industrialized countries that musculoskeletal disorders are costing industry and the community dearly, both in human and financial terms.

In industrialized countries, low back pain is estimated to account for more than 50 percent of the total cost of work-related musculoskeletal disorders, amounting to many billions of dollars annually, and may represent more than 50 percent of total injury costs.[1] In the mid 1980s occupational back pain was estimated to represent over 20 percent of all reported cases of work-related disability in the United States, accounting for 32 percent of compensation payments, at a sum amounting to over $11.1 billion, and the costs have continued to rise.[2]

These figures take no account of the personal and social disruption that back pain creates for those it affects, as well as for their immediate family and friends; nor for the frustration and feelings of futility engendered in health-care and social welfare professionals who try unsuccessfully to rehabilitate the worker for a return to work. It appears that in many industrialized countries, the traditional medical approach to the management of work-related back pain has failed in a significant percentage of cases. Unfortunately, less attention and money have been directed at preventing work-related back pain than seems justified by the cost of these disorders once they occur.

Increasing reports of pain, discomfort, and dysfunction of the neck and upper extremities associated with repetitive work in fixed or awkward postures indicate that these conditions are no less a problem than back pain in terms of diagnosis and management, although there is now anecdotal evidence that prevention programs for them can be very cost effective.[2]

In the United States, the reporting of "disorders associated with repeated trauma" has more than tripled since 1984. While this category includes chronic noise-induced hearing loss as well as disorders of the neck and upper-extremity, it does not include back pain.[2] The same document points out that there were 147,000 new cases of these disorders reported in 1989, which accounted for 52 percent of all recordable occupational illnesses reported to the Occupational Safety and Health Administration (OSHA) in that year. In 1981 and 1984, noise-induced hearing loss and neck and upper-extremity disorders accounted for 18 percent and 28 percent, respectively, of occupational illnesses. It has been suggested that their real incidence rate may be 130 percent higher than the reported rate.

In Norway in the mind 1980s, it was estimated that approximately 60 percent of sick leave was attributable to musculoskeletal disorders of all kinds.[3,4] These conditions were also responsible for a significant number of early retirements and work pensions.

In 1983, statistics from the Swedish Occupational Injury Information System revealed that more than 50 percent of reported cases of occupational diseases were related to ergonomic factors in the workplace, such as physically heavy work, manual materials handling, repetitive work, and unsuitable work postures.[5] Employees exposed to these factors had up to 26 days more sick leave than other workers. Researchers have noted that repetitive jobs with unsuitable work postures have replaced more varied tasks, and that the prevalence of symptoms in the neck and shoulders seems to be increasing.[5]

HISTORY

Early Research

Ramazzini,[6] in 1713, described disorders in craftsmen, tradesmen, scribes, and notaries that resembled musculoskeletal complaints of today. Apart from Ramazzini's observations, comparatively little was published on work-related musculoskeletal disorders before the 1970s. One notable exception to this was the literature generated by the perplexing problem of craft palsies or occupational cramp.[7] In 1959, Hunter[8] listed 49 different occupational groups in which the hands could be affected by such cramps. The causes of these conditions are not well understood, and although they seem less prevalent now, they undoubtedly still exist.

From the 1920s to the 1960s, papers were published describing the clinical aspects of work-related musculoskeletal disorders of the upper limb and shoulder girdle, with authors speculating on their causes.[9–15] The work factors listed as the probable causes of the conditions described were speed and intensity of muscle effort; persistent strain; overuse of muscles; unaccustomed work often occurring after a change of job or equipment, or on returning from a vacation; and trauma. One researcher suggested that the conditions appeared to increase in frequency during periods of economic stress, such as during the Great Depression.[15] The medical conditions were described with care, but their prevention in the workplace seemed to have been secondary to their identification and treatment. By the middle of the twentieth century, musculotendinous injuries, notably tenosynovitis and peritendinitis, were recognized as being induced by certain types of work in workers' compensation legislation in most industrialized countries.

Gradually, attempts were made to identify the disorders more precisely, and suggestions were made for their prevention, particularly in relation to the growing and costly problem of low back pain. In 1970, Van Wely[16] reported that a team of health and safety professionals demonstrated that they could predict, with reasonable accuracy, which tasks and work postures would lead to symptoms in operators, and what parts of the worker's body would be affected. Van Wely also described how these disorders might have been prevented, emphasizing two approaches: the ergonomic design of tools, furniture, and equipment; and the thorough training of workers in correct postures and work techniques. These observations and recommendations were a turning point in the study and prevention of work-related musculoskeletal disorders.

In 1976, Herberts and Kadefors[17] in Sweden demonstrated fatigue electromyographically in the shoulder muscles of welders, thereby supporting the belief that fatigue was an important factor in the etiology of the shoulder pain commonly experienced by older welders. An earlier electromyographic (EMG) study[18] showed that excessive loads were being placed on the shoulder and arm muscles of workers using pneumatic hammers and bolt guns. It was tempting to assume that such loads, over a period of time, could lead to early degenerative changes in the musculoskeletal structures involved.

In Japan, the study of a wide range of work-related disorders of the neck and upper extremity, known in that country as occupational cervicobrachial disorders (OCD), began in the late 1960s in groups as diverse as cash-register operators, industrial workers, film rollers, creche attendants, nurses, keyboard operators, telephone operators, and clerks writing with ballpoint pens.[19–26]

Japanese research has formed the basis of many of the descriptive studies of work-related disorders in other countries. Maeda and his coworkers were the first to develop a system of collecting subjective data on symptoms of OCD,[27] using body charts. They also extensively researched various factors associated with the signs and symptoms of OCD.[28] Much of their approach and progress in identifying factors associated with the development of OCD was made possible by the early work of the Japan Association of Industrial Health. It defined OCD and outlined causative factors, clinical features, and stages of such disorders and the health services required to control them.

Awareness of work-related musculoskeletal disorders in Australia came with the work of Perrot.[29] Using a biomechanical model of injury and its prevention, he described how unnecessary movement, shear strain, torsion, and muscle imbalance could be minimized.

Peres[30] described injuries resulting from chronic fatigue resulting from intense effort, monotony, and the lack of variety of work. He emphasized the detrimental effects of a static muscle load resulting from poor posture and recommended a preventive strategy based on the redesign of work practices, early reporting of symptoms, redeployment, and task alternation. Peres recognized that most cases of injury from process work occurred in women and suggested that this was due to their weaker musculature and the greater number of women engaged in process work. However, he pointed out that men were not immune to such injury, and described overuse conditions in male canecutters, metal workers, milkers, and carpenters.

In Australia, much of the pioneering work on the association between work postures, repetitive manual work, and symptoms of neck, arm, trunk, and leg discomfort was done by Ferguson.[7,31–35] Asked to investigate an outbreak of unspecified upper-limb injuries in 77 women working in an electronics factory, Ferguson analyzed injury records, examined the subjects, and undertook task analysis. He found that the injuries fell into two broad groups: well-defined clinical syndromes such as supraspinatus tendonitis and tennis elbow; and ill defined symptom complexes. The latter group comprised the majority of cases seen, yet this was the first time such injuries had been reported in the literature in Australia.

Interestingly, Ferguson described the conditions in his subjects, and postulated the causes for them in much the same way as the Japanese researchers, although there was no contact between the two groups at that time. Ferguson broadened the view of these injuries from tenosynovitis and peritendinitis crepitans to a wide variety of musculo-tendinous injuries in the arm, which he called "repetition injuries." Later the term "strain" was added by another chronicler of these disorders in Australia,[36] and the term *repetition strain injury* (RSI) replaced tenosynovitis as the umbrella term used for a range of neck and upper-limb disorders believed to be associated with work.

In further work Ferguson examined personality, social, and work organization factors and associated medical conditions in relation to the etiology of the disorders he was investigating as well as intervention and prevention procedures for them.[33–35]

In a study of telephone operators,[34] it was concluded that the frequent complaints of discomfort, aching, and other symptoms were due to static loads on joints and muscles resulting from the fixed forward bending postures determined by the nature and design of the visual, auditory, and manipulative tasks of these peoples' work.

Ferguson drew attention to the long recovery periods in many cases of RSI, postulating a number of reasons for this, but reached no firm conclusions. However, he felt that malingering was unlikely in these cases, since most workers exhibited a desire to return to work for financial reasons. He took a broad view of the prevention of RSI, suggesting that social and work organization as well as biomechanical factors were important. He stressed the need for the adequate investigation of injuries and for epidemiologic studies, and pointed out that musculoskeletal injuries were very costly whether or not they were responsible for lost time.

Recent Research

For the past 20 years, the increasing numbers of complaints of disorders of the neck and upper extremities being reported by workers in an increasing range of industries around the world has prompted a more systematic approach to research. It is now well accepted that repetitive work with the hands and/ or the feet can lead to these complaints. The use of high forces and the need for fixed postures compound the effects on the workers.

Two groups of disorders have emerged: the more clearly defined and diagnosable conditions, most particularly of the elbow, lower arm, and hand, that are commonly associated with heavy, repetitive work with the hands; and the less well defined shoulder/neck disorders seen in workers who undertake light repetitive work in fixed postures, such as computer operators, as well as those who do heavy work.

Repetitive manual activities required continuous stabilizing around the shoulder girdle by muscles such as the trapezius. In cases in which this load is increased by the need to use force or to sit fixed in one position for long periods, the load and rate of fatigue are increased manyfold. With an increased variety of movements within a job, the effects of muscle fatigue can be substantially diminished. The less variety the greater the risks of fatigue, discomfort, pain, and injury.

The jobs listed in the following section are manually repetitive for a large percentage of the working day, and are likely to load the musculature of the upper limbs, upper trunk, and neck to a degree that requires frequent rest breaks to enable recovery and prevent premature fatigue.

In some jobs the taking of rest breaks can occur routinely within the work cycle; in others such breaks may have to be imposed through a reorganization of work. Such breaks are necessary to offset fatigue. When they do not occur (often coinciding with increased workloads and an increasing pace of work that require an increased frequency and length of breaks), workers will begin to experience symptoms of fatigue that may eventually lead to injury in the more susceptible.

Work Factors

Substantial evidence now indicates that various risk factors, present in different forms and different combinations in many jobs, do lead to higher than expected frequencies of neck and upper extremity disorders. The untrained observer can deduce that jobs involving heavier work such as press operations, sewing machining, packaging, meat and poultry processing, and assembling are strenuous and potentially harmful even for the capable and skilled individual.

The difficulties of so-called "light" work involving continuous, high speed, repetitive hand and finger movements, often in fixed and awkward postures, are not as obvious as those of heavier jobs. However, in contrast to the case for much of the repetitive and physically demanding work in industry, there has been an exponential increase in the numbers of these "light" jobs and in the percentage of workers undertaking them. This in itself should be ample justification for paying more attention to the potential health hazards of such work. The causes of occupational musculoskeletal conditions arising from "light," white collar jobs are complex, and there may be a need to reclassify these conditions. They also appear to be less amenable to simple preventive strategies than the better known, more traditionally identified conditions described in the orthopedic literature.

Among white collar workers, and particularly office workers performing keyboard-based tasks, it is likely that the increased prevalence of musculoskeletal disorders is due to the following factors:

1. The rapid introduction of computer technology without due regard for how human operators will work within such systems.
2. A concomitant, increasingly repetitive and fixed nature of tasks that were formerly more varied in terms of postures and movements.
3. Increasing awareness by workers of occupational health and safety issues, without the concomitant changes in attitude required by planners and managers to meet increasingly better standards of working conditions and services to workers.

In Australia, an unprecedented number of disorders of the upper limb and neck were reported in the office workforce in the mid-1980s.[37,38] Whereas there had been an endemic level of shoulder, arm, and hand disorders in the manufacturing, food processing, and garment making industries before this time, there arose a growing number of white collar workers reporting symptoms from what had previously been considered light, relatively undemanding work. These complaints reached epidemic proportions in 1985–1986 and brought much attention to the previously unrecognized problems of the shoulder/neck region. While there was much speculation about the causes of these problems, and debate about the nature of the resulting disorders, researchers in many parts of the world are only now reaching plausible hypotheses and explanations for the occurrence of these phenomena. An excellent review of research literature on shoulder-neck complaints, as well as Guidelines for Practitioners in managing these complaints, have recently been published.[39,40]

Associations between work and an increased prevalence of neck and upper extremity disorders have been found in engineering assembly and process work[18,31,41-53]; meat and poultry workers[54-61]; food packing[62]; sewing machinists and garment workers[63-66]; cashiers, accounting machine operators, and key punchers[67-72]; video data terminal (VDT) and data entry operators[73-86]; mail workers[87-88]; and musicians.[89]

Most researchers now agree that physical loading of the musculoskeletal system, sometimes in conjunction with psychological stress, precipitates the initial symptoms of such disorders, which may resolve spontaneously, come and go intermittently without further development, or gradually or rapidly progress to the point at which the individual cannot continue to work under the same conditions. The progression of such disorders is likely to relate to the extent of physical loading they impose, both acutely and cumulatively; to psychological factors such as personal or work stresses; and to the adequacy with which their causes and symptoms are addressed both within and outside the workplace.

Individual Factors

Individuals exposed to hazards in occupational situations react differently to them. This also can be said of individuals' reactions to stressful and/or repetitive movements and prolonged fixed postures. An operation that is difficult and even damaging for one person may not constitute a risk for another. The higher the levels of physical stress, the greater will be the numbers who succumb to injury. Susceptibility to strain appears to be a continuum, with the highly susceptible at one end and the highly resilient at the other. If so, there is an argument for screening out susceptible individuals before permitting them to work at jobs known to cause symptoms; but this is not easy, nor is it usually acceptable. There must be some understanding of why some people are resilient and others are not.

While there appears to be no strong recent evidence that personal (individual) factors might influence this resilience, writers of some of the earlier papers on work-related musculoskeletal injury did speculate that anatomic, physiologic, and psychological factors were associated with the development of disorders of the neck and upper limb. For instance, it was suggested that the anatomy of the wrist in some people might have a bearing on the way in which stresses are transmitted within and through it.[14] Physiologically, deficiencies in the peripheral circulation were considered by some investigators as being the direct cause of fatigue and subsequent strain,[90] while others considered muscle strength to be responsible for these effects.[19] Psychological factors such as personality, anxiety, and mood have also been implicated in the reduced capacity to withstand stress.[30,80,91]

However, much more evidence is needed in the area of personal factors before they can be used to determine which individuals may be at greater risk of developing musculoskeletal disorders as the result of their work. On the other hand, scientific evidence increasingly points to links between certain types of work and workplaces, and to differences in individual methods of work[50,85] and the incidence of disorders of the neck and upper extremities.

It seems that any individual has an increased risk of strain when new demands are made on the individual; the individual habitually works beyond his/her capacity; personal, social or environmental factors reduce the individual's tolerance to physical stress.

The relationship between physical workload and its effects on functional capacity and on the development and severity of symptoms appears to be modified by temporal factors, such as the length of the working day, periods worked without breaks, and the percentage of the working day spent doing repetitive activities in fixed postures. Additionally, personality, mood, the perception of load, work pressures, job satisfaction, and other personal factors may alter the individual's response to early signs of fatigue and discomfort.

The following factors need to be considered in preventing these disorders[85]:

1.   External load factors (task and workplace design and work organization) required by a task, including number of movements; static muscle work; force; work postures determined by equipment and furniture; and time worked without a break.

2.   Factors that influence load but which may vary between individuals, including work postures adopted; static muscle work used; unnecessary force used; number and duration of pauses taken; and speed and accuracy of movements.

3.   Factors that alter the individual's response to a particular load (workplace, individual, and social factors), including age; sex; physical capabilities; environmental factors such as vibration, cold, noise, and other contaminants; previous repetitive work and job experience; and psychosocial variables.

A CLASSIFICATION OF DISORDERS AND THEIR SIGNS AND SYMPTOMS

Three main groups of musculoskeletal or soft tissue disorders give rise to neck and upper extremity pain in workers. These are traumatic, degenerative, and abusive use syndromes (Table 18–1).

Traumatic

Traumatic disorders, while not as common as degenerative or abusive use syndromes, constitute a group of disorders which, under Australian Workers' Compensation law,[92] may be regarded as work-induced injuries. These disor-

Table 18-1. A Classification of Disorders Associated with Neck and Upper Extremity Pain in Workers

Traumatic	Degenerative	Abusive Use
Acute soft tissue injury	Intervertebral disc disease	Postural overload
Fracture	Cervical spondylosis	syndrome
Dislocation	Arthrosis	Overuse syndrome
Subluxation	Seronegative	Environmental condition
Laceration	spondyloarthropathy	syndromes
Traumatic arthritis	Rheumatoid arthritis	
Traumatic bursitis	Inflammatory joint disease	
Reflex sympathetic	Soft tissue disease	
dystrophy	Bony necrosis	
Burns		

ders are characterized by their causal relationship to a discrete traumatic incident. Such an incident may be unrelated to a work process and may occur at or on the way to or from the workplace. Typical examples are cervical spine injuries in "journey accidents" and soft-tissue injuries or fractures resulting from falls or other accidents during the work period.

It may be argued that these musculoskeletal injuries were not caused by the work process, but they are generally considered as work related.

They may result in a temporary or permanent, total or partial, painful disability for the worker. This may cause economic and other loss and hardship to both the worker and employer. Often it is difficult for the traumatically injured worker to remain at work or to return to work after a substantial absence.

Table 18–2 provides an expanded list of commonly encountered traumatic disorders leading to neck and upper extremity pain in the workplace. It is not within the scope of this chapter to describe these traumatic disorders in detail. This has been adequately done in many orthopedic texts.[93–97] However, it is important to point out that acute soft-tissue injuries of the cervical spine often have a devastating effect on the worker when he or she returns to work, despite an absence from work during which the final symptoms of such injuries may have resolved.

Once a return-to-work program has commenced, it is essential that care be taken to protect the worker's cervical spine from work-induced postural strain and/or trauma. This requires that management personnel, supervisors, line foremen, fellow workers, and health-care professionals recognize that the worker has a physical disability. The worker who returns with a serious preexisting injury and without having for some time experienced the rigors of work suffers well-recognized symptoms. Adding work and production pressures to this person's daily activities puts the injured soft tissue at risk, and increased static and dynamic loading on ligaments and muscles may aggravate symptoms of the injury.

Table 18-2. Commonly Seen Traumatic Disorders Leading to Neck and Upper-Extremity Pain in the Workplace.

Acute cervical spine soft tissue injuries	Ruptured or lacereated tendons of the wrist and/or hand
Fracture in the cervical and cervicothoracic spine	Trapeziometacarpal joint instability
Cervical radiculopathy	Scapholunate dissociation
Axillary nerve compression	Scaphoid fracture
Suprascapular nerve entrapment	Pisiform fracture
Fracture and fracture dislocation in the upper limb and shoulder girdle	Hook of hamate fracture
Glenohumeral instability	Distal radioulnar joint subluxation
Shoulder bursitis	Extensor carpi ulnaris subluxation
Acute tear of the rotator cuff mechanism of the shoulder joint	Injuries or degeneration of the triangular fibrocartilage complex
Shoulder impingement syndrome	Tears at the lunotriquetral joint
Distal biceps or longhead of biceps rupture	Mid-carpal instability
Triceps tendon rupture	Volar plate injuries in the hand
Fracture at the elbow	Ligamentous and capsular injuries of the fingers
Traumatic arthritis of the elbow	Sesamoiditis at the metacarpophalangeal joint of the thumb
Traumatic bursitis at the elbow	Fingertip injuries
Traumatic ulnar nerve neuritis at the elbow	Reflex sympathetic dystrophy following trauma
Ulnar nerve entrapment at the elbow or wrist	Amputations and stump pain
Traumatic arthritis at the wrist	
Ligamentous strain or rupture at the wrist	

Degenerative Musculoskeletal Disorders

The group of disorders degenerative musculoskeletal disorders is typified by clinical, radiologic, or electromyographic (EMG) evidence of degenerative changes in the joints or soft tissues of the musculoskeletal system. Notwithstanding their not being work-induced disorders, they are often pre-existing conditions, the symptoms of which may be precipitated or aggravated by incidents at work or which may predict the onset of a work-related injury. These conditions may lead to neck and upper extremity pain in workers.

The significant difference between the degenerative and the traumatic group of musculoskeletal disorders is in the time and nature of their onset. The onset of a traumatic disorder is usually sudden and related to a specific incident, whereas the onset of a degenerative disorder is usually insidious and not incident related. Again, it is not within the scope of this chapter to discuss the management of these disorders. Degenerative disorders commonly related to neck and upper extremity pain in the workplace include:

Cervical spinal intervertebral disc lesions
Cervical spondylosis and related disorders

Cervical spinal zygapophyseal joint arthrosis
Thoracic outlet syndrome
Disease (e.g., rheumatoid arthritis, ankylosing spondylitis)
Frozen shoulder
Tennis elbow, golfer's elbow, medial or lateral humeral epicondylitis
Olecranon bursitis
Olecranon-trochlear arthritis
Aspetic necrosis of the lunate bone
Arthrosis of the trapezio–first metacarpal joint
Compression syndromes (e.g., carpal tunnel syndrome)
Tenosynovitis (e.g., rheumatoid or De Quervain's stenosing tenosynovitis)
Trigger finger
Dupuytren's disease
Ganglion
Osteoarthritis of the scapho-trapezial-trapezoid joints
Scapholunate advanced collapse
Keinböch's disease
Pisotriquetral arthritis
Radiocapitellar arthritis

Abusive Use Syndromes

This group of disorders is noted for their lack of specific diagnosis. They present with widespread symptoms that include pain, paresthesiae, loss of coordination and hand function, weakness of grip, intermittent swelling and, occasionally, apparent vascular disturbance.

However, some specific conditions that may arise from abusive use of the upper limb, head, and neck include:

Flexor or extensor carpi ulnaris tendonitis
Radial or posterior interosseous nerve entrapment
Triceps tendonitis
Ulnar neuritis
Pronator syndrome: anterior interosseous and pronator teres syndrome
Biceps tendonitis
Adverse neural tension
Vibration syndrome
Cold exposure syndrome

There are three major subgroups of abusive use disorders: (1) postural overload syndromes, (2) overuse syndrome, and (3) environmental condition syndromes. Environmental condition syndromes include vibration and cold exposure.

Postural Overload Syndromes

Postural overload syndromes arise from tasks done in postures that mechanically disadvantage the muscular system. Muscles involved in these syndromes may be grouped into three categories.

1. Muscles primarily performing the tasks (prime movers).
2. Muscles synergistically contracting to facilitate the prime movers (synergists).
3. Muscles statically contracting to maintain body balance to permit the prime movers and synergists to act in the performance of the task (stabilizers).

The following example will serve to demonstrate situations in which muscles in all three categories may act at a mechanical disadvantage.

A keyboard operator who has not been taught correct keyboard techniques and posture is likely to approach the keys with the wrist kept at approximately 30° to 45° of extension. In this position, lift-off occurs in the following sequence: (1) The extensor carpi ulnaris, extensor carpi radialis longus, and brevis muscles contract statically to maintain the wrist posture, while the extensor digitorum communis extends the metacarpophalangeal joints. (2) At the same time, the flexor digitorum sublimis and profundus flex the proximal and distal interphalangeal joints. (3) The fingers then strike the keys as a result of contraction of the interossiae and lumbricals, which flex the metacarpophalangeal joints when the extensor digitorum communis relaxes. This is referred to as "hand hammer function."

The problem occurs when the prime mover for lift-off, the extensor digitorum communis, fails to relax sufficiently, or contract eccentrically, to permit efficient key striking. This is due to the maintained posture of wrist extension producing inner-range static contraction of the extensor digitorum communis, which then acts as a synergist to the wrist extensors, thus failing to fully relax during key striking. The result is inner-range dynamic and static overload of the extensor digitorum communis as: (1) a prime mover for lift-off (dynamic), and (2) a synergist to wrist extension (static).

Such long-term inner-range postural overload leads to adaptive shortening of the extensor digitorum communis. If this keyboard operator also has a chronic head forward posture with an increased cervical and thoracic spinal curvature, spinal stability will be maintained by excessive static contraction of the long extensor muscles of the spine (stabilizers). These muscles contract in their outer range for long periods, resulting in symptomatic overload.

Therefore, the keyboard operator is likely to exhibit the following symptoms and signs:

Mid-dorsal aching
Suprascapular pain
Aching of the upper cervical spine
Suboccipital pain

Headache
Pain radiating into the upper arm
Laterial epicondylar ache and pain
Posterior forearm pain
Hand pain
Loss of power grip strength
A "pins and needles" sensation in the suprascapular region and forearm
Loss of coordination and hand precision skills

The strategies for preventing these problems include maintenance of the normal curvatures of the thoracic and cervical spine, and proper adjustment of the operator's chair and sitting posture. Detailed instruction in safe keyboard operation involves adjusting keyboard/chair height relationships to permit lift-off and keystrike to occur within approximately 5° of wrist flexion. The work environment must include office furniture that is adjustable and permits optimal posture.

Overuse Syndrome

Like postural overload syndromes, overuse syndrome is also clearly de-marcated from traumatic and degenerative disorders, since it is not yet known to present with any identifiable pathology reported in clinical or research medicine. It is listed under abusive use disorders in this discussion because its symptoms appear to correlate well with the performance of specific tasks.

Overuse syndrome has been defined as "Established pain and tenderness in muscle and joint ligaments of the upper extremity, produced by hand-use intensive activity for long periods and use which is clearly excessive for the individuals affected."[98]

Overuse syndrome is not caused by repetitive use alone. It is associated with abusive use, whereby the intensity of the work performed by a muscle, multiplied by the duration of this work, exceeds the capacity of the muscle. The intensity of the work, which is the product of the force of the load and the distance through which the load is lifted, is affected by the velocity of muscle contraction. The intensity of muscle work is also affected by the quality of the muscle contraction. In ballistic movements, agonist and antagonist muscle groups co-ordinate to accelerate or decelerate a particular segment of the upper extremity.

While it is not the purpose of this chapter to discuss in detail the physiology of work, it is important to emphasize that the "ability of muscle fibers to main-tain a high tension, and the individual's subjective feeling of fatigue, are highly dependent on the blood flow through the muscle".[99]

Workers who must perform highly co-ordinated, high-velocity, intense muscular work over long periods are at risk of exceeding the reoxygenation capacity of the muscle group being used, and therefore the capacity to persist in managing work loads. Muscles may then become painful.

Symptoms. The symptoms of overuse syndrome are local pain in muscles, ligaments, and joints; weakness of the affected limb; "pins and needles" or heaviness; and loss of responsiveness (e.g., the tendency to strike wrong keys). This may be a description of loss of coordination and proprioception.

Signs. The signs of overuse syndrome are tenderness in the muscles and particular structures; swelling over the affected muscle groups; weakness of precision and power grip; and loss of coordination, particularly proprioception.

Both postural overload and overuse syndromes are related to the nature of a work method and the physical and organizational environment in which the work is done. Therefore, consideration of the interaction of biomechanical, physiologic, and psychological effects will be necessary to determine the efficiency with which work is performed.

Environmental Condition Syndromes

Exposure to vibration is a common problem when using power tools. If used for sufficiently long periods, or at high levels, such tools may cause discomfort, reduced work efficiency, and musculoskeletal complaints. There is controversy about the methods used to reduce exposure to vibration, but some standards for such exposure, albeit inadequate, are available.

The physiologic effects of vibration from a hand-held tool may include tissue strain or compression, the severity of which will depend on how the vibration is transmitted to the tissue and whether resonance or attenuation occurs.[100]

The severity of the effects of hand-transmitted vibration as a component of work is influenced by the magnitude of the vibration (frequency × amplitude); the duration of exposure per working day; rest spells and breaks; the posture of the hands and arms (i.e., wrist, elbow, and shoulder joint angles); the direction of vibration through the arms; and any predisposing health factors.

Exposure of the hand and fingers to cold profoundly affects their strength, dexterity, and sensitivity. The grip forces required to hold hand tools are significantly higher at reduced hand temperatures. Occupations such as poultry processing or boning result in frequent contact with cold objects by the gloved hand.[97] Cooling factors include the ambient temperature (0° or 5°); cold gloves and clothing, and direct contact with cold objects (0° to 2°), significantly reducing the skin temperature of the hands (0° to 5°). The frequency and duration of cold exposure are key factors is an analysis directed toward preventing its effects on the hand.

Summary

To clearly understand the etiology and consequently the management of work-related pain, a thorough understanding of the diagnostic criteria for accurately categorizing such pain is essential. For example, tenosynovitis may follow a crushing injury to the hand, may be associated with rheumatoid arthritis, or may be a consequence of postural overload syndrome. The management of primary tenosynovitis is simple and well documented, and should not present a long-term problem. However, the prevention of aggravation and recurrence of this condition depends upon its cause and the control of aggravating factors.

The categorization of discrete diagnoses of work-related injury into a collective group such as repetition strain injury (RSI),[101] occupational cervicobrachial disorders (OCD), or cumulative trauma disorder (CTD) can be misleading, and clearly is technically incorrect. It has also discouraged the correct and accurate diagnosis of these disorders and has made a complex set of signs and symptoms appear to be deceptively simple.

The classification offered in this chapter (Table 18–1) is an attempt to solve a diagnostic dilemma, to broaden our overview, and to allow us to deal with these painful disorders a little more scientifically and effectively.

PREVENTION

Despite the problems in diagnosing work-related musculoskeletal disorders, their varying classification, and difficulties treating many of the work related disorders of the neck and upper extremity, it is important to remember that many of these conditions are preventable. The complex interaction of work, personal, and social factors that may give rise to complaints related to the neck and upper extremities in workers means that ergonomics is an essential component of any program for preventing these problems.

Ergonomics considers the design of work and its organization, as well as the design of the workplace in relation to the capabilities and limitations of the worker. A range of freely available publications now deal specifically with the prevention of these disorders,[102–110] all of which outline different strategies for accomplishing this, including the extensive application of principles of ergonomics.

Where unavoidable problems arise, appropriate case management should aim at minimizing the severity of a condition and returning the patient to work, with necessary, modifications, as soon as possible.

The prevention of work-related musculoskeletal disorders can be considered under the three main headings of:

Primary prevention. Aiming at eliminating or minimizing risks to health or well being.

Secondary prevention. Alleviating the symptoms of ill health or injury, minimizing residual disability, and eliminating or at least minimizing factors that may cause recurrence.

Tertiary prevention. Rehabilitating patients with disabilities to the fullest possible function, and modifying the workplace to accommodate any residual disability.

The effective implementation and evaluation of measures for preventing musculoskeletal disorders in the workplace may require a multidisciplinary approach involving ergonomics, occupational health, epidemiology, engineering, administration, and management. A prevention program will require co-operation, organization, and commitment, most particularly from senior management. It may be expensive in the short term, because of the need to purchase new equipment or rearrange the work and/or the workplace, and it may temporarily reduce production. Often there is a reluctance on the part of management to accept short-term costs and organizational upheaval for the long-term benefit of a prevention program. Nevertheless, such an approach may be necessary for the successful long-term control of work-related musculoskeletal disorders and their associated costs.

Ergonomic Analyses in the Workplace

To avoid mismatches between workers and their jobs, there must be some understanding of the demands of a particular kind of work and the capacity of each worker to meet those demands. Measurement of workload and its effects on individuals and groups is for physical therapists one of the more challenging aspects of the management of neck and upper extremity disorders.

Measurement can be accomplished in the following areas: workplace measurement and assessment, task analysis; workload measurement (individuals or groups); symptom recording.

Workplace Measurement and Assessment including Task Analysis

Workplace measurement and assessment techniques measure or assess the adequacy of the workplace and ability of the required tasks to accommodate workers' physical and mental capabilities and limitations. Many well-known methods are described and discussed in a number of text books on ergonomics. Several are particularly useful for physical therapists.[109,111,12] A wide range of techniques is available, but each may need tailoring to local requirements and conditions. Some training in ergonomics for physical therapists is essential if they are to develop measurement methods that are valid, reliable, and usable.

Measurement of Workload

Again, many of the techniques are described in detail in the textbooks previously mentioned. They attempt in different ways to record and analyse loads on the body during work. Two better known methods are Posture Targeting and Ovako Working Postures Analysing System (OWAS).[111] Another method recently developed especially for the assessment of loads on the upper limbs is called Rapid Upper Limb Assessment (RULA). This method is easy to use and is described in detail, along with worksheets and score cards.[109]

Symptom Recording

Body charts are a practical method for collecting information about symptoms of neck and upper-extremity disorders in the workplace.

Although specific conditions of the neck and upper extremities have been identified as being associated with particular types of work, growing numbers of workers, especially those engaged in so-called "light," highly repetitive work, such as VDT operators, are complaining of ill-defined symptom complexes, the causes of which are not yet fully determined. These conditions are seldom adequately defined or described; however, many may be manifestations of local muscle fatigue and overload of related structures. Others appear to result from postural overloading, particularly of the neck, and may involve referred symptoms. In the absence of specific diagnoses, the delineation of these conditions can be aided by the use of body charts that a worker or clinician may complete.

Body charts have enabled researchers and those concerned with control of musculoskeletal disorders in the workplace to gain a clearer picture of symptom patterns and their prevalence without having to categorize them as medical conditions. Further, it has enabled a systematic approach to the prevention of such disorders by identifying occupational groups with a high prevalence of symptoms in the neck and upper extremities, and by pinpointing elements of these groups' jobs that may be associated with symptom development.[85,113]

Functional Capacity Assessments

Mismatches often occur between the demands of a job and the worker's capacity to undertake the work safely. Therefore, medical practitioners and physical therapists must understand in some detail the demands of various tasks (workload measurement or assessment) and the capabilities of individual workers to perform these tasks (assessment of functional capacity), and must appreciate that these capabilities are likely to change over time.

In cases in which particular work puts unreasonable demands on workers, it is vital that advice be given on how risks of injury can be reduced through better workplace layout or design, more adequate training, or more efficient work organization. Consideration will have to be given to modification of work to accommodate individuals with reduced physical capacity. As a last resort it may be necessary to advise people who are physically unsuited for certain work against undertaking that work and seeking a less demanding job.

Specific Task Training and Education in Ergonomics

Most jobs can be done in a variety of ways and one way will usually be less stressful and fatiguing than others. It is important that the most efficient methods be identified for each job, and that these methods be taught only to new employees and those learning a new job or using new equipment. Even with training, however, employees may slip into inefficient practices, and these should be monitored and corrected by on-the-job supervision.

For the development of correct work techniques and postures, together with training and on-the-job supervision, supervisors should be consulted to help define these factors. Wherever possible, training should be organized and run by a training officer or someone else skilled in teaching others.

Education is an especially important aspect of ergonomics. If money, time, and expertise are used to produce an ergonomically sound workplace, then employees should understand why it has been so designed and how it can best be used.

Task Variation and Job Rotation

Task variation or multi-skilling is highly desirable, and can be achieved through job enlargement, which requires careful job and task design to enable a number of different types of activities to be incorporated into a job description; or (less effectively) through job rotation.

Job rotation is a ready way of spreading the load of particularly stressful jobs among a large group of employees, but it does have drawbacks. It works only in settings in which jobs are sufficiently different to provide physical and mental variety. Moreover, many employees do not like rotating for a number of reasons, even when it is in their best interests to do so. Furthermore, job rotation can mask the real causes of the problems created by a particular kind of work, and may only prolong the period before such problems arise. Job rotation also means that employees have to learn more skills, and therefore require more training and supervision. Consequently, rotation should be seen only as a temporary solution while engineering, work design, and organizational problems are being resolved.

Job enlargement (enrichment) is a much more acceptable alternative for providing task variation, but requires careful planning and longer training periods.

Work Rates

Human performance varies between individuals and over time, and work rates should therefore be realistic, accommodating the physical and psychological capacities of the slowest workers. This is particularly important in machine-paced work.

Minimizing Aggravating Factors

Organizational difficulties of various kinds can arise in any enterprise. Mechanical and technical breakdowns and inefficiencies can have a disruptive effect on employees, and usually involve periods of extra load to make up production or output. Poor quality control may require reworking of a product or product component without additional productivity. Therefore, machine and equipment adjustment and maintenance are most important in the smooth and efficient operation of any system. Other organizational factors, such as the need for overtime, shift work, and peak loading, as well as bonus payment and other incentive schemes, often require higher outputs than the employees of an organization can safely manage, and should be avoided with careful planning.

Pause Exercises

Pause exercises (pause gymnastics), originally a Scandinavian concept,[114] are increasingly gaining acceptance in other countries.[115] They are rhythmic, free, or set movements performed during the working day to help alleviate the effects of fixed work postures and repetitive movements. They usually include a series of full-range movements, sometimes done to music, designed to meet the needs of particular working groups. Set movements should vary from time to time to avoid boredom, and should be performed moderately slowly and carefully to ensure maximum benefit. Since the nature of work varies a great deal from time to time and between different groups of people, pause exercise movements should be designed to take this into account. They should be supervised initially and at regular intervals by a professional trained in anatomy and exercise physiology, such as a physical therapist. Such a person can also ensure that movements are performed correctly, and can identify individual difficulties so that they can be investigated and treated early.

Pause exercises programs aim to:

Encourage changes of posture from those adopted for the majority of the work day.
Strengthen and stretch muscles that might be weak or tight.
Stimulate circulation and help reduce feelings of fatigue at the end of the working day.

A comprehensive review of the safety and effectiveness of a range of exercise programs for VDT/office workers has recently been published.[116]

Work Pauses

The importance of pauses during physical activity is widely acknowledged. Although there is little information about the benefits of work pauses, there is sufficient evidence to suggest that they are essential in certain tasks in order to avoid unnecessary fatigue.[117,118] They can be self-regulated or fixed and supervised, but to be effective their duration and frequency must be appropriate to the levels of activity and fatigue experienced by the persons using them. For example, more frequent, longer breaks may be required at the end of a day or a week, and the system must be flexible in order to accommodate different circumstances. Individually regulated breaks are the most desirable, but workers often have to be encouraged to pause from work even when they are tired. They must be positively discouraged from accumulating breaks.

Pause exercises and regulated work pauses are only temporary solutions in alleviating the effects of fixed, repetitive, or demanding work. In the long-term, work should be designed to allow variation in tasks and movements, and regular pauses throughout the day.

Evaluation of Prevention Programs

As mentioned above, a number of publications produced by government agencies,[102–108] universities,[109] and journals[110] address the prevention, control, and management of neck and upper limb disorders. All deal with the identification of potentially harmful workloads; methods for measuring these workloads and/or assessing their impact; and control or prevention procedures suitable for different types of work. Nearly all of these publications recommend monitoring of the effectiveness of such prevention programs, although the criteria for monitoring are not discussed. Methods by which a formal evaluation of quite extensive programs might be undertaken have not been addressed at all in any of the publications, and this seems to be a glaring oversight. When so many resources and so much time can be devoted to controlling these disorders, it would seem important to build some sort of evaluation into a prevention program, if only to help sell it to increasingly cost-conscious managers.

Some attempts have been made to evaluate the outcome of programs for preventing neck and upper extremity disorders, the most notable of which was undertaken in Norway and included a cost-benefit analysis.[119] In 1975, an intervention study was initiated in a Norwegian electronics factory in response to an unusually high rate of sick leave in the preceding 2 years, and increasing complaints of musculoskeletal disorders of the upper limb, neck, shoulder, and back.[120] This study attempted to respectively discover the reasons for the increasing rates of complaints and to evaluate the impact of ergonomic changes undertaken at the factory from 1975 onward.

It proved more difficult to argue that the ergonomic changes led directly to a reduction in musculoskeletal disorders than to show that the former work situations at the factory contributed to the occurrence of the disorders. Nevertheless, there was evidence that the changes had a positive influence on health and were associated with decreasing complaints of symptoms. However, a more recent study of assembly workers in Sweden demonstrated the effectiveness of instruction in correct work techniques to new workers in reducing the numbers of days lost through arm-neck-shoulder complaints.[51] This highlights an important area that has had little attention in the literature, namely, the beneficial effects of training and education of workers, supervisors, and managers in what they can do for themselves to control musculoskeletal disorders arising from work.

A group of investigators in the United States attempted with some degree of success to establish an intervention program in a manufacturing industry.[121] Although the statistical analyses were never reported, complaints of disorders appeared to decrease, while the productivity in some jobs increased significantly. The changes implemented by the program included organizational rearrangements, such as the introduction of job rotation in selected areas and the provision of gloves to some workers; and engineering controls, such as the introduction of rotatable jigs and suspended tool retractors, and the redesign of components. Many of the researchers' recommendations were rejected as being not feasible, but some of the easier, less costly changes were made. In addition to this, some workers modified or redesigned tools that helped decrease injuries and increase productivity. Generally, the changes that proved most successful were those in which the front line supervisor participated and acted upon recommendations.

More recently, an American company reported in a commercial newsletter on a program that is applying the OSHA Guidelines for Meatpacking Plants[108] to a baking company. However, while it seems that the response to the program has been positive, no evaluation has been undertaken at this stage. A common feature of intervention programs such as this is occupational health professionals' interest and participation in them. In the program described above, these professionals provided statistical and epidemiologic surveillance of injuries and complaints, and thereby provided the mechanism by which the success of the program could be measured, however imprecisely.

The difficulties of measuring the effects of changes in ergonomics or of any preventive health care program in the workplace are not insurmountable, but it is impossible to eliminate the influence of other factors that may alter the way in which people work or perceive their work. In the case of musculoskeletal disorders, part of the problem is related to the "Hawthorne Effect" (a change in performance of subjects merely because they are part of a study), part is related to the ubiquitous and ill-defined nature of the conditions being studied, and part is related to the numerous sources of bias and confounding variables that arise in the workplace. Nevertheless, as increasing numbers of work-related musculoskeletal disorders are reported, there is an urgent need to convincingly demonstrate that certain preventive measures are effective against them.

REHABILITATION

The general concept of medical rehabilitation is of well-established, institutionalized care given by large, multidisciplinary centers and usually associated with mainstream health-care systems. Worker rehabilitation may be included in the services offered by these centers, but only when an injury or illness has become chronic. Specialist on-site worker rehabilitation centers providing occupational health services and funded by employers, or centers funded privately or by the government and located in nearby areas, are now common in many countries. These centers cater to the particular needs of workers to enable them to return to work as early as possible and with a minimum of disability. This involves not only an understanding of occupationally related medical conditions and their treatment, but also a consideration of workplace factors that may have led to a worker's condition and which may have to be modified before a return to work is possible. Such an approach requires liaison with managers and supervisors, and a knowledge of the individual client's work and work process. Consequently, it is desirable for professionals working in occupational health services or worker rehabilitation centers to be trained in occupational health and safety.

In general terms, it may be estimated that a workforce of 300 or more full-time employees in a manufacturing company would justify the employment of a part-time physical therapist, visiting doctor, and full-time occupational health nurse, although this would vary according to the nature of the industry and its occupational health and safety programs.

Worker rehabilitation can be considered as having two stages: therapeutic intervention and vocational rehabilitation.

Therapeutic Intervention

The treatment of many of the conditions listed in Table 18–1 has been detailed in textbooks of physical therapy and medicine, and will not be described here. Injuries at the worksite largely affect the musculoskeletal system and soft tissue, and require attention as soon as possible after they occur. It is preferable that primary care for such injuries occur at the workplace and in accordance with the statutory regulations of relevant legislation, such as occupational health and safety and workers' compensation acts.

An occupational health nurse is the most appropriate person to undertake immediate primary care; where this is not possible, it may be necessary to refer the worker to an appropriate health service. Workers in most countries are not compelled to attend the employer's chosen health service, but may instead attend one of their own choice. This may be a general practitioner or family physician, hospital, community health center, or alternative practitioner such as a chiropractor or acupuncturist. Whatever the choice, it is preferable that the practitioner have some training and/or experience in occupational health and safety. Physical therapy, occupational therapy, and medical review may follow immediate primary care.

Vocational Rehabilitation

The objective of vocational rehabilitation is the return of the injured worker to as full and productive a life as possible from an occupational point of view. The realization of this objective is a multifaceted process including attention to therapeutic rehabilitation and activities of daily living; workplace and job analysis; co-ordination of all medical, legal, and medicolegal activities; administrative and production demands; psychological factors; matters of workers compensation; rehabilitation counseling; vocational assessment; work trial assessment; vocational counseling; job placement; redeployment placement; funded work trials; interaction with other employment and rehabilitation agencies; constant monitoring and documentation of progress; manipulation of criteria for progress; reporting; and other factors.

The injured worker should be referred to a vocational rehabilitation consultant as soon as the worker's medical advisers believe, on medical grounds, that the worker can perform some duties within his or her physical and emotional capacity. This occurs before the worker is fit to return to normal duties. The usual timing of such a referral is within 21 days of a medical assessment in which it is determined that a return to full recovery will be protracted and that it is in the worker's best interests to return to some productive work in the interim period. This may be referred to as ''early referral to a rehabilitation consultant.''

Upon referral, the rehabilitation consultant visits the worker to assess the latter's current physical and emotional status and ability to perform activities of daily living. The consultant confirms this assessment by contacting all health personnel concerned with the worker.

It is important at this stage to establish the worker's remaining employment profile: the summation of the worker's functional capabilities. This is best achieved by using a functional-capacity assessment, which should be undertaken by physical or occupational therapists experienced in such assessments.

The tools and technology for functional-capacity assessment vary tremendously, but some universal criteria are essential, including high validity and reliability; standardized equipment and protocols; ability to assess the level of worker participation; ability to assess workday endurance; and ability to assess static, dynamic, and mobility tolerances; weighted activities, and specific upper limb function in terms of frequency, duration, and intensity.

This is followed by a job analysis at the workplace to assess whether the worker can return to the duties previously performed. Should normal duties not be appropriate, alternative duties will have to be found. These may be of a transitional nature, thereby allowing the worker to undertake certain duties for short periods.

It is the rehabilitation consultant's responsibility to recommend suitable modifications in the workplace to the worker's employer, and to ensure that these modifications are made, in order to avoid exacerbation of the worker's pre-existing condition or the creation of a new injury. These changes include those of an ergonomic nature, with particular attention to the biomechanical aspects of work methods, and those of an administrative nature, including work flow and incentive schemes. In this way, the rehabilitation consultant is responsible for actively preventing injury within the workplace.

A successful return to work will depend on the consultant's manipulating the major criteria of the frequency, duration and intensity of work-related operations. Space does not allow a detailed consideration of these criteria, but they can be manipulated in a variety of ways. The method of performing duties is modified in accordance with the categories set out above. In this way, using the example cited earlier in the chapter, a keyboard operator would be instructed in correct task performance in order to avoid particular forms of pathomechanical operation. For example, postures will be corrected to avoid postural overload syndromes, techniques will be modified to avoid overuse syndromes, and so on. The worker will return to work after the medical advisor has issued an appropriate certificate permitting such duties as are set out in a rehabilitation plan prepared by the rehabilitation consultant. The rehabilitation consultant will attend the workplace at the time the worker returns to work, so as to supervise the induction. The program will be recorded and given to the worker, the medical advisers, the employer, the worker's legal representatives, and any other personnel necessary for the smooth management of the program. The program will be modified according to the criteria previously outlined, at times coincidentally with the medical review of the worker. In this way the person responsible for certifying the worker's fitness to perform certain duties will be informed prospectively of the changes to be made in the rehabilitation program as progress is achieved. Ideally, this should also permit the worker to progress through a program of transitional alternative duties to normal duties, although in some cases the progression may be permanently to alternative duties.

The process described above takes place under the watchful eye of the rehabilitation consultant, who monitors progress and documents changes in the program. It is necessary for the consultant to regularly review the worksite situation.

Success in the occupational placement of injured workers is directly related to the time of their referral. Early referral should be considered mandatory, since it has been shown that when a worker's final recovery will be protracted, and the worker can perform some physical duties, the earlier the referral the better the outcome of both treatment and placement.

The interaction between those who provide vocational and those who provide therapeutic rehabilitation is not only essential, but is the most efficient and effective way of ensuring a comprehensive return-to-work program for an injured worker.

REFERENCES

1. Nachemson AL: Models of prevention-early care programmes. p. 27. In: Abstracts of the Second International Conference on Musculoskeletal Injuries in the Workplace. Copenhagen, May 27–29, 1986
2. Occupational Safety and Health Administration (OSHA), U.S. Department of Labor. Federal Register/Proposed Rules. 57:149, August 3, 1992
3. Westgaard RH, Aarås A: Static muscle load and illness among workers doing electro-mechanical assembly work. A report. Institute of Work Physiology, Oslo, 1980
4. Westgaard RH, Aarås A: Postural muscle strain as a causal factor in the development of musculo-skeletal illnesses. Appl Ergonom 15:162, 1984
5. Kilbom Å: Occupational disorders of the musculoskeletal system. Newsletter of

the National Board of Occupational Safety and Health 4/82, 1/83: p. 6, Stockholm, 1983

6. Ramazzini B: DeMorbis Artificum. (Diseases of Workers) 1713. Wright WC (Trans). University of Chicago Press, Chicago, 1940
7. Ferguson D: An Australian study of telegraphists' cramp. Br J Ind Med 28:280, 1971
8. Hunter D: Health in Industry. Penguin, London, 1959
9. Blood W: Tenosynovitis in industrial workers. Br Med J (Clin Res) 2:468, 1942
10. Flowerdew RE, Bode OB: Tensosynovitis in untrained farm workers. Br Med J (Clin Res) 2:637, 1942
11. Howard NJ: Peritendinitis crepitans. A muscle-effort syndrome. J Bone Joint Surg 19:447, 1937
12. Reed JV, Harcourt AK: Tenosynovitis: an industrial disability. Am J Surg 62:392, 1943
13. Smiley JA: The hazards of rope making. Br J Ind Med 8:265, 1951
14. Thompson AR, Plewes LW, Shaw EG: Peritendinitis crepitans and simple tenosynovitis: A clinical study of 544 cases in industry. Br J Ind Med 8:150, 1951
15. Conn HR: Tenosynovitis. Ohio State Med J 27:713, 1931
16. Van Wely P: Design and disease. Appl Ergonom 1:262, 1970
17. Herberts P, Kadefors R: A study of painful shoulders in welders. Acta Orthop Scand 47:381, 1976
18. Carlsöö S, Mayr J: A study of the load on joints and muscles in work with a pneumatic hammer and a bolt gun. Scand J Work Environ Health 11:32, 1974
19. Komoike Y, Horiguchi S: Fatigue assessment on key punch operators, typists and others. Ergonomics 4:101, 1971
20. Onishi N, Nomura H, Sakai K: Fatigue and strength of upper limb muscles of flight reservation system operators. J Hum Ergol (Tokyo) 2:133, 1973
21. Nishiyama K, Nakaseko M, Hosokawa M: Cash register operators' work and its hygienical problems in supermarket. Sangyo Igaku 15:229, 1973
22. Ohara H, Aoyama H, Itani T: Health hazard among cash register operators and the effects of improved working conditions. J Hum Ergol (Tokyo) 5:31, 1976
23. Onishi N, Nomura H, Sakai K et al: Shoulder muscle tenderness and physical features of female industrial workers. J Hum Ergol (Tokyo) 6:87, 1976
24. Onishi N, Sakai K, Itani T et al: Muscle load and fatigue of film rolling workers. J Hum Ergol (Tokyo) 6:179, 1976.
25. Ono Y, Masuda K, Iwata M et al: Fatigue and health problems of workers in a home for mentally and physically handicapped persons. Proceedings of the Eighth International Ergonomics Association Congress. p. 158. Tokyo, 1982
26. Nakaseko M, Tokunaga R, Hosokawa M: History of occupational cervicobrachial disorder in Japan. J Hum Ergol (Tokyo) 11:7, 1982
27. Maeda K: Concept and criteria of occupational cervicobrachial disorder in Japan. Proceedings of Seminar on Ergonomics and Repetitive Tasks, Nordic Council of Ministers. Helsinki, October 19–23, 1981
28. Maeda K, Horiguchi S, Hosokawa H: History of the studies on occupational cervicobrachial disorder in Japan and remaining problems. J Hum Ergol (Tokyo) 11: 17, 1982
29. Perrott JW: Anatomical factors in occupational trauma. Med J Aust 1:73, 1961
30. Peres NJC: Process work without strain. Australian Factory, July, 1, 1961
31. Ferguson D: Repetition injuries in process workers. Med J Aust 2:408, 1971
32. Ferguson D, Duncan J: A study of the effect of equipment design on posture. Scientific Proceedings of the Australian and New Zealand Society of Occupational Medicine. Melbourne, p. 56, October 1972

33. Duncan J, Ferguson D: Keyboard operating posture and symptoms in operating Ergonomics 17:651, 1974
34. Ferguson D: Posture, aching and body build in telephonists. J Hum Ergol (Tokyo) 5:183, 1976
35. Ferguson D, Duncan J: A trial of physiotherapy for symptoms in keyboard operating. Aust J Physiother 22:61, 1976
36. Repetition Strain Injury in the Australian Public Service. Task Force Report. Australian Government Publishing Service. Canberra, 16, 1985
37. Worksafe Australia: Repetition Strain Injury (RSI). A Report and Model Code of Practice. Australian Government Publishing Service. Canberra, 1986
38. Stone W. Occupational repetition strain injuries. Aust Fam Physician 13:9, 1984
39. Winkel J, Westgaard R: Occupational and individual risk factors for shoulder-neck complaints. I: Guidelines for the practitioner. Int J Indust Ergonom 10:79, 1992
40. Winkel J, Westgaard R: Occupational and individual risk factors for shoulder-neck complaints. II: The scientific basis (literature review) for the guide. Int J Indust Ergonom 10:85, 1992
41. Kuorinka I, Koskinen P: Occupational rheumatic diseases and upper limb strain in manual jobs in a light mechanical industry. Scand J Work Environ Health 5, suppl. 3:39, 1979
42. Herberts P, Kadefors R, Andersson G et al: Shoulder pain in industry: an epidemiological study on welders. Acta Orthop Scand 52:299, 1981
43. Kvarnstrom S: Occurrence of musculoskeletal disorders in a manufacturing industry with special attention to occupational shoulder disorders. Scand J Rehabil Med, suppl. 8:1, 1983
44. Kvarnstrom S: Diseases of the musculo-skeletal system in an engineering company. Scand J Rehabil Med, suppl. 8:61, 1983
45. Kvarnstrom S: Occupational cervicobrachial disorders in an engineering company. Scand J Rehabil Med, suppl. 8:77, 1983
46. Kvarnstrom S: Occupational cervicobrachial disorder—a case-control study. Scand J Rehabil Med, suppl. 8:101, 1983
47. Silverstein BA, Fine LJ, Armstrong TJ: Hand-wrist cumulative trauma disorders in industry. Br J Ind Med 43:779, 1986
48. Silverstein BA, Fine LJ, Armstrong TJ: Occupational factors and carpal tunnel syndrome. Am J Ind Med 11:343, 1987
49. Christensen H: Muscle activity and fatigue in the shoulder muscles of assembly plant employees. Scand J Work Environ Health 12:587, 1986
50. Kilbom Å, Persson J, Jonsson BG. Disorders of the cervicobrachial region among female workers in the electronics industry. Int J Indust Ergonom 1:37, 1986
51. Jonsson BG, Persson J, Kilbom Å: Disorders of the cervicobrachial region among female workers in the electronics industry. Int J Indust Ergonom 3:1, 1988
52. Parenmark G, Engvall B, Malmkvist A-K: Ergonomic on-the-job training of assembly workers. Arm-neck-shoulder complaints drastically reduced amongst beginners. Appl Ergonom 19:143, 1988
53. Ohlsson K, Attewell R, Skerfving S: Self-reported symptoms in the neck and upper limbs of female assembly workers. Scand J Work Environ Health 15:75, 1989
54. Armstrong TJ, Foulke J, Joseph B et al: Investigation of cumulative trauma disorders in a poultry processing plant. Am Ind Hyg Assoc J 43:103, 1982
55. Viikari-Juntura E: Neck and upper limb disorders among slaughterhouse workers. Scand J Work Environ Health 9:283, 1983
56. Falck B, Arnio P: Left-sided carpal tunnel syndrome in butchers. Scand J Work Environ Health 9:291, 1983

57. Roto P, Kivi P: Prevalence of epicondylitis and tenosynovitis among meatcutters. Scand J Work Environ Health 10:203, 1984
58. Streib EW, Sun SF: Distal ulnar neuropathy in meat packers. J Occup Med 26: 842, 1984
59. Finkel ML: The effects of repeated mechanical trauma in the meat industry. Am J Ind Med 8:375, 1985
60. Magnusson M, Ortengren R, Andersson G et al: An ergonomic study of work methods and physical disorders among professional butchers. Appl Ergonom 18: 43, 1987
61. Magnusson M, Ortengren R: Investigation of optimal table height and surface angle in meatcutting. Appl Ergonom 18:146, 1987
62. Luopajärvi T, Kuorinka I, Virolainen M et al: Prevalence of tenosynovitis and other injuries of the upper extremities in repetitive work. Scand J Work Environ Health 5, suppl. 3:48, 1979
63. Punnett L, Robins JM, Wegman DH et al: Soft tissue disorders in the upper limbs of female garment workers. Scand J Work Environ Health 11:417, 1985
64. Brisson C, Vinet A, Vezina M et al: Effect of duration of employment in piecework on severe disability among female garment workers. Scand J Work Environ Health 15:329, 1989
65. Sokas RK, Spiegelman D, Wegman DH: Self-reported musculoskeletal complaints among garment workers. Am J Ind Med 15:197, 1989
66. Westgaard RH, Janus T: Individual and work-related factors associated with symptoms of musculoskeletal complaints. II: Different risk factors among sewing machine operators. Br J Ind Med 49:154, 1992
67. Maeda K, Hünting W, Grandjean E: Localised fatigue in accounting machine operators. J Occup Med 22:810, 1980
68. Hünting W, Grandjean E, Maeda K: Constrained postures in accounting machine operators. Appl Ergonom 11:145, 1980
69. Hünting W, Laubli T, Grandjean E: Postural and visual loads at BDT workplaces. I: Constrained postures. Ergonomics 24:917, 1981
70. Nishiyama K, Nakaseko M, Hosokawa M: Cash register operators' work and its hygienical problems in supermarket. Sangyo Igaku 15:229, 1973
71. Ohara H, Aoyama H, Itani T: Health hazard among cash register operators and the effects of improved working conditions. J Hum Ergol (Tokyo) 5:31, 1976
72. Margolis W, Kraus J: The prevalence of carpal tunnel syndrome symptoms in female supermarket checkers. J Occup Med 12:953, 1987
73. Smith M, Cohen B, Stammerjohn L: An investigation of health complaints and job stress in video display operations. Hum Factors 23:387, 1981
74. Grandjean E, Hünting W, Nishiyama K: Preferred VDT workstation setting, body posture and physical impairments. J Hum Ergol 11:45, 1982
75. Grandjean E, Hünting W, Piderman M: VDT workstation design: preferred settings and their effects. Hum Factors 25:161, 1983
76. Grandjean E: Postures and the design of VDT workstations. Behav Informat Technol 3:301, 1984
77. Kukkonen R, Luopajärvi T, Riihimaki V: Prevention of fatigue among data entry operators. p. 28. In Kvalseth TO (ed): Ergonimics of Workstation Design. Butterworths, London, 1983
78. Ong CN: VDT workplace design and physical fatigue: a case study in Singapore. p. 484. In Grandjean E (ed): Ergonomics and Health in Modern Offices. Taylor and Francis, London, 1984

79. Sauter SL: Predictors of strain in VDT-users and traditional office workers. p. 129. In Grandjean E (ed): Ergonomics and Health in Modern Offices. Taylor and Francis, London, 1984
80. Björkstén M: Musculoskeletal disorders among medical secretaries. p. 31. Abstracts of the XXI International Occupational Health Congress. Dublin, September 9–14, 1984
81. Hagberg M, Sundelin G: Discomfort and load on the upper trapezius muscle when operating a word processor. Ergonomics 29:1637, 1986
82. Rossignol A Morse E Summers V et al: Video display terminal use and reported health symptoms among Massachusetts clerical workers. J Occup Med 29:112, 1987
83. Jeyaratnam J, Ong CN, Kee WC et al: Musculoskeletal symptoms among VDU operators. In Smith MJ, Salvendy G (eds): Work with Computers: Organizational, Management, Stress and Health Aspects. Elsevier Science Publishers, Amsterdam, 1989
84. Linton SJ, Kamwendo K: Risk factors in the psychosocial work environment for neck and shoulder pain in secretaries. J Occup Med 31:609, 1989
85. McPhee BJ: Musculoskeletal complaints in workers engaged in repetitive work in fixed postures. p. 51. In Bullock M (ed): Ergonomics. The Physiotherapist in the Workplace. Churchill Livingstone, Edinburgh, 1990
86. Kamwendo K, Linton SJ, Mortiz U: Neck and shoulder disorders in medical secretaries. Scand J Rehabil Med 23:57, 1991
87. Wells JA, Zipp JF, Schuette PT et al: Musculoskeletal disorders among letter carriers. J Occup Med 25:814, 1983
88. Jørgensen K, Fallentin N, Sidenius B: The strain on the shoulder and neck muscles during letter sorting. Int J Indust Ergonom 3:243, 1989
89. Fry HJH: Overuse syndrome of the upper limb in musicians. Med J Aust 144:4, 182, 1985
90. Welch R: The measurement of physiological predisposition to tenosynovitis. Ergonomics 16:665, 1973
91. Welch R: The causes of tenosynovitis in industry. Ind med 41:16, 1972
92. Workers' Compensation Act of South Australia. Section 9. 1971
93. Cyriax J: Textbook of Orthopaedic Medicine. 7th Ed. Vol. 1 Bailliere Tindall, London, 1978
94. Grieve, GP: Common Vertebral Joint Problems. Churchill Livingstone, Edinburgh, 1981
95. Watson-Jones R: Fractures and Joint Injuries, Churchill Livingstone, Edinburgh, 1962
96. Holh M: Soft tissue neck injuries. p. 282. In The Cervical Spine Research Society Editorial Sub-Committee (eds): The Cervical Spine. JP Lippincott, Philadelphia, 1983
97. Millender LH, Louis DS, Simmons BP (eds): Occupational Disorders of the Upper Extremity. Churchill Livingstone, New York, 1992
98. Fry HJH: Overuse syndrome of the upper limb in musicians. Med J Aust 144:4, 182, 1985
99. Astrand PO, Rohdahl K: Physiological bases of exercise, p. 118. In: Textbook of Work Physiology. 2nd Ed. McGraw-Hill, New York, 1977
100. Kjelberg A, Wickstrom B: Whole-body vibration; exposure time and acute effects—a review. Ergonomics 28:3, 535, 1985
101. Browne CD, Nolan BM, Faithfull DK: Occupational repetition strain injuries. Guidelines for diagnosis and management. Med J Aust 3:329, 1984

102. Worksafe Australia: National Code of Practice for the Prevention and Management of Occupational Overuse Syndrome. Australian Government Publishing Service, Canberra, 1990 (First published 1986)

103. Worksafe Australia: Guidance Note for the Prevention Occupational Overuse Syndrome in Keyboard Employment. Australian Government Publishing Service, Canberra, 1989

104. Worksafe Australia: Guidance Note for the Prevention Occupational Overuse Syndrome in the Manufacturing Industry. Australian Government Publishing Service, Canberra, 1992

105. New Zealand Department of Labour: Occupational Overuse Syndrome: Guidelines for Prevention. OS&H, Department of Labour, Wellington, 1991

106. New Zealand Department of Labour: Occupational Overuse Syndrome. Treatment and Rehabilitation. A Practitioner's Guide. OS&H, Department of Labour, Wellington, 1992

107. Health and Safety Executive (UK): Work Related Upper Limb Disorders—A Guide to Prevention. Her Majesty's Stationery Office, London, 1990

108. US Department of Labor (Occupational Safety and Health Administration): Ergonomics Program Management Guidelines for Meatpacking Plants. 1991 (Reprinted)

109. McAtamney L, Corlett EN: Reducing the Risks of Work Related Upper Limb Disorders. A Guide and Methods. Institute for Occupational Ergonomics, University of Nottingham, UK, 1992

110. Luopajärvi T: Ergonomic analysis of workplace and postural load. p. 51. In Bullock M (ed): Ergonomics. The Physiotherapist in the Workplace. Churchill Livingstone, Edinburgh, 1990

111. Wilson JR, Corlett EN: Evaluation of Human Work. Taylor and Francis, London, 1990

112. Kuorinka I, Jonsson B, Kilbom Å et al: Standardised Nordic questionnaires for the analysis of musculoskeletal symptoms. Appl Ergonom 18:233, 1987

113. McPhee B: Report to the National Health and Medical Research Council on a Travelling Fellowship. Commonwealth Institute of Health, Sydney, 1980

114. Gore A, Tasker D: Pause Gymnastics. CCH, Sydney, 1986

115. Lee K, Swanson N, Sauter S et al: A review of physical exercises recommended for VDT operators. Appl Ergonom 23:387, 1992

116. Rohmert W: Problems of determining rest allowances. I: Appl Ergonom 4:91, 1973

117. Rohmert W: Problems of determining rest allowances. II: Appl Ergonom 4:158, 1973

118. Spilling S, Eitrheim J, Aaråas A: Cost benefit analysis of work environments. Investment at STK's telephone plant at Kongsvinger. In Corlett EN, Wilson J, Manenica I (eds): The Ergonomics of Working Postures. Taylor and Francis, London, 1986

119. Westgaard RH, Aaråas A: The effect of improved workplace design on the development of work-related musculoskeletal illnesses. Appl Ergonom 16:91, 1985

120. McGlothlin JD, Armstrong TJ, Fine LJ, et al: Can job changes initiated by a joint labor-management task force reduce the prevalence and incidence of cumulative trauma disorders of the upper extremity? p. 336. Proceedings of the 1984 International Conference on Occupational Ergonomics. Toronto, 1984

121. King B: Strategies to combat carpal tunnel syndrome. Ed Welch on Workers' Compensation. (bimonthly newletter, undated) East Lansing, Michigan, 1992

19 | Manual Therapy: Science, Art, and Placebo

Ruth Grant

MANUAL THERAPY-THROWING DOWN THE GAUNTLET

In his editorial in the special issue of *Physical Therapy* on manual therapy (December, 1992), Jules Rothstein wrote very critically of manual therapy.[1] He stated that although manual therapy for the management of musculoskeletal problems had become a part of the curriculum of every physical therapy program in the United States, and "for some the raison d'etre for much of their practice," it has stayed the same. Manual therapy, said Rothstein, "is still primarily justified by arguments based on anatomy and by the testimony of true believers, experts of varying credentials. In the many years since I first learned techniques of manual therapy," he added, "there has been little maturation and very little scientific development in this area. It has been as if popular opinion precluded the necessity of research and refinement."[1]

Strong words indeed. We cannot, however, let them pass without critical reflection. What might be an agreed index of the maturation of manual therapy? The critical evaluation of assumptions underlying the practice of manual therapy and the commitment to share this critical evaluation with the professional community. One indication of such maturation is the growing body of literature and the growing debate about the ability of manual therapists of whatever persuasion to reliably detect "stiffness" in a spinal segment, and to describe such altered compliance.[2-4] Manual examination of spinal joints is a key component of the manual therapist's physical diagnosis of joint dysfunction in patients with spinal pain. But what are the cues that signal dysfunction to the manual therapist, and how reliable are therapists in using such cues? How accurate are manual therapists at selecting the pathognomonic segment when assessed against a "gold standard"?

Clinically, the cues that manual therapists use to differentiate a pathognomonic from an asymptomatic spinal segment are a combination of abnormal displacement, abnormal tissue resistance to displacement, and the provocation of pain by the testing procedure.[5] As with all reliability studies, intra-therapist reliability of passive intervertebral movement has been shown to be better than inter-therapist reliability.[2,6,7,8] Indeed, where "stiffness" or altered compliance alone has been assessed, results have been poor, and certainly less reliable than when pain provocation has been taken alone or in combination with other factors when reaching a clinical decision.[2,4] Matyas and Bach[2] and Maher and Latimer[4] have proposed that manual therapists rely upon the provocation of pain by a specific testing procedure (namely, verbal pain cues from the patient), and that it is these cues that account for the ability of manual therapists to detect the pathognomonic segment. Maher and Latimer have gone even further, arguing for a major reliance on pain cues in manual examination of the spine, given that changes in tissue compliance and their recognition by therapists have proven to have poor reliability. However, a major reliance on pain cues is also fraught with the danger of false positive findings in assessing the pathognomonic segment in patients with spinal pain, given the widespread pain and referred tenderness common to many patients with spinal pain.

Jull and colleagues[9] have therefore tested the hypothesis that pain provocation on manual palpation is one, but not the only cue to a spinal source of pain. These authors posed the question "can a manual therapist detect and differentiate symptomatic segmental dysfunction from asymptomatic spinal segments without any knowledge or reliance upon the subject's report of pain provocation during the manual testing procedure?" A single-blind study of cervical joint dysfunction in 12 patients with post-concussional headache and a normal control group constituted their study sample. The results showed that when the examiner rated a joint as normal and painless, the subject agreed that it was painless in 98 percent of cases. Furthermore, there was 94 percent agreement for the presence of painful joint dysfunction between the manual therapist and the subjects. This important study therefore does not support the contention of Matyas and Bach and Maher and Latimer that reliance on a verbal report of pain is required[2,4] and demonstrates that mechanical variables in tissue stiffness, in the form of abnormal displacement and abnormal tissue resistance to displacement, can be detected and related to symptomatology.

Critical evaluation of manual palpation has also given rise to the development of instrumentation for measuring the mechanical properties of the spine in vivo. Specifically, instrumentation that simulates the postero-anterior glide of the spinal motion segment has been developed by manual therapists in association with bioengineers.[10-12] This has enabled manual therapists not only to delineate that manual examination is a measure of the mechanical properties of the viscoelastic tissues of the spinal motion segment, but also that increased muscle activity (as determined by electromyography) may at least partly explain the increase in postero-anterior tissue stiffness observed clinically in patients with low back pain on manual examination.[12]

Experimental and case studies suggest that manual examination is a reliable method for detecting the segment at fault in patients with spinal pain.[5,13-15] But how accurate are manual therapists at selecting the pathognomonic segment when assessed against a gold standard? The results of the following two studies are most instructive. In both cases the gold standard was a spinal anaesthetic block used to determine the pathognomonic segment. In the cervical spine, Jull and colleagues[5] showed a 100 percent accuracy in selecting the intervertebral segment responsible for the patient's symptoms (n = 21), and in the lumbar spine in a prospective study of 15 patients, Phillips and Twomey[16] also reported 100 percent accuracy in determining the pathognomonic segment.

This brief overview of research on manual palpation has been presented to indicate the maturation and scientific development that is occurring in this area of manual therapy.

We need to guard against negativity in evaluations of research in physical therapy, and against a devaluing of papers based on clinical deductions. Constructive criticism is invaluable and stimulating, while negativity stifles growth, divides people, and drains confidence. We must encourage our experienced clinicians, our lateral thinkers, and our "armchair theorists" to express themselves, knowing that ideas, theories, or models may only be partially formulated when initially shared with others. Furthermore, in casting aspersions on those who best exemplify the art of manual therapy, we need to take care that the clinical theories they espouse are not, as a consequence, given less careful consideration and less critical evaluation than they deserve.

Personal observation, attention to detail, and contemplation or reflection are most important components of the therapist's approach to the management of the patient, and a substantial part of the best literature on physical therapy has dealt with personal observation, from which clinical theories have been derived. Clearly, such an approach is crucial to best practice. If, however, it should become the only source of justification for best professional practice, it falls short of the mark.

It may be said that people who choose such active practice-based avenues of work as physical therapy are often impatient with the notion of theory as the basis of practice. Manual or manipulative physical therapists, both in practice and as postgraduate students, are no different, in that they seek to absorb the kind of information that is "clinically relevant" and can be put to immediate use. Thus, like most practitioners of physical therapy, they are on the lookout for good ideas and new treatment approaches that can be applied immediately to the practice setting. Like most practicing physical therapists also, they are primarily interested in how to effect the desired results and less interested in the theoretical bases for such results.

LINKING ART, THEORY AND CLINICAL REASONING
IN MANUAL THERAPY

If the number of short continuing education courses advertised in physical therapy journals around the world is any guide, the art of manual therapy is very much alive. However, while it might be argued that the art will not be lost, there is no question that it must be refined by clinical reasoning (Ch. 6 exemplifies this) and substantiated by a sound theory and science basis.

But what is theory? Tammivaara and Shepard[17] stated that "Theory is a word encompassing two concepts: contemplation and observation. (The Greek thea, meaning "a viewing," is also the root for theater)." Thus, contend these authors, observation and contemplation give rise to theories or ideas about how things relate.

It could indeed be said that observation and contemplation were and are hallmarks of the work of a number of major clinical contributors to the field of manual therapy. A number of examples follow. As one example, observation and contemplation, reflecting upon experience, led to the theory of irritability of a condition; the theory of grades of movement, their definition and their application, and the theoretical basis for the movement diagram (Maitland[18,19]); for Robin McKenzie,[20] a treatment approach based on the patient's response to repeated movement; and for Brian Edwards,[21] the theory of regular and irregular patterns of movement, with recognizable patterns in patients with mechanical disorders of spinal movement. Sahrmann[22] has proposed a theory of movement system balance and a classification of low back pain syndromes based on spinal alignment, relative flexibility, and the symptom-producing changes in spinal alignment that occur with motion of the extremities.

A number of these theories have been and are being exposed to rigorous scrutiny.

Theories can develop in a number of ways. The ones I have described developed through the additive effects of experience. That is, by reflecting on experience (the contemplation component), it is possible to note patterns that can be developed into systematic ideas about phenomena. Glaser and Strauss[23] were the first to call this kind of theory development "grounded theory". A grounded theory may be defined as "one that is inductively derived from the study of the phenomenon it represents."[24] Glaser and Strauss stressed the importance of theory grounded in reality for the development of a discipline or profession.

Many scientific theories have developed through logical speculation about some problematic situation. By definition, these are not grounded in experience.[17] However, as Louis Pasteur once remarked, "chance favors the prepared mind." Once developed, a theory or system of ideas is subjected to testing in the "real world" and is subsequently refined and redefined. Perhaps one of the best known examples of this process is the gate-control theory of pain as proposed by Melzack and Wall in 1965.[25]

When a treatment does not work as expected, a physical therapist who is aware of the power and usefulness of theory might—after ruling out more immediate causes—ask whether the conditions under which the treatment is supposed to work (i.e., the theory underlying it) have been met.

One of the best known theories in research design—the Hawthorne effect—came about as a result of the conspicuous failure of the hypothesis being tested. This happened between 1927 and 1932 at the Hawthorne factory of the Western Electric Company in the United States. The researchers were investigating the level of lighting in the factory on fatigue and efficiency among the workers. As the study progressed, the researchers discovered that no matter what they did to alter the lighting, production went up and the workers reported being less tired. From this failed experiment arose a powerful theory that Elton Mayo and his colleagues subsequently substantiated: that the knowledge that one is under observation may significantly change one's behavior.[26] This knowledge in effect ushered in the need for a control group in research.

When we are surprised by a clinical problem that does not respond in the way in which we expect, it may be that we have been selectively attentive, having noted only the positive cues in the patient's subjective and physical examination, which fit the particular syndrome we have diagnosed. Schön[27] suggested that such selective attention is evidence that the practitioner may have "over-learned" what she or he knows, thus tending to become narrow, rigid, and prone to burnout.

Practitioner reflection or contemplation can serve to correct such rigidity and over-learning by retracing the steps through which particular features of the patient's problem were built up, in order to find the assumptions that were made. Significantly, this takes us right back to the two concepts fundamental to a definition of theory: contemplation and observation. In clinical practice we are testing theories all the time, yet how often do physical therapists consider their clinical practice in this light?

Schön links art, science and clinical reasoning most tellingly when he sees, as the aim of best practice, "technical problem-solving within a broader context of reflective enquiry where the art of practice . . . is linked to the scientist's art of research."[27]

GROWTH AND DEVELOPMENT IN MANUAL THERAPY—AN ANTIPODEAN VIEW

Let us return to Rothstein's statement that "In the many years since I first learned techniques of manual therapy, there has been little maturation and very little scientific development in this area," and let us take an Antipodean view. Over the two decades that have passed since the introduction of the first Graduate Diplomas in Advanced Manipulative Therapy in South Australia and Western Australia, there has been a dramatic increase in the reporting of research in manual therapy, as evidenced by the number and breadth of research studies published in proceedings of the biennial national conferences of the Manipulative Physiotherapists Association of Australia (MPAA) and the growing number of papers and abstracts of research published in the *Australian Journal of Physiotherapy*.

A fascinating kaleidoscope of the developing emphasis on research in manual therapy is contained in the proceedings of the seven biennial conferences of the MPAA that have taken place since 1978. It is acknowledged that these are non-refereed papers, many of which are only available in these proceedings. Nonetheless, they provide an interesting collage of the growing maturity and scientific basis of manual therapy in Australia. It should also be remembered that in many cases the research work described in these papers was subsequently published elsewhere.

Only one example will be delineated in detail. However, the reader is encouraged to follow to completion, by way of a second example, the development of a model for dynamic stabilization of the lumbar spine.[28–32]

The example delineated is that of the theory of adverse tension in the nervous system. In the early MPAA conference proceedings, the concept of neural tension as an important component that should be considered in the examination of the patient was presented by Maitland[33] with respect of the slump test, while Elvey[34] presented this same concept with respect to the upper limb tension test (ULTT), then referred to as the brachial plexus tension test. Taking the ULTT as the example, the theory of adverse tension was defined more specifically with propositions in terms of anatomy and pathology.[34–36] The theory and the test were further delineated with research into responses in normal subjects.[36] Concomitantly, the discriminative validity and reliability of the test were established[37] and the responses of patient groups delineated.[37,38] The refining of the theory of adverse neural tension has continued through modifications of the ULTT designed to selectively apply tension to neural structures so as to produce, for example, a radial nerve bias. Normal responses were reported and data for patients with tennis elbow were analyzed.[39,40]

Theoretical considerations are now being extended to the sympathetic nervous system. Butler and Slater (see Ch. 15) hypothesize that loss of normal movement and of the tension requirements of the sympathetic nervous system may be another mechanism for sympathetically maintained pain. As a first step in attempting to resolve this issue, Slater and associates[41] have reported "the sympathetic slump" technique for selectively loading the sympathetic trunk. The effects of this maneuver were studied in a randomized, double blind, placebo-controlled study of normal volunteers, employing repeated measures. The loading technique was associated with a significantly greater increase in digital skin conductance as compared to control and placebo procedures, and a significant decrease in digital skin temperature as compared to control values. (These dependent variables were measured via the thumb and index fingers of both hands in the subjects studied).

Concomitant with the later development and testing of the theory of adverse neural tension has been a redefinition, by Butler, of the theoretical basis of adverse tension in the nervous system. The emphasis has moved intraneurally, to a consideration of the ramifications of altered axoplasmic flow in neurons.[42,43] In order to maintain a healthy chemical connection between the cell body, the axon, nerve terminals, and target cells, there normally exists a well-developed axonal transport system. Some human axons are four feet long, traverse mobile parts of the body, encounter tight spaces and tunnels, and receive a different blood supply along the way. Adverse tension in the nervous system presents real potential for altering axoplasmic flow. However, the hypothesis that improvement following manual therapy might be due to a normalization of axoplasmic flow remains to be tested.

THE PLACEBO EFFECT

Although this section will consider the placebo effect "generically," the relevance for manual therapists will be abundantly clear.

Patrick Wall,[44] in an excellent article on the placebo effect, stated that:

> "There are at least four reasons why this subject provokes a shudder of discomfort like a cold hand in the dark. First, the phrase has an aura of quackery, particularly when practitioners have the chutzpah to charge for it. Second, it is seen as a tiresome and expensive artefact which prolongs and complicates the demonstration of the 'true' effect of a therapy. Third, the very mention of the placebo effect is taken as a hostile questioning of the validity of the logic on which a therapy is based. Last and most fundamental, we all trust our sensation as a reflection of objective reality, and yet the placebo changes the sensation without affecting the objective reality. The placebo therefore has an eerie aspect because it seems to shake our belief in the reliability of our sensory experience."

The placebo effect has been studied extensively. Gallimore and Turner,[45] after reviewing 1,500 articles and books on the subject, concluded that the characteristics of the physician (we may read "manual therapist" of whatever persuasion), rather than of the patient, are critical in producing the placebo response. There is evidence that a therapist who shows concern and support, is friendly and reassuring, and conveys expertise and trustworthiness may evoke a strong placebo response.[46-50] This information comes as no surprise to us, and the diminution or relief of pain that accompanies the therapist–patient relationship is in actuality an important aspect of physical therapy and needs to be seen for what it is: communication and the creation of a therapeutic environment that may elicit the physiologic responses expected from application of the treatment procedure itself.

A classic example suffices to illustrate the strength of the placebo response. Hashish and colleagues[51] used a double-blind study to measure swelling, trismus, pain, and serum C-reactive protein (an index of inflammation) before and after treating patients who had had wisdom teeth removed. The 150 patients were assigned to five groups: a control group that received no treatment and four groups that received ultrasound therapy. Three of these patient groups were treated with different dosages of therapeutic pulsed ultrasound (0.1, 0.5, and 1.5 watts/cm^2), while the fourth group was a mock ultrasound group. Wishing to determine the effective dose, the researchers found that the ultrasound machine was effective whether or not it was turned on, provided that both the patient and the therapist believed that it was emitting sound. The importance of the research, however, was that although all of the treatment groups improved as compared to the control group, the mock ultrasound produced better results in all four measures used in the study than did the true ultrasound dosage of 1.5 watt/cm^2. Thus, the placebo treatment significantly changed factors deemed to be local expressions of tissue damage.

Endorphin release has been shown to be a placebo reaction and may assist in explaining these results. However, placebo-mediated endorphin release is by no means the only physiologically induced placebo effect to have been observed. Among those recorded in the literature are improvements in the shape of electrocardiograms, depression of cholesterol levels, control of diabetes, and changes in gastric acidity.[44,50]

What are the ramifications of such findings? Namely, that improvement in the patient's condition following treatment cannot ipso facto be taken as evidence of the accuracy of the theory on which the treatment is based, nor indeed as evidence of the efficacy of the specific technique used. This is thought provoking, and reminds us again of the remarkably strong and indistinguishable links between psyche and soma.

For an informed discussion of the placebo effect (and here I draw heavily on Wall[44]), it is instructive to consider some of the myths surrounding the placebo response. Each of these has been refuted. First, that placebo responders have nothing wrong with them in the first place, "but suffer a somatic hallucination." Second, that there is a fixed fraction (one-third) of the population who respond to placebos. This myth has arisen through the misreading and misquoting of Beecher's classic work of 1955.[52] Wall, in scanning a large series of double-blind studies, showed that the fraction of placebo responses could vary from 0 percent to 100 percent, depending on the circumstances of the trial. A third myth is that placebo responders suffer some personality defect (neurosis, introversion, extroversion, suggestibility) that explains the response. A fourth myth is that giving a placebo is the same thing as doing nothing. Wall has emphasized that the placebo response is a phenomenon quite distinct from spontaneous improvement in a condition.

What are the hypotheses on which the mechanism of the placebo effect is based? Wall has identified three. The first is that the effect results from a decrease in anxiety on the part of the patient. This seems very reasonable but currently lacks validation. The second hypothesis is that the expectation of benefit leads to a "cognitive readjustment of appropriate behaviour." White and colleagues,[53] in their book on the subject, provided considerable evidence that the placebo responder to a particular technique or drug can be identified by simply asking that person what is expected. This applies as much to the therapist (or doctor or nurse) as to the patient. The third hypothesis is that the placebo effect is a classical conditioned Pavlovian response. The work by Voudouris and co-workers[54,55] is used to support this last hypothesis and to illustrate it with an example. In the first stage of these workers' experiments, the tolerance thresholds of normal subjects to iontophoretic pain were established. The subjects' responses were then compared with and without the application of a placebo cream. In one group of subjects the placebo cream was applied and the subjects were informed that it was a powerful analgesic. As expected, some subjects showed placebo responses. In another group the cream was applied and the intensity of the iontophoretic pain stimulus was reduced without the subjects' knowledge. These subjects who had experienced an apparently truly analgesic effect of the cream, subsequently became strong placebo responders.

These results have relevance for research involving placebos, and particularly for studies within subject crossover design. The results suggest that subjects who receive a placebo before the administration of a particular treatment may well not be equivalent to subjects who receive the placebo after the treatment. Voudouris and associates[55] also suggested that their findings may help to explain a worsening of symptoms sometimes observed in chronic pain patients when a variety of short-term palliative treatments are tried and then discontinued.

CONCLUSION

Science, art, and placebo are all important components of manual therapy. The art has been much described and is widely promulgated. If the scientific and theoretical basis of manual therapy is to continue to grow, it is likely that an upsetting of established beliefs will be an integral part of the critical analysis that is now taking place and which must continue to take place. Finally, in the words of Voudouris and co-workers,[55] "until the underlying mechanisms of the placebo response are better understood, our potential for maximizing the effectiveness of all therapies will remain underutilized."

REFERENCES

1. Rothstein JM: Manual therapy: A special issue and a special topic. Phys Ther 72: 839, 1992
2. Matyas TA, Bach TM: The reliability of selected techniques in clinical arthrometrics. Aust J Physiother 31:175, 1985
3. Haas M: The reliability of reliability. J Manip Physiol Ther 14:199, 1991
4. Maher C, Latimer J: Pain or resistance—the manual therapists dilemma. Aust J Physiother 38:257, 1992

5. Jull G, Bogduk N, Marsland A: The accuracy of manual diagnosis for cervical zygapophyseal joint pain syndromes. Med J Aust 148:233, 1988

6. Kaltenborn F, Lindahl O: Reproducerbarheten vid rorelseundersokning av enskilda kotor. Lakartidningen 66:962, 1969

7. Gonnella C, Paris S, Kutner M: Reliability in evaluating passive intervertebral motion. Phys Ther 62:436, 1982

8. Panzer DM: The reliability of lumbar motion palpation, J Manip Physiol Ther 15:518, 1992

9. Jull G, Treleaven J, Versace G: Manual examination of spinal joints: Is pain provocation a major diagnostic cue for dysfunction? Australian Journal of Physiotherapy (in press)

10. Lee M, Svensson N: Measurement of stiffness during simulated spinal physiotherapy. Clin Phys Physiol Measure 11:201, 1990

11. Lee R, Evans J: Load-displacement-time characteristics of the spine under posteroanterior mobilisation. Aust J Physiother 38:115, 1992

12. Shirley D, Lee M: A preliminary investigation of the relationship between lumbar postero-anterior mobility and low back pain. J Manual Manip Ther 1:22, 1993

13. Behrsin J, Andrews F: Lumbar segmental instability: Manual assessment findings supported by radiological assessment. Aust J Physiother 37:171, 1991

14. Janos S, Ray C: Mechanical examination of the lumbar spine and mechanical discography/facet joint injection. p. A92. Proceedings of the International Federation of Orthopaedic Manipulative Therapists Fifth International Conference, Vail, Colorado, 1992

15. Hides JA, Stokes MJ, Saide M et al: Evidence of lumbar multifidus wasting ipsilateral to symptoms in patients with acute/subacute low back pain. Spine 19:105, 1994

16. Phillips DR, Twomey LT: Comparison of manual diagnosis with a diagnosis established by a uni-level lumbar spinal block procedure. p. 55. Proceedings of the Eighth Biennial Conference of the Manipulative Physiotherapists Association of Australia, Perth, November 24–27, 1993

17. Tammivaara J, Shepard KF: Theory: The guide to clinical practice and research. Phys Ther 70:578, 1990

18. Maitland GD: Peripheral Manipulation. 1st Ed. Butterworths, London, 1970

19. Maitland GD: Vertebral Manipulation. 5th Ed. Butterworths, London, 1986

20. McKenzie RA: The Lumbar Spine: Mechanical Diagnosis and Therapy. Spinal Publications, Waikanae, New Zealand, 1981

21. Edwards BC: Manual of Combined Movements. Churchill Livingstone, Edinburgh, 1992

22. Sahrmann SA: Movement as a cause of musculoskeletal pain. p. 69. Proceedings of the Eighth Biennial Conference of Manipulative Physiotherapists Association of Australia, Perth, 1993

23. Glaser B, Strauss A: The Discovery of Grounded Theory. Aldine Publishing Company, Chicago, 1967

24. Strauss A, Corbin J: Basics of Qualitative Research. Sage Publications, Newbury Park, CA, 1991

25. Melzack R, Wall PD: Pain mechanisms: A new theory. Science 150:971, 1965

26. Payton OD: Research: The Validation of Clinical Practice. F.A. Davis, Philadelphia, 1979

27. Schön DA: From technical rationality to reflection-in-action. In Dowie J, Elstein A (eds): Professional Judgement. Cambridge University Press, Cambridge, 1988

28. Jull G, Comerford M, Richardson C: Strategies for the initial activation of dynamic lumbar stabilization. p. 71. Proceedings of the Seventh Biennial Conference of the Manipulative Physiotherapists Association of Australia, Blue Mountains, 1991

29. Jull GA, Richardson CA, Toppenberg R, et al: Towards a measurement of active muscle control for lumbar stabilization. Aust J Physiother 39:187, 1993

30. Richardson C, Toppenberg R, Jull G: An initial evaluation of eight abdominal exercises for their ability to provide stabilization for the lumbar spine. Aust J Physiother 36:6, 1990

31. Richardson C, Jull G, Toppenberg R, Comerford M: Techniques for active lumbar stabilization for spinal protection. Aust J Physiother 38:105, 1992

32. Wohlfahrt D, Jull G, Richardson C: The relationship between the dynamic and static function of the abdominal muscles. Aust J Physiother 39:9, 1992

33. Maitland GD: Movement of pain sensitive structures in the vertebral canal in a group of physiotherapy students. p. 37. Proceedings of the Inaugural Congress of the Manipulative Therapists Association of Australia, Sydney, 1978

34. Elvey R: Abnormal brachial plexus tension signs. p. 67. Proceedings of the Second Biennial Conference of the Manipulative Therapists Association of Australia, Adelaide, 1980

35. Elvey R: The pathophysiology of radiculopathy. p. 406. Proceedings of the Fifth Biennial Conference of the Manipulative Therapists Association of Australia. Melbourne, 1987

36. Kenneally M, Rubenach H, Elvey R: The Upper Limb Tension Test: The SLR test of the arm, p. 167. In Grant R (ed): Physical Therapy of the Cervical and Thoracic Spine. Churchill Livingstone, New York, 1988

37. Selvaratnam PJ, Matyas TA, Glasgow EF: Noninvasive discrimination of brachial plexus involvement in upper limb pain. Spine 19:26, 1994

38. Young L, Bell A: The Upper limb Tension Test Response in a group of post Colles' fracture patients. p. 226. Proceedings of the Seventh Biennial Conference of the Manipulative Therapists Association of Australia, Blue Mountains, 1991

39. Yaxley GA, Jull GA: A modified upper limb tension test: An investigation of responses in normal subjects. Aust J Physiother 37:143, 1991

40. Yaxley GA, Jull GA: Adverse tension in the neural system: A preliminary study of tennis elbow. Aust J Physiother 39:15, 1993

41. Slater H, Wright A, Vicenzino B: Physiological effects of the 'sympathetic slump' on peripheral sympathetic nervous system function. p. 94. Proceedings of the Eighth Biennial Conference of Manipulative Physiotherapists Association of Australia, Perth, 1993

42. Butler DS: Mobilisation of the Nervous System. Churchill Livingstone, Melbourne, 1991

43. Butler DS: Axoplasmic flow and manipulative physiotherapy. p. 206. Proceedings of the Seventh Biennial Conference of the Manipulative Physiotherapists Association of Australia, Blue Mountains, 1991

44. Wall PD: The placebo effect: An unpopular topic. Pain 52:1, 1992

45. Gallimore RG, Turner JL: Contemporary studies of placebo phenomena. In Jarvik ME (ed): Psychopharmacology in the Practice of Medicine. Appleton-Century-Crofts, New York, 1977

46. Lesse S: Placebo reaction in psychotherapy. Dis Nerv Syst 23:313, 1962

47. Liberman R: An analysis of the placebo phenomenon. J Chron Dis 15:761, 1962

48. Shapiro AK: A contribution to a history of the placebo effect. Behav Sci 5:109, 1960

49. Ben-Sira Z: The function of the professionals' affective behaviour in client satisfaction: A revised approach to social interaction theory. J Health Soc Sci 17:3, 1976
50. Gielen F: Discussion of placebo effect in physiotherapy based on a noncritical review of literature. Physiother Can 41:210, 1989
51. Hashish I, Harvey W, Harris M: Anti-inflammatory effects of ultrasound therapy: Evidence for a major placebo effect. Br J Rheumatol 25:77, 1986
52. Beecher HR: The powerful placebo. JAMA 159:1602, 1955
53. White L, Tursky B, Schwarz GE: Placebo: Theory Research and Mechanisms. Guilford Press, New York, 1985
54. Voudouris NJ, Peck GL, Coleman G: Conditioned response models of placebo phenomena. Pain 38:109, 1989
55. Voudouris NJ, Peck GL, Coleman G: The role of conditioning and verbal expectancy in the placebo response. Pain 43:121, 1990

Index

Page numbers followed by an f *indicate figures, and those followed by a* t *indicate tables.*

Abduction tests, shoulder, 211–212, 211f
Abusive use syndromes, work-related, 387t, 389–392
Accessory movements, passive, examination of, 142–143, 248–250
Active movement tests, 124–134
  in cervical headache, 268
  of cervical spine, 126–127, 128f
  combined movements in, 125, 131, 131f
  compression, 133–134
  differentiation of movement in, 124–126
  distraction, 133–134
  extension
    of cervical spine, 128f
    of thoracic spine, 127, 129f
  flexion, of thoracic spine, 127, 129f–130f
  functional provoking activity, 124–126
  neural tensioning procedures with, 131–132
  physiologic movements in, 126–127, 128f–130f, 129
  repeated movements in, 133
  rotation, of thoracic spine, 127, 130f
  speed of movements in, 133
  sustained position in, 132–133, 132f
  symptom provocation in, 133
  of thoracic spine, 127, 129, 129f–130f
Adverse neural tension tests, 95, 134–135.
    See also Upper limb tension test.
  theoretical development of, 414–415
Allodynia, 228
Analgesic use, history of, in subjective examination, 116
Angina pectoris, vs. pain referred from thoracic spine, 84, 85f, 86, 321
Ankylosing spondylitis, pain in, 83
Anteroposterior oscillatory pressures, on joints, 142–143

Anticoagulant therapy, history of, in subjective examination, 116
APA. *See* Australian Physiotherapy Association.
Arachnoid mater, thoracic, pain in, 319
Arm(s)
  crossing behind neck, in hypermobility, 213
  pain in
    in cervical nerve root compression, 308–311
    in zygapophyseal arthropathy, 290
Arthralgia, of zygapophyseal joint, case study of, 294–298, 296f–297f
Arthritis, rheumatoid, of thoracic spine, 83
Arthrokinematics, definition of, 49t
Aspirin therapy, history of, in subjective examination, 116
Atlantoaxial joint
  active movement testing at, 268
  anatomy of, 10–12, 11f, 167–168
  articular surfaces of, 168
  axial rotation of, 29–31, 30t, 34t
  biomechanics of, 29–31, 30t, 34t
  combined movement tests of, 169, 171, 172f–174f, 173
    palpation in, 175, 177, 177f–181f
    treatment based on, 182
  hypermobility of, 31
  innervation of, 67, 67f
  motion of, 29–31, 30t, 37–38, 168
  palpation of, 141, 175, 177, 177f–181f
Atlanto-occipital joint
  active movement testing at, 268
  anatomy of, 7–8, 8f, 167–168
  articular surfaces of, 168
  biomechanics of, 28–29, 28t, 34t

Atlanto-occipital joint *(Continued)*
  combined movement tests of, 168–169,
    169f–171f
    palpation in, 173, 174f–176f, 175
    treatment based on, 181–182
  dislocation of, 8
  innervation of, 67, 67f
  motion of, 28–29, 28t, 37–38, 168
  palpation of, 141, 173, 174f–176f, 175
Atlas. *See also* Atlanto-occipital joint;
    Atlantoaxial joint.
  anatomy of, 7–9, 8f, 11f
  motion of, 29
  palpation of, 141
Australian Physiotherapy Association,
    premanipulative testing protocol of,
    151–157, 152f–153f, 155f
  evaluation of, 157–161, 157t, 158f–160f
  history of, 146
  research on, 161–162
Autonomic nervous system. *See also*
    Sympathetically maintained pain.
  in abnormal pain response, 104, 228–229
Axes of rotation
  of cervical spine, 39–42, 39f–40f, 41t
  in movement system balance, 341–342
Axial rotation
  of atlantoaxial joint, 29–31, 30t, 34t
  of cervical spine, 33–34, 33t–34t
Axillary nerve, testing of, 235
Axis. *See also* Atlantoaxial joint.
  anatomy of, 9–12, 11f
  palpation of, 141
Axoplasmic flow, normalization of, 415

Back pain, work-related, 379–380
Basilar arteries. *See also* Vertebrobasilar
    insufficiency.
  anatomy of, 14
Bending, lateral, of thoracic spine, 55–57,
    55f–57f, 63
Biomechanics
  of cervical spine, 27–45
    atlantoaxial joint, 29–31, 30t
    atlanto-occipital joint, 28–29, 28t
    axial rotation, 33–34, 33t–34t, 39–42,
      39f–40f, 41t
    extension, 32t–33t, 36–38, 36f
    flexion, 32t–33t, 36–38, 36f
    instantaneous axes of rotation, 39–42,
      39f–40f, 41t

  quality of motion, 38
  range of motion, 31–33, 32t, 36–38
  state of the art of, 42–43
  uncinate process function, 34–35,
    35f–37f
  of muscles, 201
  principles of, 27–28
  of shoulder crossed syndrome, 203
  of thoracic spine, 47–64
    degrees of motion of, 48f, 49
    extension, 53–55, 53f–54f, 62
    flexion, 49–52, 50f–52f, 62
    habitual movements, 48f, 49
    lateral bending, 55–57, 55f–57f, 63
    rotation, 58f–61f, 59–62, 63
    terminology of, 49t
    in vitro study of, 48, 48f
Body chart, for work-related symptom
    recording, 395
Butterfly vertebra, 7

Carotid artery system, evaluation of, as
    precaution, 115
Carotid tubercles, of vertebrae, 12
Cartilaginous stage, of spinal development, 4
C1-C2 joint. *See* Atlantoaxial joint.
Centralization, of pain, 365–366, 366f
Central nervous system. *See also* Spinal cord.
  in muscular control, 198–201, 200f
  pain processing in, 227–228
    abnormal, 104
Cervical collar, for discogenic pain, 303
Cervical headache, 261–285
  associated disorders with, 264
  causes of, 261, 266
  history of, 262–263
  medical history in, 265
  onset of, 265, 266
  pain referral in, 22–23
  physical examination of, 266–273
    articular, 267–270, 270f
    combined movements in, 168–169,
      169f–181f, 171, 173
    muscle function, 271–273, 274f
    neural tissues, 270–271
    palpation in, 173, 174f–181f, 175, 177
    posture, 271–273
    vertebral artery, 270
  precipitating factors for, 265
  relieving factors for, 265

subjective examination of, 262–266
symptoms of
area of, 263–264
neurologic, 264–265
quality of, 264
temporal pattern of, 262–263
treatment of, 274–279
for articular dysfunction, 275–276
combined movements in, 181–182
muscle activation and retraining in, 274f,
276–279, 277f–279f
neural tissue mobilization in, 275–276,
276f
trial, 274–275
Cervical manipulative therapy
alternatives to, in vertebrobasilar
insufficiency, 155–157
for cervical headache. *See* Cervical
headache, treatment of.
combined movements in
atlanto-occipital complex, 181–182
atlas-axis complex, 182
lower cervical spine, 193
middle cervical spine, 185–189,
187f–190f, 189, 191
complications of. *See* Vertebrobasilar
insufficiency.
for discogenic pain, 303–306, 304f–307f
for discogenic wry neck, 307
guidelines for, 156
informed consent for, 156, 159, 160f, 161
for mechanical disorders, 374–375
passive movement in, 288–294
diagnosis and, 288
direction of, 291–293
history and, 289–290
intervertebral space widening on one
side, 292
of intervertebral structures, 292–293
joint position for, 291–293
pain avoidance in, 292
pain response in, 289
referred pain in, 292
signs and, 291
stretching tissues in, 292
symptoms and, 290–291
technique performance in, 293–294
technique selection for, 291
for radicular pain, 309–311
simulated, in premanipulation testing, 152,
154, 154f, 162
testing before, 115, 136–137
APA protocol results, 157–162, 157t,
158f–160f
with dizziness history, 152f–153f,
153–155, 155f
historical aspects of, 145–146
physical examination in, 151–155,
152f–153f, 155f
recording results of, 157
subjective examination in, 151
at subsequent visits, 156
symptoms provoked in, 155
technique choice based on, 155–156
vertebrobasilar insufficiency in. *See*
Vertebrobasilar insufficiency.
for wry neck
discogenic, 307
from zygapophyseal joint locking,
299–300
for zygapophyseal joint arthralgia,
295–298, 296f–297f
for zygapophyseal joint locking
acute, 299–300
recurrent, 300
Cervical nerve root compression, 19–20, 20f
case study of, 308–311
in cervical headache, 264–265, 270–271,
275–276, 277f
pain in, 65, 70, 72–75
treatment of, 275–276, 277f
Cervical spinal movements
anatomic considerations in, 14–21
in degenerative pathology, 19–21, 20f
nucleus pulposus, 14–16
uncinate processes, 16, 17f, 18
zygapophyseal joints, 18–19
at atlantoaxial joint, 29–31, 30t, 37–38, 168
at atlanto-occipital joint, 28–29, 28t,
37–38, 168
axial rotation, 33–34, 33t–34t
balance of. *See* Movement system balance.
biomechanics of. *See* Cervical spine,
biomechanics of.
combined
of atlanto-occipital complex, 168–169,
169f–171f, 173, 174f–176f, 175,
181–182
of atlas-axis complex, 169, 171,
172f–174f, 173, 175, 177,
177f–181f, 182

Cervical spinal movements *(Continued)*
    of lower cervical spine, 191–193,
        191f–192f
    of middle cervical spine, 182–191,
        187f–190f
    extension
        active movement, 128f
        biomechanics of, 32t–33t, 36–38, 36f
        injury in, 21
        in premanipulative testing, 152–154,
            152f
    flexion
        biomechanics of, 32t–33t, 36–38, 36f
        lateral, 188–189, 187f–190f
        therapeutic, 188–189, 187f–190f
        vertebral positions in, 19
    innervation for, 22
    instantaneous axes of rotation, 39–42,
        39f–40f, 41t, 341–342
    in muscle balance evaluation, 351
    pain in
        end-of-range, 289
        instantaneous axis of rotation and,
            41–42, 41t
        through-range, 289
    patterns of
        irregular, 185, 186
        regular, 184, 186
    quality of, 38
    range of, 31–33, 32t, 36–38
    rotation
        in craniovertebral junction instability, 115
        instantaneous axes of, 39–42, 39f–40f,
            41t, 341–342
        with lateral flexion, 182–183, 186
        in premanipulative testing, 152–154,
            153f, 155f
        therapeutic, 187–189, 187f–190f
    uncinate process in, 34–35, 35f–37f
Cervical spine. *See also* Atlantoaxial joint;
        Atlanto-occipital joint.
    anatomy of, 7–21
        atlantoaxial joint, 10–12, 11f, 167–168
        atlanto-occipital joint, 7–8, 8f, 167–168
        atlas, 7–9, 8f, 11f
        axis, 9–12, 11f
        in injury, 21
        innervation, 22, 66–68, 66f–68f
        motion segments, 14–21, 15f, 17f–18f,
            20f

    nucleus pulposus, 15–16
    vertebrae, 12–14, 13f–14f
    vertebral arteries, 14
anomalies of, 6–7
biomechanics of, 27–45
    atlantoaxial joint, 29–31, 30t, 34t
    atlanto-occipital joint, 28–29, 28t, 34t
    axial rotation, 33–34, 33t–34t
    extension, 32t–33t, 36–38, 36f
    flexion, 32t–33t, 36–38, 36f
    instantaneous axes of rotation, 39–42,
        39f–40f, 41t
    quality of motion, 38
    range of motion, 31–33, 32t, 36–38
    state of the art of, 42–43
    uncinate process function, 34–35,
        35f–37f
degenerative disease of, 19–21, 20f
development of, 2–6, 3f–4f
    nucleus pulposus, 15–16
extension of. *See under* Cervical spinal
    movements.
flexion of. *See under* Cervical spinal
    movements.
functions of, 1–2
growth of, 5–6
injury of
    extension, 21
    flexion, 21
    work-related, 387
innervation of, 22, 66–68, 66f–68f
intervertebral discs of. *See* Intervertebral
    discs.
joints of. *See* Joints.
laxity of, in craniovertebral junction
    instability, 115
lordosis of, 6
    muscle function in, 347, 348, 350
manipulation of. *See* Cervical manipulative
    therapy.
movements of. *See* Cervical spinal
    movements.
ossification of, 4–5
pain syndromes of. *See under* Pain.
palpation of, 140–141
physical examination of. *e* Physical
    examination.
range of motion of, 31–33, 32t, 36–38
rotation of. *See under* Cervical spinal
    movements.

stability of, 18
    assessment of, 114–115
    vs. thoracic spine, 1–2
"Cervical spondylosis," 288
Cervical vertigo, 150–151
Cervico-encephalic syndrome, 23
Cervicogenic nerves
    injury of, 320. *See also specific nerves.*
    weakness of, 325
Cervicothoracic junction, of sympathetic
    trunk, injury of, 322
Chemical pain, 361
Chest pain
    referred from cervical spine, 68–70,
        71f–72f
    referred from thoracic spine, 84, 85f, 86,
        321
Children, muscle imbalance in, 203
Chin tuck test, in cervical headache, 273, 274f
Chordoma, 7
Chronic paroxysmal hemicrania, headache in,
    263
Clinical reasoning in physical therapy,
    89–108
    biomedical concepts in, 97–98
    vs. clinical reasoning in medicine, 90–91
    data collection in, 92f, 93. *See also*
        Physical examination; Subjective
        examination.
    decision making in, 92f, 94
    expertise level and, 96–98
    hypothesis categories in, 99–105
        contributing factors, 101
        management, 102
        mechanism of symptoms, 103–105
        patient presentation, 99–100
        precautions to therapy, 101
        prognosis, 102
        symptom mechanisms, 103–105
        symptom source, 100–101
    illness scripts in, 98
    information perception and interpretation
        in, 92–93, 92f
    instance scripts in, 98
    knowledge base for, 95–99, 96f, 97t
    linked to art and science, 413
    metacognition in, 94
    model for, 92–94, 92f
    schemas in, 95–96, 96f, 97t
    search and scan strategies in, 93–94

Cluster headache, 263, 264
Cold temperature, work-related pain from,
    392
Collar, cervical, for discogenic pain, 303, 304
Combined movements, 167–193
    of atlanto-occipital complex
        in examination, 168–169, 169f–171f
        palpation of, 173, 174f–176f, 175
        treatment based on, 181–182
    of atlas-axis complex
        in examination, 169, 171, 172f–174f,
            173
        palpation of, 175, 177, 177f–181f
        treatment based on, 182
    of lower cervical spine, 191–193
        in examination, 191–192, 191f–192f
        treatment based on, 193
    of middle cervical spine, 182–191
        in examination, 183
        palpation of, 185
        patterns of, 184–185
        in prediction of treatment response, 189,
            191
        treatment based on, 185–189, 187f–190f
    pain provocation in, 228
    in physical examination, 131, 131f
        of cervical headache, 168–169,
            169f–181f, 171, 173, 175, 177
Communication
    in data collection, 93
    in passive movement examination, 249
Compression
    cervical pain in, 289
    as cervical spinal movement pattern,
        184
    nerve root. *See* Nerve root compression.
Compression tests, 133–134
Computed tomography
    of atlantoaxial joint, 31
    of cervical spine, 34, 34t
Connective tissue, remodeling of, mechanical
    factors in, 369–371
Constitutional hypermobility, 212–213
Contraction
    in dysfunction syndrome, 362–364
    stretching of, 292
Convergence mechanism, in referred pain, 69
Corticosteroid therapy, history of, in
    subjective examination, 116
Costolamellar ligament, innervation of, 79f

Costotransverse joints
  ankylosing spondylitis of, 83
  innervation of, 79f, 80
  movement of
    in lateral bending, 57, 57f
    in rotation, 60, 61f, 62
    in spinal extension, 54–55, 54f
    in spinal flexion, 51, 51f
  as pain source, 82, 83, 86
  rheumatoid arthritis of, 83
Costotransverse ligament, 79f
Costovertebral joints
  movement of
    in rotation, 60, 61f, 62
    in spinal extension, 53, 54f
    in spinal flexion, 52, 52f
  osteophytes of, sympathetic pain in, 317
Coupled motion, definition of, 49t
Craniomandibular dysfunction, cervical
    headache in, 272
Craniovertebral junction
  instability of, signs of, 114–115
  testing at
    in cervical headache, 268–269
    for stability, 137–138
Cumulative microtrauma, in movement
    system imbalance, 340

Data collection, in clinical reasoning, 92f, 93
Decision making, in clinical reasoning, 92f,
    94
Defense behavior, muscle imbalance in,
    199–200, 200f
Deformation, mechanical, pain in. *See*
    Mechanical diagnosis and therapy.
Degenerative disease
  of cervical spine, 19–21, 20f
  of thoracic spine, 83
  work-related pain in, 387t, 388–389
Dens (odontoid process), anatomy of, 8, 8f, 9,
    11–12
Derangement syndrome, 364–368
  centralization phenomenon in, 365–366,
    366f
  conceptual model for, 367–368
  exercise in, 374
  manipulation in, 374–375
  patient profile in, 364–365
  peripheralization in, 366
  treatment of, 367–368

Dermatomes, of intercostal nerves, 325
Diagnosis. *See also specific disorders and tests.*
  clinical. *See* Clinical reasoning in physical
    therapy.
  examination in. *See* Physical examination;
    Subjective examination.
  mechanical. *See* Mechanical diagnosis and
    therapy.
Differentiation, of movement, 124–126
Digastric muscle, tightness of, 202, 205–206
Discs, intervertebral. *See* Intervertebral discs.
Distraction tests, 133–134
Dizziness
  in cervical headache, 264
  differential diagnosis of, 154, 155f
  premanipulative testing with, 153–155
  types of, 150–151
  vertebrobasilar insufficiency and, 149–151
  vestibular (cervical/reflex vertigo),
    150–151
Dorsal rami
  in cervical spine innervation, 66, 66f
  in thoracic spine innervation, 78, 79f–81f,
    80
  injury of, 320
Double crush hypothesis, in nerve
    compression, 224–225, 226
Drugs, history of, in subjective examination,
    116
Dura mater
  innervation of, 67, 67f, 79f
  pain in, 226
  stress on, in upper limb tension test, 223
  thoracic, 314, 314f
    as pain source, 82, 319
Dysfunction syndrome, 362–364
  conceptual model of, 364
  exercise in, 373
  manipulation in, 374

Education
  in ergonomics, 396
  for self-treatment, 371–372
Elbow
  extension of
    in hypermobility, 213
    in upper limb tension test, 230t,
      232–233, 232f
  flexion of, in upper limb tension test,
    232–233, 234f

Electromyography
  in cervical headache, 273
  of neck muscles, 201
  in work-related pain, 381
Emotion, in pain response, 104–105
Environmental condition syndromes, 392
Ergonomics. *See* Work-related pain,
    prevention of.
Examination
  neurologic, 134–135. *See also* Neural
      tension tests; Upper limb tension test.
    in cervical headache, 270–271
  physical. *See* Physical examination.
  subjective. *See* Subjective examination.
Exercise
  for cervical headache, 276–279, 277f–279f
  for derangement syndrome, 374
  for discogenic pain, 305, 306, 306f–307f
  for dysfunction syndrome, 373
  for muscle strengthening, 354–355
  pause, in work-related pain prevention, 397
  for postural syndrome, 372
  for zygapophyseal arthralgia, 295, 297, 298
  for zygapophyseal joint locking, 300
Extension and extension tests
  active movement, 127, 128f–129f
  of cervical spine
    active movement, 128f
    biomechanics of, 32t–33t, 36–38, 36f
    injury in, 21
    in premanipulative testing, 152–154, 152f
  of elbow
    in hypermobility, 213
    in upper limb tension test, 230t, 232,
        232f
  passive movement, 140
  in premanipulative testing, 152–154, 152f
  with rotation
    of atlantoaxial joint, 171, 173,
        173f–174f, 177, 179f–181f
    of atlanto-occipital complex, 169,
        170f–171f, 175, 176f
  of thoracic spine
    active movement, 127, 129f
    biomechanics of, 53–55, 53f–54f, 62
  of thumb, 213
Eye movements, neck muscle function and,
    198

Facet joints. *See* Zygapophyseal joints.

Fatigue, prevention of, in workplace, 397–398
Flexibility
  of muscles, evaluation of, 206–207,
      207f–209f, 209, 347–349
  relative, movement and, 344–346, 345f
Flexion and flexion tests
  active movement, of thoracic spine, 127,
      129f–130f
  of cervical spine, 188–189, 187f–190f
    biomechanics of, 32t–33t, 36–38, 36f
    with rotation, 182–183, 191f–192f, 192
    therapeutic, 188–189, 187f–190f
    vertebral positions in, 19
  of elbow, in upper limb tension test,
      232–233, 234f
  head, 209–210, 210f
  lateral
    in middle cervical spinal disorders,
        188–189, 187f–190f
    with rotation, of middle cervical spine,
        182–183
  neck, in thoracic neuropathy, 326
  passive movement, 140
  with rotation
    of atlantoaxial joint, 169, 171, 172f, 175,
        177, 177f–179f
    of atlanto-occipital complex, 168–169,
        169f–170f, 173, 174f–175f, 175
    in lower cervical spinal disorders,
        191f–192f, 192
    therapeutic, in middle cervical spinal
        disorders, 188–189, 187f–190f
  of thoracic spine, biomechanics of, 49–52,
      50f–52f, 62
Fracture, of thoracic spine, meningeal
    tethering in, 335
Functional capacity assessment, in work-
    related pain prevention, 395

Gothic shoulders, 205
Growth plates, 4–5

Hands, touching behind neck, in
    hypermobility, 213
Hawthorne effect, 413
Head
  flexion tests of, 209–210, 210f
  posture of
    in cervical headache, 272
    in discogenic pain, 301, 302f

Head *(Continued)*
    in lower body asymmetry, 200–201
    neck pain and, 197
    in standing, 206
    rotation tests of, in hypermobility, 213
Headache
    cervical. *See* Cervical headache.
    in chronic paroxysmal hemicrania, 263
    cluster, 263, 264
    migraine, vs. cervical headache, 262–265
    physical examination in, 132–133, 132f
    school, 203
    sympathetic nervous system contribution
        to, treatment of, 333, 334f, 335
    tension, 197, 262
Hemivertebra, 6
High arm cross test, in hypermobility, 213
Hip, dislocation of, remodeling after,
        368–369, 369f–370f
History
    in passive movement treatment planning,
        289–290
    in subjective examination, 117–118
Hyoid muscles, headache related to, 201
Hyperalgesia, in neural injury, 238
Hypermobility, of muscles, 212–213
Hypothesis categories, in clinical reasoning.
        See under Clinical reasoning in
        physical therapy.
Hypothetico-deductive reasoning, in clinical
        reasoning, 90–91

Iliocostalis cervicis muscle, innervation of, 66
Iliocostalis muscles, innervation of, 80
Informed consent, for cervical manipulative
        therapy, 156, 159, 160f, 161
Instantaneous axes of rotation
    of cervical spine, 39–42, 39f–40f, 41t
        abnormal, 41–42, 41t
    in movement system balance, 341–342
Instrumentation, for spinal mechanical
        properties, 411
Intercostal nerves
    anatomy of, 314, 314f
    dermatomes of, 325
    injury of, 320, 321
        evaluation of, 325, 330
        treatment of, 333, 334f
Interscapular space, flattening of, 204, 204f
Interspinalis muscle, innervation of, 66

Intertransversarii muscles, innervation of, 66f
Intervertebral discs
    cervical
        anatomy of, 14–16, 15f
        bipartite, 18
        degeneration of, 18, 19
        herniation of, 16
        innervation of, 22, 67–68, 68f
        as pain source, 300–306, 302f,
            304f–307f
        derangement of. *See* Derangement
            syndrome.
    thoracic
        herniation of, 83
        injury of, 318
        innervation of, 80f–81f, 82
        as pain source, 82–83, 84, 85f, 86
Intervertebral space, opening one side of, 292
Interview. *See* Subjective examination.
Irritability, 95
    vs. nonirritability, 291
    vs. pathology, 239–240, 240t
    in upper limb tension test, 223–224
Isokinetic testing, of muscle strength,
        350–351

Job-related pain. *See* Work-related pain.
Joints
    dysfunction of. *See also* Movement system
        balance.
        in cervical headache, 267–270, 270f, 275
        treatment of, 275
    examination of, in cervical headache,
        267–270, 270f
    instability of, in constitutional
        hypermobility, 212–213
    internal disorders of, passive movement
        treatment of, 258–259
    movement of, muscle control in, 343–344
    muscle function and, 195–196
    nerve compression in, 222
    peripheral, examination of, 138
    position of, in passive movement treatment,
        291–293
    pressure on, in examination, 142
    relative stiffness of, movement and,
        344–346, 345f
    soft tissue crossing, abnormalities of,
        muscle imbalance in, 342
    stretching of, 292

surfaces of, in instantaneous axis of
rotation, 341–342
uncovertebral
anatomy of, 16, 17f, 18
osteophytes in, 20, 20f
zygapophyseal. *See* Zygapophyseal joints.
Jones model for clinical reasoning in physical
therapy, 92–94, 92f

Keyboard operators, work-related pain in,
384–385, 390–391
Kinematics. *See* Biomechanics.
Kinetics, in movement system balance theory,
346
Knowledge base, for clinical reasoning, 92f,
95–99, 96f, 97t

Lateral flexion tests
in middle cervical spinal disorders,
188–189, 187f–190f
with rotation, of middle cervical spine,
182–183
of thoracic spine, 127, 130f
Latissimus dorsi muscle
innervation of, 80
tightness of, 205, 205f
Layer (stratification) syndrome, 203
Leg-length asymmetry, upper body muscle
action in, 200–201
Leg raise test, in thoracic neuropathy, 327
Levator scapulae muscles
function of, in shoulder movement, 348
innervation of, 22
overactivity of, in cervical headache, 272
tightness of, 202, 205, 207, 208f
Limbic system, in muscular control, 198–199
Longissimus capitis muscle, innervation of, 66
Longissimus cervicis muscle, innervation of, 66
Longissimus thoracis muscle, innervation of,
79f
Longus cervicis muscle
as stabilizer, 347
testing of, 350
Lordosis, cervical, muscle function in, 347,
348, 350
Lower cervical syndrome, 23
Low load test, for muscle balance, 273, 274f
Lung, disorders of, sympathetic dysfunction
in, 317
Luschka, joints of. *See* Uncovertebral joints.

McKenzie system. *See* Mechanical diagnosis
and therapy.
Maitland concept, 245
Manual therapy, 409–420. *See also* Cervical
manipulative therapy; Thoracic
manipulative therapy; *specific
disorder and technique.*
as art, 412–413
criticism of, 409
in mechanical disorders, 374–375
pain provocation in, 410
placebo effect and, 415–417
research on, 411–415
theories of, 412–413
Masseter muscle, tightness of, 202
Mechanical diagnosis and therapy, 359–377
anatomic regional differences in, 375
of cervical spine vs. thoracic spine, 375
conditions inappropriate for, 360–361
of derangement syndrome, 364–368, 374
centralization phenomenon in, 365–366,
366f
of dysfunction syndrome, 362–364, 373
exercise in, 372–374
manipulation in, 374–375
pain mechanisms and, 361
of postural syndrome, 362, 363f, 372
principles of, 360–361
self treatment philosophy and, 371–372
of thoracic spine vs. cervical spine, 375
tissue repair and remodeling and, 368–371,
369f–370f
Mechanical pain. *See* Mechanical diagnosis
and therapy.
Mechanical stimuli, symptom response to, 113
Median nerve
entrapment of, 222
testing of, with upper limb tension test,
230, 230t, 231f
Medical evaluation, consideration of, in
subjective examination, 116–117
Meninges
stress on, in upper limb tension test, 223
thoracic
pain in, 319
tethering of, treatment of, 335
Mesoderm, in spinal development, 3–4, 4f
Metacognition, in clinical reasoning, 94
Microtrauma, cumulative, in movement
system imbalance, 340

Migraine headache, vs. cervical headache, 262–265
Mobilization
  vs. manipulative therapy, 291
  of nerves
    in cervical headache, 275–276, 277f
    in thoracic neuropathy, 332–333
    in upper limb tension test, 239–240, 240t
  of ribs, 333, 334f
Momentary pain, in passive movement treatment, 258
Motion, of cervical spine. *See* Cervical spinal movements.
Movement system balance, 339–357
  assessment of, 346–353
    flexibility, 347–349
    movement patterns, 347–349
    muscle strength, 349–351
    posture, 346–347
    protocol for, 351–353
  factors in, 340
    cumulative microtrauma, 340–341
    instantaneous axes of rotation, 341–342
    joint surface shape, 341–342
    kinetics, 346
    motor control, 343–344
    muscle length, 342–343
    relative stiffness, 344–346, 345f
    soft tissue condition, 342
  treatment principles based on, 353–355
  underlying premise of, 340
Multifidi muscles, innervation of, 66, 66f, 78, 79f
Multiple crush hypothesis, in nerve compression, 224–225
Muscles
  altered movement patterns of, 201–203
    evaluation of. *See subhead*: evaluation of.
  antagonists of, testing of, 349
  biomechanics of, 201
  central nervous system regulation of, 198–201
  dominance of, 343–344
    testing of, 349–350
  electromyography of, 201
    in cervical headache, 273
  evaluation of, 136, 203–212, 346–353
    antagonists, 349
    in cervical headache, 271–273, 274f

flexibility testing in, 206–207, 207f–209f, 209, 347–349
  in hypermobility, 213
  isokinetic testing in, 350–351
  length, 347
  movement patterns, 209–212, 210f–211f, 347–349
  performance testing, 136
  posture, 346–347, 351–352
  protocol for, 351–353
  in standing, 204–206, 204f–206f
  strength testing in, 209–212, 210f–211f, 349–351
  synergists, 349
flexibility of, testing of, 206–207, 207f–209f, 209, 347–349
functions of, 390
hypermobility of, 212–213
imbalance of. *See also* Movement system balance.
  altered movement patterns in, 201–203
  in cervical headache, 271–273, 274f, 276–279, 277f–279f
  in children, 203
  evaluation of. *See subhead*: evaluation of.
  in postural overload syndromes, 390–391
  in shoulder crossed syndrome, 200f, 202–203
  treatment of, 214–215, 274f, 276–279, 277f–279f
joint function and, 195–196
length of
  adaptation to, 342–343
  evaluation of, 347
limbic system effects on, 198–199
motor control of, 343–344
movement patterns of, evaluation of, 209–212, 210f–211f
neck
  defensive responses of, 199–200
  eye movements and, 198
  innervation of, 66–67, 66f
  in lordosis, 347
  lower body position effects on, 200–201
  proprioceptive function of, 198
  reflex influence on, 198–200
  shoulder motion effects on, 197
  shoulder muscle function with, 197

spasm of, 196–197, 198–199
in standing, 205–206, 206f
tightness of, 207, 209, 209f
in walking, 201
weakness of, 205–206, 206f, 209–210, 210f
nerve compression in, 222
overuse of, 391–392
in pain pathogenesis, 196–201
as prime movers, 390
reflex influence on, 198–200
regional groups of, 197
retraining of, 353–355
shortened, adaptation of, 342–343
shoulder, 197
central nervous system regulation of, 198–199
in standing, 204–205, 204f–206f
tightness of, 202–203, 206–207, 207f–208f
weakness of, 210–212, 210f–211f
spasm of, 196–197, 198–199
treatment of, 214
as stabilizers, 390
strength of
at cold temperatures, 392
evaluation of, 209–212, 210f–211f, 349–351
exercises for, 354–355
stress effects on, 199
stretching of, 354
synergists of, 390
testing of, 349
thoracic
pain originating in, 82–83
as pain source, 83
tightness of, 202
in constitutional hypermobility, 212
evaluation of, 206–207, 207f–209f, 209
training of, 213–215
trigger points in, 197, 206
weakness of, 202
evaluation of, 209–212, 210f–211f
in long-lasting tightness, 202
Musculocutaneous nerve
entrapment of, 222
testing of, 233–234
Mylohyoid muscle, weakness of, 202

Nausea, in cervical headache, 264

Neck
muscles of. *See under* Muscles.
pain in. *See also* Work-related pain.
head posture and, 197
whiplash injury of. *See* Whiplash injury.
wry
in children, 203
discogenic, 307
from zygapophyseal joint locking, 298–300
Nerve(s)
cervicogenic. *See also specific nerves.*
injury of, 320
weakness of, 325
compression of
double crush hypothesis and, 224–225, 226
external forces in, 223
in joints, 222
in muscle tissue, 222
connective tissue of, irritation of, in upper limb tension test, 223
ectopic pacemakers in, 223–224
injury of
in thoracic region. *See* Thoracic neuropathy.
types of, 317–318
irritability of
vs. pathology, 239–240, 240t
in upper limb tension test, 223–224
mobilization of
in cervical headache, 275–276, 276f
in thoracic neuropathy, 332–333
in upper limb tension test, 239–240, 240t
palpation of, 135
stretching of, pain in, 226
Nerve conduction, tests for, 134
Nerve root(s), thoracic, anatomy of, 314, 314f
Nerve root compression
cervical, 19–20, 20f
case study of, 308–311
in cervical headache, 264–265, 270–271, 275–276, 277f
pain in, 65, 70, 72–75
radicular pain with, 74–75
treatment of, 275–276, 277f
in derangement syndrome, 367
thoracic, 320–321
treatment of, 333, 334f

Nervous system
  autonomic, in pain response. *See*
    Sympathetically maintained pain.
  physical examination of, 134–135
    in cervical headache, 270–271
  testing of. *See* Neural tension tests; Upper
    limb tension test.
Neural tension tests, 95, 131–132. *See also*
    Upper limb tension test.
  definition of, 218
  slump test, 135, 327, 328f–331f, 331
  of sympathetic trunk, 135
Neural tube
  defects of, 6
  development of, 2–3, 3f, 5–6
Neurodynamics, definition of, 314
Neurogenic pain, mechanisms of, 218–219
Neurogenic symptoms, definition of, 314
Neuroma, pain in, 224
Neuropathic pain, definition of, 315
Neuropathy, thoracic. *See* Thoracic
    neuropathy.
Night pain, 226
  evaluation of, 113
Nociception. *See also* Pain.
  patterns of, 103–104
Nociceptive pain, definition of, 315
Nonsteroidal anti-inflammatory drug therapy,
    history of, in subjective examination,
    116
Nostalgia paresthetica, 325
Notochord, development of, 2–4, 3f–4f, 5–6
Nucleus pulposus, development of, 15–16

Oblique muscles
  innervation of, 66f
  tightness of, 202, 207, 209, 209f
Observation, in physical examination, 124
Occipitoatlantal joint. *See* Atlanto-occipital
    joint.
Occiput-C1 joint. *See* Atlanto-occipital joint.
Occupational cervicobrachial disorders,
    381–382
Occupational disorders, pain in. *See* Work-
    related pain.
Odontoid process (dens), anatomy of, 8, 8f, 9,
    11–12
Office workers, work-related pain in,
    384–385, 390–391
Oscillatory pressures, on joints, 142–143

Ossification, of spine, 4–5
Osteokinematics, definition of, 49t
Osteophytes
  of costovertebral joints, sympathetic pain
    in, 317
  nerve root compression and, 20, 20f
  spinal cord compression and, 20–21
Overuse syndrome, work-related, 391–392

Pacemakers, neural, 223–224
Pain. *See also* Headache.
  affective mechanisms in, 104–105
  arm, in cervical nerve root compression,
    308–311
  assessment of, 110–113, 111f
  autonomic mechanisms in, 104, 228–229
  avoidance of, in passive movement, 292
  body chart for, 111–112, 111f
  centralization of, 365–366, 366f
  central patterns of, 104, 227–228
  cervical, 65–76
    combined states in, 74–75
    compression, 289
    end-of-range, in passive movement, 289
    instantaneous axis of rotation and,
      41–42, 41t
    local, 289
    radicular, 65, 70, 72–75
    referred, 68–70, 71f–72f, 289
    somatic, 65, 66–70, 66f–68f, 71f–72f,
      74–75
    in stretching, 289
    through-range, in passive movement, 289
  character of, 112
  chemical, 361
  chest
    referred from cervical spine, 68–70,
      71f–72f
    referred from thoracic spine, 84, 85f, 86,
      321
  constant, passive movement treatment with,
    293
  definition of, 105
  depth of, 112
  description of, 226
  discogenic, 82–83, 84, 85f, 86
    case study of, 300–306, 302f, 304f–307f
  in dysfunction syndrome, 362–364
  emotional component of, 104–105
  exaggerated, 228

in manual examination, 410–411
mechanical. *See* Mechanical diagnosis and
therapy.
from mechanical stimuli, 113
mechanisms of, 103–105, 218–219, 361
in thoracic spine, 315–317, 316f
mild, passive movement treatment with,
293–294
momentary, in passive movement
treatment, 258
muscle spasm from, 196–197
muscular, treatment of, 214–215. *See also*
Movement system balance.
musculoskeletal movement alterations in,
355
neck. *See also* Work-related pain.
head posture and, 197
neurogenic, mechanisms of, 218–219
in neuroma, 224
neuropathic, definition of, 315
night, 113, 226
nociceptive, definition of, 315
nonspecific, mechanical diagnosis and
therapy of. *See* Mechanical diagnosis
and therapy.
in passive movement, 255–259, 289, 292,
293
pathogenesis of, muscles in, 196–201, 200f
pathologic, mechanisms of, 315
peripheralization of, 366
peripherally evoked, 103, 225–226
physiologic, mechanisms of, 315
placebo effect on, 415–417
in postural syndrome, 362, 363f
radicular, 65, 70, 72–75
case study of, 308–311
with somatic pain, 74–75
referred
by cervical nerves, 267
from cervical spine, 22–23, 68–70,
71f–72f
in passive movement, 289, 292
from thoracic neuropathy, 321
from thoracic spine, 84, 85f, 86,
324–326
in reflex sympathetic dystrophy, 229
severity of, 112–113
shoulder
in cervical nerve root compression,
308–311

work-related. *See* Work-related pain.
sites of, 110–112, 111f
suboccipital, in cervical headache, 263–264
sympathetically maintained. *See*
Sympathetically maintained pain.
symptoms of, 226
terminology of, 218
thoracic, 77, 82–86. *See also* Thoracic
neuropathy.
in meningeal irritation, 319
pain patterns in, 84, 85f, 86
sources of, 82–84
twenty-four-hour pattern of, 114
upper limb tension test and, 225–229
autonomic patterns of, 228–229
central patterns of, 227–228
peripherally evoked patterns of, 225–226
work-related. *See* Work-related pain.
in wry neck
from acute zygapophyseal joint locking,
298–300
discogenic, 307
in zygapophyseal joints, case study of,
294–298, 296f–297f
Palpation, 140–141
of atlanto-occipital complex, 173,
174f–176f, 175
of atlas-axis complex, 175, 177, 177f–181f
in cervical headache, 173, 174f–176f, 175,
177, 177f–181f
efficacy of, 410–411
of lower cervical spine, 191–193,
191f–192f
of middle cervical spine, 185
of muscles, 203–204
of nerves, 135
of ribs, in lower cervical spinal disorders,
191–192, 192f
of soft tissues, 140–141
of vertebrae, 12, 141
of zygapophyseal joints, in shoulder
abduction, 348
Paresthesia
in craniovertebral junction instability, 114
in nerve root compression, 73
Passive movement (evaluative), 139–143,
247–253
accessory movements in, 142–143,
248–250
case study of, 252

Passive movement (evaluative) *(Continued)*
in cervical headache, 168–169, 169f–174f, 171, 173
combined movements in
of atlanto-occipital complex, 168–169, 169f–171f
of atlas-axis complex, 169, 171, 172f–174f, 173
of lower cervical spine, 191–192, 191f–192f
of middle cervical spine, 183–185
communication in, 249
diagram of, 249
full, 252–253
guidelines for, 246–247
information sources for, 246–247
limited, 250–251
movements used in, 248–250
pain response to, technique selection and, 289
physiologic movements in, 140
significance of, 249–250
in thoracic neuropathy, 326
Passive movement (therapeutic), 253–259, 288–294
in atlanto-occipital complex disorders, 181–182
in atlas-axis complex disorders, 182
combined movements in
in atlanto-occipital complex disorders, 181–182
in atlas-axis complex disorders, 182
in lower cervical spinal disorders, 193
in middle cervical spinal disorders, 185–189, 187f–190f, 191
direction of, 291–293
factors affecting technique selection
diagnosis, 288
history, 289–290
pain response, 289
signs, 291
symptoms, 290–291
technique effects, 291
firmness of, 254
grades of, 254–255, 255f
information sources for, 246–247
joint position for, 291–293
in lower cervical spinal disorders, 193
in middle cervical spinal disorders, 185–189, 187f–190f, 191

with pain, 255–256
constant, 293
mild, 293–294
and tissue resistance, 257–259
pain mechanisms and, 254
principles of, 254
resistance in, 254–259, 255f
technique performance in, 293–294
with tissue resistance, 256–257
Pathologic pain, mechanisms of, 315
Pattern recognition, in clinical reasoning, 91
Pause exercises, in work-related pain prevention, 397
Pectoralis muscles
overactivity of, in cervical headache, 272
tightness of, 202, 205, 205f, 207, 208f
Pelvis, asymmetry of, upper body muscle action in, 200
Peripheralization, of pain, 366
Physical examination, 118–143
active movement tests in. *See* Active movement tests.
assessment during, 132
in cervical headache, 266–273
articular function, 267–270, 270f
combined movements in, 168–169, 169f–174f, 171, 173
muscle function, 271–273, 274f
neural tissues, 270–271
posture, 271–273
vertebral artery, 270
combined movements in
atlanto-occipital complex, 168–169, 169f–171f, 173, 174f–176f, 175
atlas-axis complex, 169, 171, 172f–181f, 173, 175, 177
lower cervical spine, 191–192
middle cervical spine, 183–185
communication in, 93, 249
components of, 123–124
of craniovertebral junction, 137–138
in dizziness, 153–155
extension tests in. *See* Extension and extension tests.
flexion tests in. *See* Flexion and flexion tests.
full, 120–121, 252–253
hypotheses generation during. *See under* Clinical reasoning in physical therapy.
instrumentation for, 411

limited, 118–120, 250–251
manual techniques in, 410–411
muscle evaluation in. *See* Muscles, evaluation of.
of nervous system, 104, 134–135. *See also* Neural tension tests; Upper limb tension test.
  in cervical headache, 270–271
observation in, 124
palpation in. *See* Palpation.
passive, 139–143, 247–253. *See also* Palpation.
  accessory movements in, 142–143, 248–250
  full, 252–253
  guidelines for, 246–247
  limited, 250–251
  movements used in, 248–250
  physiologic movements in, 140
of peripheral joints, 138
of peripheral pulses, 137
physical signs of potential involvement in, 122–123
planning, 118–121, 250–251
posture evaluation in, 124, 346–347, 351–352
precautions in, 101–102, 118–120, 136–138
after provocation, 124–126, 133, 139
rotation tests in. *See* Rotation and rotation tests.
search and scan strategies in, 93–94
slump test in, 135, 327, 328f–331f, 331, 332
of soft tissues, 140–141
structures included in, 122
of sympathetic trunk, 135
in thoracic neuropathy, 323–332
  conduction patterns, 324–326
  individual nerve tests in, 330
  multistructural considerations in, 331
  neurodynamics, 326–330, 328f–331f
  passive neck flexion in, 326
  slump test in, 327, 328f–331f, 331
  straight leg raise in, 327
  structural differentiation in, 331–332
  tension tests in, 331–332
  test response clarification in, 332
  upper limb tension test in, 326–327
in thoracic outlet syndrome, 137

upper limb tension test. *See* Upper limb tension test.
of vascular system, 136–137, 152–155, 152f–153f, 155f
of vertebrae, 141
of viscera, 138–139
Physiologic pain, mechanisms of, 315
Pia mater, thoracic, pain in, 319
Placebo effect, of manual therapy, 415–417
Plexus, in thoracic spinal innervation, 82
Posteroanterior oscillatory pressures, 142–143
  in discogenic pain, 303–305, 304f
  in middle cervical spinal disorders, 188, 189, 190f
  in wry neck, 299–300
  in zygapophyseal arthralgia, 295–298, 296f–297f
Postural syndrome, 362, 363f
  exercise in, 372
  work-related, 390–391
Posture
  anomalies of, in cervical headache, 271–273, 276–279, 277f–279f
  correction of, 353–354, 372
  evaluation of, 124, 346–347, 351–352
  head
    in cervical headache, 272
    in discogenic pain, 301, 302f
    in lower body asymmetry, 200–201
    neck pain and, 197
    in standing, 206
  improvement of, in muscle imbalance, 215
  reflexes involved in, muscle function and, 199–200
  sitting, 346–347, 351
  standing, 206, 346–347, 351
Posture targeting method, for workload measurement, 394
Precautions to examination and management
  physical examination for, 136–138, 151–155, 152f–153f, 155f
  in physical examination planning, 118–121, 250–251
  subjective examination for, 101–102, 114–117, 151
    carotid artery system, 115
    general health, 115–116
    medical findings in, 116–117
    pharmacologic status, 116
    spinal cord function, 115

Precautions to examination and management
(*Continued*)
structural stability, 114–115
vertebrobasilar system, 115
in upper limb tension test, 240–241
Prehension pattern, muscle action in, 200
Pressure sensor, for neck flexor strength
training, 277f, 279
Prevertebral muscles, innervation of, 66
Problem solving. *See* Clinical reasoning in
physical therapy.
Proprioception
deficits of, in cervical headache, 272
neck muscles in, 198
Provocation, of symptoms
in active movement tests, 124–126, 133
in passive movement tests, 139
Proximal (shoulder) crossed syndrome, 200f,
202–203
Pulses, peripheral, evaluation of, 137
Push up test, 210–211, 211f

Radial nerve
entrapment of, 222, 223
testing of, with upper limb tension test,
230, 230t, 232, 232f–233f
Radicular pain, cervical, 65, 70, 72–74
case study of, 308–311
with somatic pain, 74–75
Radiography
of atlantoaxial joint, 29–30
of cervical spine, 33, 33t
Rapid upper limb assessment method, for
workload measurement, 394–395
Recti muscles, tightness of, 202, 207, 209,
209f
Rectus capitis anterior major muscle
function of, 347
testing of, 350
Rectus capitis muscle, innervation of, 66f
Referred pain. *See under* Pain.
Reflexes, muscular function and, 198–200,
200f
Reflex sympathetic dystrophy, 229
Reflex vertigo, 150–151
Rehabilitation, in work-related pain, 399–402
return to work after, 387
services for, 399–400
therapeutic interventions for, 400
vocational, 400–402

Relative stiffness, movement and, 344–346,
345f
Remodeling, of tissue, mechanical factors in,
368–371, 369f–370f
Repetition strain injury, 382–383
Research, on manual therapy, 411–415
Resistance, tissue, in passive movement
treatment, 254–255, 255f, 256–259
Rest, in mechanical disorders, 371
Rheumatoid arthritis, of thoracic spine, 83
Rhomboid muscles
innervation of, 22, 80
weakness of, 202, 204, 204f
Ribs
hypermobility of, thoracic neuropathy in,
320
mobilization of, 333, 334f
movement of
in lateral bending, 56–57, 56f–57f, 63
in spinal extension, 53–55, 54f, 62
in spinal flexion, 49–51, 51f, 62
palpation of, in lower cervical spinal
disorders, 191–192, 192f
Rotation and rotation tests
active movement, 127, 130f
of atlas, 29–30, 30t
axes of, 39–41, 39f–40f, 341–342
of cervical spine
axes of, 39–41, 39f–40f
in craniovertebral junction instability,
115
with lateral flexion, 182–183, 186
in premanipulative testing, 152–154,
153f, 155f
therapeutic, 187–189, 187f–190f
with extension
of atlantoaxial joint, 171, 173,
173f–174f, 177, 179f–181f
of atlanto-occipital complex, 169,
170f–171f, 175, 176f
with flexion
of atlantoaxial joint, 169, 171, 172f, 175,
177, 177f–179f
of atlanto-occipital complex, 168–169,
169f–170f, 173, 174f–175f, 175
in lower cervical spinal disorders,
191f–192f, 192
head, in hypermobility, 213
with lateral flexion, of middle cervical
spine, 182–183, 186

passive movement, 140
shoulder, in upper limb tension test, 219f,
  230t, 231f, 232, 234f
therapeutic, in middle cervical spinal
  disorders, 187–189, 187f–190f
of thoracic spine, 127, 130f
biomechanics of, 58f–61f, 59–63
Rothstein, Jules, on manual therapy scientific
  development, 409

Scalene muscles
  innervation of, 67
  overactivity of, in cervical headache, 272
  tightness of, 202
Scapula
  elevation of, in adverse neural tension,
    348–349
  position of, in muscle balance evaluation,
    351–352
  stability of, testing of, 210–211, 211f
Scapular nerve, dorsal
  evaluation of, 330
  injury of, 320
Scapulohumeral muscles, innervation of, 22
Scapulothoracic joint, as base of movement,
  350
Scar tissue
  dysfunction syndrome from, 364
  muscle imbalance from, 342
Schemas, in clinical reasoning, 95–96, 96f,
  97t
School headache, 203
Sclerotomes, referred pain and, 70, 71f–72f
Scoliosis
  neck muscle adaptation to, 200
  thoracic neuropathy in, 320
  upper body muscle action in, 200
Search strategies, in clinical reasoning, 93–94
Segmentation, of spine, 6–7
Self-treatment philosophy, 371–372
Semispinalis muscles
  cervical, innervation of, 66, 66f
  thoracic
    anatomy of, 79f
    innervation of, 78
Sensorimotor stimulation program, in muscle
  imbalance, 214–215
Serratus anterior muscle, weakness of, 202,
  205
  scapular winging in, 210

Shoulder
  abduction of, 211–212, 211f
    in flexibility evaluation, 348
    in upper limb tension test, 219f, 230t,
      232f, 235f
  depression of, in upper limb tension test,
    230, 230t, 231f, 234f
  gothic, 205
  muscle groups of, 343–344
  pain in
    in cervical nerve root compression,
      308–311
    work-related. *See* Work-related pain.
  rotation of, in upper limb tension test, 219f,
    230t, 231f, 232, 234f
Shoulder (proximal) crossed syndrome, 200f,
  202–203
Sinuvertebral nerves
  anatomy of, thoracic, 81–82
  structures innervated by
    cervical, 67–68, 67f–68f
    thoracic, 79f, 80f–81f, 82
Sitting posture, evaluation of, 346–347, 351
Sleep, symptom behavior during, 113
Slump test, 135, 327, 328f–331f, 331, 332
Somatic pain syndromes
  cervical, 65, 66–70, 66f–68f, 71f–72f
    with radicular pain, 74–75
  referred, 68–69
Somites, in spinal development, 2–3, 3f
Spasm, muscular, 196–197, 198–199
  treatment of, 214
Spinal cord
  cervical
    anatomy of, 20–21
    osteophytes affecting, 20–21
  compression of, in derangement syndrome,
    367
  dysfunction of, in craniovertebral junction
    instability, 115
  growth of, 6
  pain processing in, 227
  stress on, in upper limb tension test, 224
  thoracic
    evaluation of, 324–325
    injury of, 318–319, 324–325
Spinal nerves, in thoracic spine innervation,
  78, 79f, 80
Splenius capitis muscle, innervation of, 66
Splenius cervicis muscle, innervation of, 66

Spondylosis, cervical, 288
Standing
    muscle evaluation in, 204–206, 204f–206f
    postural evaluation in, 346–347, 351
Sternocleidomastoid muscle
    innervation of, 22, 67
    overactivity of, in cervical headache, 272
    predominance of, 209–210, 210f
    shortening of, 347
    tightness of, 202, 205, 206f, 207
Stiffness
    in passive movement treatment, 254–255,
        255f, 256–259
    relative, movement and, 344–346, 345f
Straight leg raise test, in thoracic neuropathy,
    327
Stratification (layer) syndrome, 203
Strength. *See under* Muscles.
Stress
    on muscles, 199
    muscular adaptation to, 342
    in upper limb tension test, 223, 224
    work-related pain in, 381, 385–386
Stretching
    cervical pain in, 289
    as cervical spinal movement pattern, 184
    of contracted tissue, 292, 373
    of muscles, exercises for, 354
    of nerves, pain in, 226
Subclavian artery, occlusion of, testing for,
    137
Subjective examination, 110–117
    case study of, 99–105
        contributing factors, 101
        management hypotheses based on, 102
        patient presentation, 99–100
        precautions for physical therapy, 101
        prognosis hypotheses based on, 102
        symptom mechanism hypotheses based
            on, 103–105
        symptom source in, 100–101
    of cervical headache, 262–266
    communication techniques in, 93
    contributing factors in, 101
    of general health, 115–116
    goals of, 110
    history taking and, 117–118
    hypotheses generation during, 99–105
    initial patient encounter in, 93, 99–100
    irritability assessment in, 95

    management hypotheses based on, 102
    mechanical stimuli response in, 113
    medical record in, 116–117
    night pain in, 113
    of pharmacologic status, 116
    in physical examination planning, 118–121,
        250–251
    for precautions to physical therapy, 101,
        114–117, 151
    prognosis hypotheses based on, 102
    search and scan strategies in, 93–94
    of structural stability, 114–115
    symptom evaluation in
        behavior, 113–114
        characteristics, 110–113, 111f
        sources, 100–101
    symptom mechanism hypotheses based on,
        103–105
    twenty-four hour symptom patterns in, 114
    of vital structures, 115
Suboccipital muscles
    innervation of, 66
    shortening of, in cervical headache, 272
Suboccipital pain, in cervical headache,
    263–264
Subscapular nerve, injury of, 320
Suprahyoid muscle, weakness of, 202
Suprascapular nerve
    evaluation of, 330
    injury of, 320, 325
    testing of, 235
Sweating, in sympathetic neuropathy,
    325–326
Swimming, muscle testing in, 350
Sympathetically maintained pain, 104, 229
    clinical features of, 325–326
    definition of, 315
    in headache, treatment of, 333, 334f, 335
    mechanisms of, 315–317, 316f
Sympathetic nervous system, anatomy of,
    321, 322f–323f
"Sympathetic slump," 327, 330, 330f, 414
Sympathetic trunk
    anatomy of, 314, 314f, 321, 322f–323f
    injury of, 321–323
    tension tests for, 135, 327, 330, 330f

Temporalis muscle, tightness of, 202
Temporomandibular dysfunction, cervical
    headache in, 272

Tension headache, 197
  vs. cervical headache, 262
Tension tests, neural. *See* Neural tension tests.
Test movements
  active. *See* Active movement tests.
  combined. *See* Combined movements.
  extension. *See* Extension and extension
    tests.
  flexion. *See* Flexion and flexion tests.
  neural tension. *See* Neural tension tests;
    Upper limb tension test.
  passive. *See* Passive movement
    (evaluative).
  rotation. *See* Rotation and rotation tests.
Theories, of manual therapy, 412–413
Thoracic manipulative therapy, 332–333
  in headache, with sympathetic component,
    333, 334f, 335
  in intercostal nerve entrapment, 333, 334f
  in mechanical disorders, 374–375
  in meningeal tethering, 335
  in nerve root compression, 333, 334f
  in thoracic neuropathy, 332–335, 334f
Thoracic nerve, long
  evaluation of, 330
  injury of, 320, 325
Thoracic neuropathy, 313–338
  anatomic considerations in, 314, 314f
  intercostal nerve, 333, 334f
  meninges, 319
    physical examination of, 324
  nerve roots, 320–321
    physical examination of, 325
    treatment of, 333, 334f
  pain mechanisms in, 315–317, 316f
  peripheral, 319–320
    physical examination of, 325
  physical examination in, 323–332
    conduction patterns, 324–326
    individual nerve tests in, 330
    multistructural considerations in, 331
    neurodynamics, 326–330, 328f–331f
    passive neck flexion in, 326
    slump test in, 327, 328f–331f, 331
    straight leg raise in, 327
    structural differentiation in, 331–332
    tension tests in, 331–332
    test response clarification in, 332
    upper limb tension test in, 326–327
  spinal cord, 318–319

  physical examination of, 324–325
  sympathetic, 315–317, 316f, 321–323,
    322f–323f
    physical examination of, 325–326
    treatment of, 333, 334f, 335
  terminology of, 314–315
  treatment of, 332–335
    in intercostal nerve entrapment, 333,
      334f
    in nerve root entrapment, 333, 334f
    in sympathetic nerve involvement, 333,
      334f, 335
  types of injury in, 317–318
Thoracic outlet syndrome, testing for, 137
Thoracic spinal movements
  active testing of. *See* Active movement
    tests.
  balance of. *See* Movement system balance.
  biomechanics of. *See* Thoracic spine,
    biomechanics of.
  degrees of motion of, 48f, 49
  extension, 53–55, 53f–54f, 62
  flexion, 49–52, 50f–52f, 62
  habitual, 48f, 49
  lateral bending, 55–57, 55f–57f, 63
  rotation, 58f–61f, 59–62, 63
Thoracic spine
  anatomy of, neural tissues, 314, 314f
  anomalies of, 6–7
  biomechanics of, 47–64
    degrees of motion of, 48f, 49
    extension, 53–55, 53f–54f, 62
    flexion, 49–52, 50f–52f, 62
    habitual movements, 48f, 49
    lateral bending, 55–57, 55f–57f, 63
    rotation, 58f–61f, 59–62, 63
    terminology of, 49t
    in vitro study of, 48, 48f
  vs. cervical spine, 1–2
  embryology of, 2–5, 3f–4f
  fracture of, meningeal tethering in, 335
  functions of, 1–2
  growth of, 5–6
  innervation of, 78, 79f–81f, 80–82
  intervertebral discs of. *See* Intervertebral
    discs.
  movement of. *See* Thoracic spinal
    movements.
  neural tissues of, anatomy of, 314, 314f
  ossification of, 4–5

Thoracic spine *(Continued)*
  pain syndromes of, 77, 82–86
    patterns of, 84, 85f, 86
    sources of, 82–84
  palpation of, 140–141
  physical examination of. *See under*
    Thoracic neuropathy.
Thoracodorsal nerve, injury of, 320, 325
Thrust manipulation, in wry neck, 299
Thumb, hyperextension of, 213
Torticollis. *See* Wry neck.
Traction, cervical
  in discogenic pain, 303
  in radicular pain, 309, 310
Transverse ligament, anatomy of, 8, 8f
Transverse pressures, on joints, 142
Trapezius muscles
  evaluation of, 352
  innervation of, 22, 67, 80
  overactivity of, in cervical headache, 272
  tightness of, 202, 205, 205f, 207, 207f
  training for, in cervical headache, 277–278,
    279f
  weakness of, 202, 204, 204f
    in cervical headache, 272
Traumatic disorders, work-related pain,
    386–387, 387t–388t
Trigeminocervical nucleus, 22–23
Trigger points, in muscles, 197, 206
T4 syndrome, 321

Ulnar nerve
  entrapment of, 222, 223
  testing of, with upper limb tension test,
    230t, 232–233, 234f–235f, 326
Uncinate processes
  biomechanics of, 34–35, 35f–37f
  growth of, 16, 17f, 18
Uncovertebral joints
  anatomy of, 16, 17f, 18
  osteophytes in, 20, 20f
Upper limb tension test, 135, 217–244
  analysis of, 236–238, 236f
  nerve mobilization in, 239–240, 240t
  neural tissues involved in, 219–221,
    219f–220f
  neuropathology and, 221–226
    compressive forces in, 223
    in double crush injury, 224–225
    in joints, 222

    in muscle, 222
    in neural connective tissue, 223
    in neural tissue, 223–224
  non-neural tissue in, 237–238
  pain and, 225–229
    autonomic patterns of, 228–229
    central patterns of, 226–227
    peripherally evoked patterns of, 225– 226
  positivity of, 236–237, 236f
  precautions with, 240–241
  responses to, 220, 220f
    categorization of, 237
    in central pain patterns, 228
    in peripheral neuropathy, 226
    in sympathetic pain patterns, 229
  sequence of, 219–221, 219f
  structural differentiation in, 236–237, 236f
  terminology of, 218–219
  in theory development, 414
  in thoracic neuropathy, 326–327
  treatment with, 238–241, 240t
    in radicular pain, 310–311
  variations in, 229–235, 230t
    axillary nerve bias, 235
    median nerve bias (2A), 230, 230t, 231f
    musculocutaneous nerve bias, 233–234
    radial nerve bias (2B), 230, 230t, 232,
      232f–233f
    suprascapular nerve bias, 235
    ulnar nerve bias (3), 230t, 232–233,
      234f–235f, 326
  variations of, component sequencing for, 238

Vertebrae
  anatomy of, 12–14, 13f
  anomalies of, 6–7
    palpation of, 141
  butterfly, 7
  development of, 2–6, 3f–4f
  discs between. *See* Intervertebral discs.
  intersegmental motion of, examination of,
    269–270, 270f
  thoracic, as pain source, 82–83
Vertebral arteries. *See also* Vertebrobasilar
    insufficiency.
  anatomy of, 9, 11f, 14, 147–148, 147f–148f
  blood flow in, 147–148
  injury of, 147–148
Vertebral column, growth of, 5
Vertebral joints. *See also specific joints.*

range of motion of, 140
Vertebra prominens, 12
Vertebrobasilar insufficiency, 145–165
  in cervical headache, 270
  in craniovertebral junction instability, 115
  dizziness in, 149–151
  functional, 150
  from manipulation
    historical aspects of, 145–146
    incidence of, 146–147
    mechanisms of, 147–149, 147f–148f
    predisposing factors for, 147–148, 147f
  premanipulative testing for, 115, 136–137
    APA protocol results, 157–162, 157t,
      158f–160f
    with dizziness history, 152f–153f,
      153–155, 155f
    historical aspects of, 145–146
    physical examination in, 151–155,
      152f–153f, 155f
    recording results of, 157
    subjective examination in, 151
    at subsequent visits, 156
    symptoms provoked in, 155
    technique choice based on, 155–156
  symptoms of, 149–151
Vertigo. *See* Dizziness.
Vibration, work-related pain from, 392
Viscera
  pain referred from, 84
  pain referred to, 321
  physical examination of, 138–139
Visual disturbances, in cervical headache, 264
Vocational rehabilitation, in work-related
    pain, 400–402

Walking, neck muscle activity in, 201
Whiplash injury
  self treatment of, 372
  sympathetic trunk injury in, 322
  vertebral motion in, 38
Wolf's Law, in postural malalignment, 342
Work-related pain, 379–407
  in abuse use syndromes, 387t, 389–392
  classification of, 386, 387t
  in degenerative disorders, 387t, 388–389
  economic aspects of, 379
  in environmental condition syndromes, 392
  epidemiology of, 379–380
  historical aspects of, 380–386

early research on, 380–383
  recent research on, 383–386
  individual factors in, 385–386
  in overuse syndrome, 391–392
  in postural overload syndromes, 390–391
  prevention of, 393–399
    aggravating factor control for, 397
    education in, 396
    ergonomic analyses for, 393, 394–395
    functional capacity assessment for, 395
    job rotation for, 396
    multidisciplinary approach to, 394
    pause exercises for, 397
    primary, 393
    program evaluation for, 398–399
    secondary, 393
    symptom recording for, 395
    task variation for, 396
    tertiary, 393
    workload measurement for, 394–395
    work pauses for, 397–398
    workplace evaluation for, 394
    work rate determination in, 396
  rehabilitation in, 399–402
    return to work after, 387
    services for, 399–400
    therapeutic interventions for, 400
    vocational, 400–402
  in traumatic disorders, 386–387, 387t–388t
  in white-collar workers, 384–385, 390–391
  work factors in, 384–385
Wry neck
  in children, 203
  discogenic, case study of, 307
  from zygapophyseal joint locking, case
    study of, 298–300

Zygapophyseal joints (cervical)
  anatomy of, 11f, 12–14, 13f, 18–19
  arthralgia of, case study of, 294–298,
    296f–297f
  arthropathy of, case study of, 290
  hypomobility of, case study of, 290–291
  innervation of, 22, 66, 66f
  locking of
    acute, 298–300
    recurrent, 300
  motion of, 19
  osteophytes in, 20, 20f
  pain referred from, 70, 72f

Zygapophyseal joints (cervical) *(Continued)*
  palpation of, 141
    in shoulder abduction, 348
Zygapophyseal joints (thoracic)
  ankylosing spondylitis of, 83
  innervation of, 79f, 80
  movement of
    in lateral bending, 57
    in rotation, 62
  as pain source, 82–83, 86
  palpation of, 141
  rheumatoid arthritis of, 83

HM